AF380004

Cellular and Molecular Pharmacology

Cellular and Molecular Pharmacology

Dr. Amteshwar Singh Jaggi
Assistant Professor (Pharmacology)
Pharmaceutical Sciences & Drug Research
Punjabi University, Patiala (Punjab)

Jasleen Kaur Virdi
Research Scholar, Department of Pharmaceutical Sciences and
Drug Research, Punjabi University, Patiala

Dr. Anjana Bali
Assistant Professor, Department of Pharmacology
School of Basic and Applied Sciences
Central University of Punjab, Bhatinda

Dr. Nirmal Singh
Professor, Department of Pharmaceutical Sciences and Drug Research,
Punjabi University, Patiala

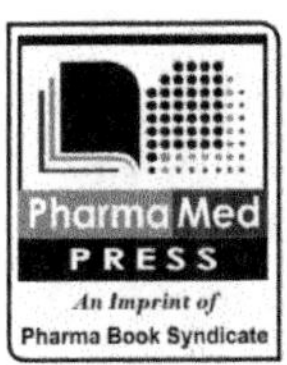

PharmaMed Press
An imprint of Pharma Book Syndicate

A Unit of BSP Books Pvt. Ltd.
4-4-309/316, Giriraj Lane,
Sultan Bazar, Hyderabad - 500 095.

Cellular and Molecular Pharmacology

by Amteshwar Singh Jaggi, Jasleen Kaur Virdi, Anjana Bali and Nirmal Singh

Published by:

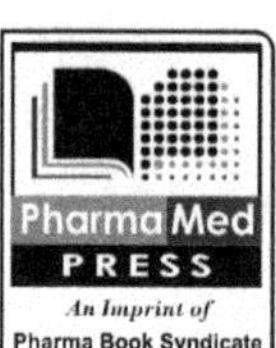

PharmaMed Press

An imprint of Pharma Book Syndicate

A Unit of BSP Books Pvt. Ltd.
4-4-309/316, Giriraj Lane, Sultan Bazar, Hyderabad - 500 095.
Phone: 040-23445600, 23445688; Fax: 91+40-23445611
E-mail: info@pharmamedpress.com
www.pharmamedpress.com/pharmamedpress.net

ISBN: 978-93-89974-34-8

PREFACE

With the advancements made in the field of Molecular Biology, the Pharmacology aspects have been unfolded at the molecular levels. To make the students aware of the recent advances made in the field of Pharmacology and Molecular biology, a new subject, "Cellular and Molecular Pharmacology," has been introduced by the Pharmacy Council of India (PCI) in the curriculum of M Pharmacy (Pharmacology) students. Cellular and Molecular Pharmacology is the first book of this type in the market for the M Pharmacy students and is written as per the new syllabus of PCI, India. The book is divided into five units and 20 chapters. The book provides key insight into topics including recombinant DNA technology, PCR, ELISA, Blotting, Gene therapy, Gene Sequencing, Autophagy, Apoptosis, MicroArray Technique, Gel electrophoresis, pharmacogenomics, Gene mapping, Genetic Variations, Proteomics. Genomics, Cell signaling pathways, Immunotherapeutics, Biosimilars, Animal Cell Culture, Assays, and Flow Cytometry. We hope the book will cater the needs of students as well as young faculty in understanding the basics of cellular and molecular pharmacology. In each chapter, the special emphasis has been made to explain the concepts of molecular biology and pharmacology in the form of figures, tables and flow charts. At the end of each chapter, review questions of both subjective as well as of objective types have been added, which will be very helpful to students as well as teachers. We hope that the book shall meet the demands of post-graduate students as well as young faculty in understanding the basic aspects related to human anatomy and physiology. The authors wish to acknowledge their family members, friends, colleagues and students for their support, love, and encouragement that helped in completing this book.

-Authors

CONTENTS

Preface .... (v)

Abbreviations .... (xix)

UNIT - 1: Cell: Biology

Chapter 1: Cell and Organelles

Plasma Membrane **4**

   Structure of Plasma Membrane (Fluid Mosaic Model) 4

   Functions of Plasma Membrane 6

Cytoplasm **6**

   Endoplasmic Reticulum (ER) 7

   Ribosomes 9

   Golgi Apparatus or Golgi Complex 9

   Mitochondria 10

   Lysosomes 11

   Peroxisomes 12

   Proteasomes 12

   Cytoskeleton 13

Nucleus **15**

Review Questions **19**

Multiple Choice Questions **20**

Chapter 2: Genome

Genome Organization **21**

   Packaging of DNA by Histone Proteins to form Chromatin 21

   Types of DNA depending on Reassociation Rate 23

   Organization of Genes 24

   Protein Coding Genes 24

   Repetitious DNA 25

Gene Expression and its Regulation **27**

(viii)

Contents

Gene Mapping 38
    Genetic Mapping 38
    Physical Mapping **40**

Review Questions 41

Multiple Choice Questions 42

Chapter 3: Necrosis and Autophagy

Necrosis 45
    Definitions and General Features 45
    Characteristic Features of Necrosis 46
    Different types of Necrosis (Morphological Patterns of Necrosis) 46
    Morphological Changes in Nucleus during Cell Death 48

Autophagy 49
    Definitions and General Features 49
    Types of Autophagy 50
    Macroautophagy 50
    Microautophagy 51
    Chaperone-Mediated Autophagy (CMA) 51
    Digestion of Cell Organelles, Endogenous Substances and Exogenous Pathogens 51
    Involvement of Genes in Autophagy 52
    Steps involved in Autophagy (Mechanism of Autophagy) 52
    Blockade of Autophagy 54

Physiological and Pathological Role of Autophagy 54

Review Questions 56

Multiple Choice Questions 57

Chapter 4: Apoptosis

Definition and General Features 59
    Morphology of Apoptosis 60

Early Stage 60

Late Stage 60
    No Inflammation during Apoptosis 60
    Characteristic Features of Apoptotic Cell Death 61
    Mechanisms of Apoptosis 62

Extrinsic (Death Receptor) Pathway 62

Intrinsic (Mitochondrial) Pathway 63

Perforin-Granzyme System 65

Execution (Common) Pathway 66

Caspases 67

Laboratory Methods to Detect Apoptosis 68

Physiological Role of Apoptosis 69

Pathophysiological Role of Apoptosis 70

Review Questions 71

Multiple Choice Questions 72

Chapter 5: Gene Sequencing

Definitions and General Features 75

Maxam–Gilbert Sequencing (Chemical Cleavage) 75

Sanger's Chain Termination Method 78

Differences between Maxam-Gilbert and Sanger Method 80

Automated Fluorescence Sequencing 81

Applications of Gene Sequencing 82

Review Questions 82

Multiple Choice Questions 83

Chapter 6: Cell Cycle and Regulation

Definitions and General Features 85

Stages of Cell Cycle 86

Interphase 86

M Phase (Mitotic Segregation) 87

Cell Cycle Control 88

Cyclins 88

Cyclin-Dependent Kinases 89

Cyclin-Dependent Kinase Inhibitors 90

Review Questions 91

Multiple Choice Questions 91

UNIT - 2: Genomic and Proteomic Tools

Chapter 7: Recombinant DNA Technology

Definition and General Features **95**

Different Steps of Recombinant DNA Technology **95**

Isolation/Extraction of Target DNA/RNA *96*

Selection of Cloning Vector *97*

Plasmids *99*

Joining the DNA Segments by Ligases *106*

Application of Recombinant DNA Technology *118*

Review Questions **120**

Multiple Choice Questions **122**

Chapter 8: Gel Electrophoresis

Introduction and General Features **125**

Basic Concepts in Electrophoresis **126**

Gels **127**

Agarose Gel *127*

Polyacrylamide Gels *130*

Horizontal vs Vertical Electrophoretic System **131**

Sample Preparation **132**

Buffer Systems **133**

Ornstein and Davis Model of Discontinuous Buffer System *133*

SDS–PAGE (Discontinuous Buffer system) *135*

Detection Methods **135**

Detection of Nucleic Acids (DNA or RNA) *135*

Detection of Proteins *136*

Isolation of Nucleic Acids or Proteins from Electrophoresis Gel **137**

Passive Diffusion *137*

Electroelution *138*

Continuous Elution *139*

Review Questions **139**

Multiple Choice Questions **140**

Chapter 9: Gene Therapy

Introduction and General Features **143**

Types of Gene Therapy **143**

In Vivo Gene Therapy 143

Ex Vivo Gene Therapy 144

Somatic Cells Gene Therapy 144

Germ Line Therapy 144

Methods of Gene Delivery **145**

Viral Vectors 145

Non-Viral Vectors 151

Applications of Gene Therapy **156**

Review Questions **161**

Multiple Choice Questions **162**

Chapter 10: Polymerase Chain Reaction

Definition and General Features **165**

Requirements for Polymerase Chain Reaction **166**

Steps Involved in Polymerase Chain Reaction **170**

Denaturation 170

Annealing 170

Extension 170

Cyclical 171

Efficiency of PCR **172**

Different Types of Polymerase Chain Reaction **172**

Reverse Transcriptase-Polymerase Chain Reaction (RT-PCR) 172

Real Time-Polymerase Chain Reaction (RT-PCR) 172

Allele Specific PCR 173

Inverse PCR (IPCR) 173

Anchored PCR 174

Asymmetric PCR 175

Applications of Polymerase Chain Reaction **175**

Review Questions **177**

Multiple Choice Questions **177**

Contents

Chapter 11: ELISA and Micro Array Technique

ELISA **179**
   Definition and General Features 179
   Types of ELISA 180

Direct ELISA **180**

Indirect ELISA **182**

Sandwich ELISA **185**

Competitive ELISA **188**
   Applications of ELISA 191

Microarray Technology **192**
   Definition and General Features 192
   Principle of Microarray Analysis 193
   Procedure of Microarray Analysis 194
   Applications of Microarray Technology 195

Review Questions **196**

Multiple Choice Questions **197**

Chapter 12: Western Blotting

Definitions and General Features **199**

Transfer Methods **200**
   Diffusion Blotting 200
   Capillary Blotting 200
   Vacuum Blotting 201
   Electrophoretic Blotting 201
   Semidry Blotting 202
   Bidirectional Blotting 203

The Blotting Procedure **203**

Membranes used for Blotting **204**

Detection Systems **205**
   Applications of Western Blotting 208

Review Questions **208**

Multiple Choice Questions **209**

UNIT - 3: Pharmaco-genomics

Chapter 13: Gene Mapping and Genetic Variations

Genes Mapping and Cloning of Genes **213**

Definitions and General Features *213*

Biochemical Approach (Functional Cloning) *214*

Positional Cloning **215**

Genetic Variations and Role in Pharmacology **216**

Definitions and General Features *216*

Genetic Polymorphism *217*

Single Nucleotide Polymorphism (SNP) *217*

Pharmacogenetics and Pharmacogenomics *219*

Potential Applications of Pharmacogenetics/Pharmacogenomics *219*

Genetic Variations in G-Protein Coupled Receptors **221**

Introduction and General Features *221*

Genetic Variations in N-terminal Domain *221*

Changes in Receptor Binding Affinity *222*

Variations in Down-Regulation of Receptors *222*

Variations in Transmembrane Domains *222*

Variations in Intracellular Loop Domains *223*

Variations in C-Terminal Domain *223*

Variations in Non-Coding Regions *224*

Review Questions **224**

Multiple Choice Questions **225**

Chapter 14: Polymorphisms Affecting Drug Metabolism and Drug Transporters

Definition and General Features **227**

Variations in Phase I Metabolism *227*

Cytochrome P450 2D6 .... *227*

Cytochrome P450 2C19 (CYP2C19) *229*

Cytochrome P450 2C9 (CYP2C9) *230*

CYP3A4 and CYP3A5 .... *230*

Variations in Phase II Metabolism *231*

N-Acetyltransferases *231*

Thiopurine Methyltransferase (TPMT) 231
UDP Glucuronyltransferases (UGTs) 231

Genetic Variations in Drug Transporters **231**
Definition and General Features 231
ABC Transporters 232
Solute Carrier (SLC) Transporters 233

Review Questions **234**

Multiple Choice Questions **235**

Chapter 15: Proteomics Sciences

Proteomics **237**
Definition and General Features 237
Types of Proteomics 238
Techniques and Steps involved in Proteomics 239
Applications of Proteomics 241

Genomics **242**
Definition and General Features 242
Genome Analysis 242
Different Areas of Genomics 243
Applications of Genomics 244

Metabolomics **245**
Definition and General Features 245
Type of Metabolites 246
Techniques and Steps involved in Metabolomics 246
Applications of Metabolomics 248

Nutrigenomics **248**
Definitions and General Features 248
Common Examples of Nutrigenomics 249
Potential Applications of Nutrigenomics 249

Functionomics **250**
Definitions and General Features 250
Potential Applications 250

Review Questions **250**

Multiple Choice Questions **251**

UNIT - 4: Immuno-therapeutics, Cell Culture and Biosimilars (Immunotheraputic Agents and Biosimilars)

Chapter 16: Immunotherapeutics and Biosimilars

Immunotherapeutic Agents **255**

Definition and General Features 255

Types of Immunotherapeutic Agents in Clinical Practice 256

Monoclonal Antibodies 256

Production of Monoclonal Antibodies 256

Humanization of Antibodies 257

Types of Monoclonal Antibodies 258

Fusion Proteins 261

Recombinant Cytokines 261

Soluble Cytokine Receptors 262

Cellular Therapy 262

Biosimilars **263**

Definitions and General Features 263

Common Biologics in Medicine 263

Approval to Market Biosimilars 263

Examples of Approved Biosimilars 264

Review Questions **265**

Multiple Choice Questions **266**

Chapter 17: Animal Cell Culture

Brief History of Animal Cell Culture **269**

Type of Animal Cells 270

Culture Systems for Cell Growth and Basic Equipments used in Cell Culture Laboratory **271**

Anchorage Dependent Culture System and Equipments 272

Anchorage Independent Culture System and Equipments 273

Types of Cell Cultures **275**

Primary Cell Cultures 275

Secondary Cell Cultures 276

Transformed Cell Cultures 277

Culture Media **278**

Counting the Cells in Animal Cell Culture **279**

    Haemocytometer *280*

    Coulter Counter *281*

Pattern of Cell Growth **282**

Storage of Cells **283**

Characterization (Monitoring) of Cell Lines **283**

    Monitoring Cell Lines for Genetic Stability *283*

    Karyotyping *283*

    Obtaining Pattern of Isozymes (Zynography) *284*

    Fluorescent Labeled Antibodies *284*

    Monitoring Cell Lines for Cell Contamination *285*

    Applications of Animal Cell Culture **285**

Review Questions **288**

Multiple Choice Questions **288**

Chapter 18: Assays and Flow Cytometry
        (Principles and Applications)

Cell Viability Assays **291**

    Definitions and General Features *291*

    Tetrazolium Reduction Assays *291*

    Resazurin Reduction Assay (Alamar Blue) *293*

    Propidium Iodide based Cell Viability Assay *294*

    Protease Activity based Viability Assay *294*

    ATP Assay *295*

    Evans Blue and Trypan Blue Test *295*

    Applications of Cell Viability Assays *296*

Calcium Influx Assays **296**

    Chemiluminescence Method *296*

    Fluorescence Method *297*

    Application of Calcium Assays *298*

Glucose Uptake Assays **298**

    Definitions and General Features *298*

    Measurement of Glucose uptake using Radiolabeled 3-o-methylglucose......*299*

    Measurement of glucose uptake using radio-labeled 2-deoxyglucose *299*

Measurement of Glucose uptake by Detecting Intensity of Fluorescence *299*
Application of Glucose uptake Assays *300*

Flow Cytometry **301**
Definition and General Features *301*
Principle *301*
Working *303*
Applications *305*

Review Questions **306**

Multiple Choice Questions **307**

UNIT - 5: Cell Signaling

Chapter 19: Receptors and Secondary Messengers

Receptors **311**

Classification of Receptor Family **312**
G-Protein Coupled Receptors *312*
Ligand Gated Ion Channels (Ionotropic Receptors) *312*
Receptor Tyrosine Kinase (Enzyme-Linked Receptor) *313*
Nuclear Receptors *314*
G-Protein Coupled Receptors *315*
Structural Features of G-Protein Coupled Receptors *315*
Signal Transduction *316*
G-Protein Coupled Effector Systems *317*

Second Messengers **318**
Inositol Trisphosphate (IP$_3$) *318*
Biosynthesis inside the Cells *318*
IP$_3$ Signaling Pathway *319*
Diacylglycerol (DAG) *319*
Signaling Pathway *319*
Clinical Uses of Protein Kinase C Modulators *320*

Nitric Oxide **320**
Introduction and Brief History *320*
Synthesis of NO by Nitric Oxide Synthase *321*
Key Targets of NO *321*

Physiological Functions of NO 322
Pathophysiological Role of NO 323
Clinical Uses of Drugs Modulating Nitric Oxide 324

Calcium Signaling **324**
Introduction and Historical Development 324
Channels and Proteins Modulating Calcium Levels inside the Cytoplasm 324
Calcium as Secondary and Tertiary Messenger 326
Intragcellular Signaling Cascade 326

Review Questions **329**

Multiple Choice Questions **330**

Chapter 20: Intracellular Signaling Pathways

cAMP **333**
Definition, Synthesis and Degradation 333
Signaling Pathway 334
Physiological Functions of cAMP 335
Clinical Uses of cAMP Modulators 336

cGMP **336**
Definition, Synthesis and Degradation 336
Signaling Pathway 337
Clinical uses of cGMP Modulators 338
JAK-STAT Signaling 338
Mechanisms Involved in JAK-STAT Signaling 339
Inhibitors of JAK-STAT Signaling 341
*Functional Significance of JAK-STAT Signaling and
Clinical uses of Inhibitors* 341
Mitogen-Activated Protein Kinase (MAP Kinase) 342

Activation Cascade of MAP Kinase (Three-Kinase Module) **342**
Inactivation of MAP Kinases 343

Types of MAP Kinases **343**
Clinical Applications of MAP Kinase Modulators 344

Review Questions **345**

Multiple Choice Questions .... **.346**

Answers 349

Index 353

ABBREVIATIONS

2-DG	:	2-Deoxyglucose
2° Ab	:	Secondary Antibody
3-MG	:	3-Methyl Glucose
AAV	:	Adeno-associated Virus
Ab	:	Antibody
ABC Transporters	:	ATP Binding Cassette Transporters
γc	:	γ-chain
ADA	:	Adenosine Deaminase
ADP	:	Adenosine Diphosphate
AFC	:	Aminofluorocoumarin
Ag	:	Antigen
AIF	:	Apoptosis Inducing Factor
AMP	:	Adenosine Monophosphate
Apaf-1	:	Apoptotic Protease Activating Factor-1
APCI	:	Atmospheric Pressure Chemical Ionization
ATP	:	Adenosine Triphosphate
BAC	:	Bacterial Artificial Chromosomes
BCRP	:	Breast Cancer Resistance Protein
BSA	:	Bovine Serum Albumin
CAD	:	Caspase Activated DNAase
CaMKIV	:	Calmodulin kinase IV
cAMP	:	Cyclic 3',5' Adenosine Monophosphate
CARE	:	Ca^{2+}-response Element
CDK	:	Cyclin-Dependent Kinases
CDKI	:	Cyclin-Dependent Kinase Inhibitors
cDNA	:	Complementary DNA
CFTR	:	Cystic Fibrosis Transmembrane Conductance Regulator
cGMP	:	Cyclic Guanosine Monophosphate
CM	:	Carboxymethyl

Abbreviations

CMD	:	Chaperone-Mediated Autophagy
CRE	:	cAMP Response Element
CREB	:	cAMP Response Element Binding Protein
CYP450	:	Cytochrome P450
DAG	:	Diacylglycerol
DBD	:	DNA-Binding Domain
ddNTP	:	Dideoxynucleotide Triphosphates
DEAE	:	Diethylaminoethyl
DISC	:	Death-Inducing Signaling Complex
DMD	:	Duchene Muscle Dystrophy
DMEM	:	Dulbecco's Minimum Essential Medium
DMS	:	Dimethyl Sulfate
DMSO	:	Dimethylsulfoxide
DNA	:	Deoxyribonucleic acid
dNTP	:	Deoxynucleotide Triphosphates
dNTPs	:	Deoxyribonucleotides
DPD	:	Dihydro Pyrimidine Dehydrogenase
DR	:	Death Receptor
dsDNA	:	Double stranded DNA
EDRF	:	Endothelium-Derived Relaxing Factor
EGFR	:	Epithelial Growth Factor Receptors
EI	:	Electron Ionization
ELISA	:	Enzyme Linked Immunosorbent Assay
EMEM	:	Eagle's Minimum Essential Medium
eNANC	:	Endothelial Nitric Oxide Synthase
eNOS	:	Endothelial Nitric Oxide Synthase
EPO	:	Erythropoietin
ERK	:	Extracellular Signal–Regulated Kinases
ESI	:	Electro Spray Ionization
FACS	:	Fluorescence-Activated Cell Sorter
FADD	:	Fas Associated Death Domain
FasL	:	Fas Ligand
FasR	:	Fas Receptor
Fc	:	Fragment Crystallizable Region
FFF	:	Field Flow Fractionation

Fura-2 AM	:	Fura-2-Acetoxymethyl Ester
G Phase	:	Gap Period
G6PDH	:	Glucose-6-Phosphate Dehydrogenase
GC	:	Gas Chromatography
GC	:	Guanylyl Cyclase
GC-MS	:	Gas Chromatography-Mass Spectrometry
G-CSF	:	Granulocyte -Colony Stimulating Factor
GEF	:	Guanine Nucleotide Exchange Factor
GF-AFC	:	Glycylphenylalanyl-aminofluorocoumarin
GLUT	:	Glucose Transporters
GM-CSF	:	Granulocyte Macrophage-Colony Stimulating Factor
GMEM	:	Glasgow's Minimum Essential Medium
GPCRs	:	G-Protein Coupled Receptors
HAMA	:	Human Anti-Mouse Antibodies
HCG	:	Human Chorionic Gonadotrophin
HeLa	:	Henrietta Lacks
HEPA	:	High Efficiency Particulate Air Filter
HITES	:	Hydrocortisone, Insulin, Transferrin, Estrogen, Selenite
HIV	:	Human Immunodeficiency Virus
HLA	:	Human Leukocyte Antigen
HPLC	:	High Performance Liquid Chromatography
HRP	:	Horseradish Peroxidase System
Hsp	:	Heat Shock Protein
IAP	:	Inhibitors of Apoptosis Proteins
IBD	:	Inflammatory Bowel Disease
IFN-γ	:	Interferon-gamma
iNANC	:	Inhibitory NANC
iNOS	:	Inducible NOS
IP$_3$	:	Inositol Triphosphate
IPCR	:	Inverse PCR
IPTG	:	Isopropyl Thio-galactoside
JAK	:	Janus Kinase
JNK	:	c-Jun N-terminal Kinases

Abbreviations

Lamp2A	:	Lysosomal associated Membrane Proteins 2A type
LH	:	Luteinizing Hormone
LINES	:	Long Interspersed Elements
LOD	:	Logarithm of Odds
LTP	:	Long Term Potentiation
LTR	:	Long Terminal Repeat
MALDI	:	Matrix Assisted Laser Detection of Desorption/ Ionization
MAP Kinase	:	Mitogen-Activated Protein Kinase
MAPK Kinase	:	MAP Kinase Kinase
MAPK	:	MAP Kinases
MAPKK Kinase	:	MAP Kinase Kinase Kinase
MDR	:	Multi Drug Resistance
MDR	:	Multi-drug Resistance Gene
MHC	:	Major Histocompatibility Complex
miRNA	:	MicroRNA
MLC kinase	:	Myosin Light Chain Kinase
MMLV	:	Moloney Murine Leukemia Virus
MOMP	:	Mitochondrial Outer Membrane Permeabilization
mPTP	:	Mitochondrial Permeability Transition Pore
MRE	:	MicroRNA Response Elements
mRNA	:	Messenger RNA
MS	:	Mass Spectrometry
MTT	:	Dimethyl Thiazolyl diphenyl Tetrazolium
NANC	:	Non-adrenergic Non-cholinergic Fibers
NFAT	:	Nuclear Factor of Activated T Cells
NIMS	:	Nanostructure-Initiator Mass Spectrometry
NMR	:	Nuclear Magnetic Resonance
NO	:	Nitric Oxide
NOS	:	Nitric Oxide Synthase
OAT	:	Organic Anion Transporter
OATP	:	Organic Anion Transporting Polypeptides
OCT	:	Organic Cation Transporter
ORI	:	Origin of Replication
PAGE	:	Polyacrylamide Gel Electrophoresis

PAGE	:	Polyacrylamide Gel Electrophoresis
PAS	:	Preautophagosomal Structure
PCR	:	Polymerase Chain Reaction
PDE	:	Phosphodiesterases
PES	:	Phenazine Ethyl Sulfate
pI	:	Isoelectric Point
PIP2	:	Phosphatidyl Inositol 4,5-Biphosphate
PKA	:	Protein Kinase A
PKC	:	Protein Kinase C
PKG	:	cGMP-dependent Protein Kinases
PLC	:	Phospholipase C
PMCA	:	Plasma Membrane Calcium ATPase
PMS	:	Phenazine Methyl Sulfate
PVDF	:	Polyvinylidenedifluoride
qPCR	:	Quantitative PCR
R Point	:	Restriction Point
RA	:	Rheumatoid Arthritis
RBC	:	Red Blood Cell
RF	:	Rheumatoid Factor
RIA	:	Radio-immuno Assay
RISC	:	RNA-Induced Silencing Complex
RNA	:	Ribonucleic Acid
Rop	:	Repressor of Primer
rRNA	:	Ribosomal Ribonucleic Acid
RT-PCR	:	Real Time-Polymerase Chain Reaction
rt-PCR	:	Reverse Transcriptase-Polymerase Chain Reaction
S Phase	:	Synthesis Phase
SCID	:	Severe Combined Immunodeficiency Disease
SCID	:	Severe Combined Immunodeficiency Disorder
SDS	:	Sodium Dodecyl Sulphate
SERCA	:	Sarcoplasmic Reticulum Ca2+ATPase
sGC	:	Soluble Guanyl cyclase
SIMS	:	Secondary Ion Mass Spectrometry
SINES	:	Short Interspersed Elements
siRNAs	:	Small Interfering RNAs

SLC Transporters	:	Solute-Carrier transporters
SLE	:	Systemic Lupus Erythematosus
SNP	:	Single Nucleotide Polymorphism
snRNA	:	Small Nuclear RNA
SOCS	:	Suppressors of Cytokine Signaling
ssDNA	:	Single Stranded DNA
SSRI	:	Selective Serotonin Reuptake Inhibitors
STATs	:	Signal Transducer and Activator of Transcription proteins
T3	:	Triiodothyronine
T4	:	Tetraiodothyronine
TAD	:	Transcriptional Activation Domain
TEMED	:	Tetramethylethylenediamine
TNF	:	Tumor Necrosis Factor
TNF-γ	:	Tumor Necrosis Factor
TPMT	:	Thiopurine Methyl Transferase
TPMT	:	Thiopurine Methyltransferase
TRADD	:	TNF Receptor Associated Death Domain
tRNA	:	Transfer RNA
TSH	:	Thyroid Stimulating Hormone
TUNEL	:	Terminal dUTP Nick End-Labeling
UGT	:	UDP Glucuronyltransferases
UTR	:	Untranslated Region
UV	:	Ultraviolet
v-ATPases	:	Vacuolar ATPases
VEGF	:	Vascular Endothelial Growth Factor
YAC	:	Yeast Artificial Chromosomes

Cell Biology

1. Cell and Organelles (Introduction and General Features) 3

2. Genome 21

3. Necrosis and Autophagy 45

4. Apoptosis 59

5. Gene Sequencing 75

6. Cell Cycle and Regulation 85

Cell and Organelles
(Introduction and General Features)

CHAPTER OUTLINE

Plasma Membrane
Structure of Plasma Membrane
(Fluid Mosaic Model)
Functions of Plasma Membrane

Cytoplasm
Endoplasmic Reticulum
Ribosomes

Golgi Apparatus or Golgi Complex
Mitochondria
Lysosomes
Peroxisomes
Proteasomes
Cytoskeleton

Nucleus

INTRODUCTION AND GENERAL FEATURES

A cell is the structural and functional unit of body. It means that the body is composed of cells. The vast array of processes and functions of body occur in a correct manner due to 200 different types of cells, which are specialized to perform a particular function. They work in collaboration to maintain the homeostasis of the body. However, all cells have some common structural and functional features, which are necessary for proper execution of their activities. For this reason, cell has been defined from decades as a complete unit bound by a membrane which contributes to the structure and function of a living being, thus, also called structural and functional unit of life.

For proper understanding of various chemical and biological processes in the body, it is a necessity to have knowledge about the basic unit of life, cell. A study of structure and functions of cell is known as 'cell biology'. A cell is composed of different intricate components known as cell organelles, which work in association with one another to enable the cell to perform its functions. To study the cell in an easy way, the cell is segregated into following parts: the plasma membrane, cytoplasm and nucleus. They are discussed as under:

PLASMA MEMBRANE

It is a flexible membrane around the cytoplasm of a cell and it acts as a barrier between the outer and the internal environment of the cell. It selectively regulates the movement of substances to and fro the cell. The lipid components of the membrane allow lipid soluble molecules (non-polar) to pass through, but block the movement of substances polar (water soluble) in nature. This particular characteristic helps in establishing and sustaining a suitable environment for carrying out the cellular functions. Plasma membrane is also important for maintaining communication amongst the cells and the environment on the outside of the cell.

STRUCTURE OF PLASMA MEMBRANE (FLUID MOSAIC MODEL)

The structure of plasma membrane has been explained through the **'Fluid Mosaic Model'** as described by S. J. Singer and G. L. Nicolson (1972). The salient features regarding the structure of plasma membrane may be explained below **(Figure 1.1)**:

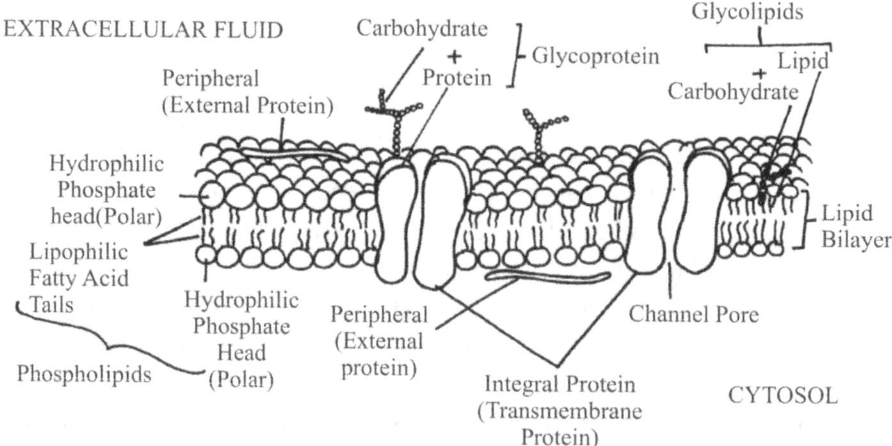

FIGURE 1.1 Fluid Mosaic Model explaining the structure of plasma membrane

1. According to this model, membrane is not rigid in nature; rather, it is fluid in nature. The structural constituents of membrane can float over the membrane.
2. Plasma membrane is mainly composed of lipids and proteins.
3. Phospholipid (75%) is the major lipid present in cell membrane. Phospholipid is amphipathic in nature as it has both hydrophilic phosphate heads and lipophilic tails.

4. Phospholipids form a lipid bilayer (two layers) in which hydrophilic phosphate heads face towards outside (face towards extracellular space) and inside (face towards intracellular space) of cell. On the other hand, two lipophilic tails face towards each other. Thus, lipophilic tails form the centre of membrane.

5. Other lipids of cell membrane include cholesterol (20%) and glycolipids (5%). Cholesterol helps in maintaining the membrane fluidity.

6. Within lipid bilayer, the membrane proteins are arranged.

7. Integral proteins (internal proteins) extend through into the bilayer and are embedded in the membrane. Most of the transmembrane proteins are integral proteins. They extend from extracellular fluid to the cytoplasm. These proteins cannot be isolated without breaking cell membrane. Most of these proteins function as ion channels through which molecules can enter inside or move outside **(Table 1.1)**.

8. Peripheral proteins (external proteins) are less firmly attached to the membrane. Mostly, these are located on the outer surface of plasma membrane. These can be easily removed from cell membrane without damaging the membrane. These mainly function as receptors **(Table 1.1)**.

TABLE 1.1 Key differences between integral and peripheral proteins of cell membrane

S.No.	Integral Proteins	Peripheral Proteins
1.	These are present inside the lipid bilayer	These are located on the outer surface of plasma membrane
2.	These are firmly attached to membrane	These are less firmly attached to membrane
3.	These proteins cannot be isolated without breaking cell membrane.	These can be easily removed from cell membrane without damaging the membrane.
4.	Most of these proteins function as ion channels	Most of these proteins mainly function as receptors.

9. Glycoproteins are also membrane proteins and these carry carbohydrate groups at their ends. These are also present on the outer surface of membrane i.e., these extend into the extracellular fluid. These glycoproteins are important markers for cell identification (cell recognition) and antigenic determination.

10. The glycoproteins are present on the extracellular surface. Similarly, the carbohydrate portions of glycolipids are also exposed on the outer face of the plasma membrane. Accordingly, the surface of the cell is covered by a carbohydrate coat, known as the 'glycocalyx', which is formed by glycolipids and glycoproteins.

FUNCTIONS OF PLASMA MEMBRANE

Plasma membrane serves many functions and these include:

1. It protects the cell and organelles of the cell
2. The cell membrane supports the cell and helps in maintaining the shape of the cell.
3. The lipid bilayer is semi-permeable and it selectively regulates the movement of substances to and from the cell
4. It acts as a site for receptors, transporters, channels. These functions are performed by proteins of plasma membrane.
5. Glycocalyx helps in cell recognition and antigenic determination.

CYTOPLASM

It is clear, gel like material present in between the plasma membrane and nucleus of the cell. It serves as a space in which cell organelles are present and most of the cellular reactions take place in cytoplasm. Cytoplasm is composed of cytosol (fluid portion) and the organelles (solid part). The cell organelles are surrounded by cytosol.

CYTOSOL

It is also known as 'Intracellular fluid' and it makes up approximately 55% of total volume of the cell. The composition of the cytosol varies in different cells. It is mainly made up of water (75-90%) along with various other particles suspended in water such as electrolytes, amino acids, glucose, ions, ATP, lipids, fatty acids, waste products and proteins.

ORGANELLES

These are small, specialized components of cells with characteristic structures. These perform specific functions, which are vital for the cell either individually or in collaboration with other cells. These organelles are suspended in the cytosol. All organelles contain certain characteristic enzymes depending upon the function attributed to them. Their number in different cells depends on the function of the particular cell. These organelles include endoplasmic reticulum, mitochondria, nucleus, ribosomes etc.

ENDOPLASMIC RETICULUM (ER)

The characteristic features of endoplasmic reticulum may be discussed as below:

1. The flattened sacs, tubules and vesicles exist in the form of a network in the cytoplasm to form endoplasmic reticulum **(Figure 1.2)**.

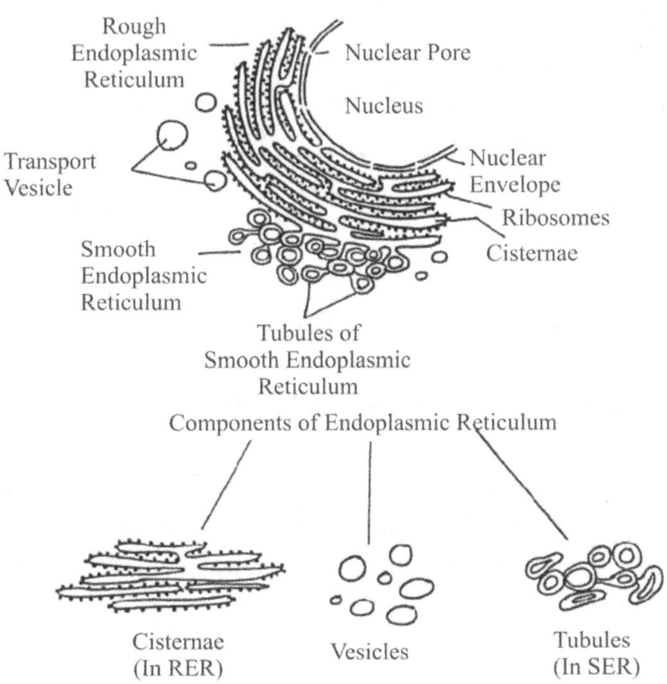

FIGURE 1.2 Structure of endoplasmic reticulum showing its different parts such as cisternae (present in RER), vesicles and tubules (present in SER)

2. The composition of its wall (membrane) is similar to that of the cell membrane i.e., lipid bilayer membranes containing large quantity of proteins.

3. Another characteristic feature of endoplasmic reticulum is its very large surface area and its total surface area may be more than that of plasma membrane of the cell. In hepatocytes, the surface area of endoplasmic reticulum may be even 30 to 40 times of the area of the cell membrane. Therefore, an extensive amount of area in cytoplasm is occupied by endoplasmic reticulum.

4. Endoplasmic reticulum is connected to the nuclear envelope all around the nucleus. Sometimes, it may extend even up to the cell membrane.

5. The vesicles and tubules of endoplasmic reticulum contain a fluid of watery consistency called endoplasmic matrix.

6. There are two types of endoplasmic reticulum depending on their structure and function. Rough ER (RER) and smooth ER (SER) **(Table 1.2)**.

TABLE 1.2 Key differences between RER and SER

S. No	Rough endoplasmic reticulum	Smooth endoplasmic reticulum
1.	The outer surface is covered with ribosomes.	The outer surface is not covered with ribosomes.
2.	The outer surface is rough due to presence of ribosomes	The outer surface is smooth due to absence of ribosomes
3.	It is responsible for production and processing of proteins.	It synthesizes of fatty material, detoxifies drugs and acts as calcium store

7. Rough endoplasmic reticulum (granular ER) is covered with granular structures called ribosomes, which are present on its outer membrane. Ribosomes are made up of RNA and proteins and these are exclusively responsible for synthesizing proteins. The proteins synthesized by the ribosomes move inside the rough ER, where it undergoes processing for becoming functional. For example, proteins formed from ribosomes move inside the ER, where proteins are attached to carbohydrates to form glycoproteins.

8. The major function of RER includes production and processing of various proteins essential for carrying out different functions in the cells such as, secretory proteins, organelle proteins, membrane associated proteins, etc.

9. Smooth ER (agranular ER) does not possess ribosomes on its membrane and these are called smooth because of its appearance.

10. The functions of SER include:
    (i) Synthesis of fatty acids and steroids (estrogen, testosterone)
    (ii) Detoxification of drugs or substances in SER of hepatocytes
    (iii) Smooth ER present in skeletal muscles is called as 'Sarcoplasmic reticulum'. It is store house of calcium and it releases Ca^{2+} ions from its stores during muscle contraction.

RIBOSOMES

The characteristic features of ribosomes may be described as follows:

1. These are the minute, spherical structures present in the cells for the synthesis of proteins. Therefore, these are also termed as protein factories. Indeed, ribosomes link amino acids in a specific order as specified by messenger RNA (mRNA). In other words, these are involved in the process of translating mRNA into protein.

2. It is made up from ribosomal RNA (rRNA) and protein. Therefore, it is also termed as 'ribonucleoprotein'.

3. The unit of measurement of ribosomes is the 'Svedberg' unit, which measures the rate of sedimentation in centrifugation.

4. Eukaryotic ribosomes are of 80 S type, which is in contrast to 70 S type of ribosomes in prokaryotes. In eukaryotes, 80 S ribosomes have a small (40S) and large (60S) subunit. The smaller ribosomal subunit reads the mRNA, and the large subunit joins amino acids to form a polypeptide chain.

5. Ribosomes may be present on the outer surface of the ER as in RER. However, these may also exist independently in the cytosol.

6. During active protein synthesis, a number of ribosomes may be attached over mRNA to form 'polysomes'.

GOLGI APPARATUS OR GOLGI COMPLEX

The characteristic features of Golgi apparatus may be discussed below:

1. It is a cup-like membranous organelle consisting of tubules, vesicles and flattened sac like structures called 'cisternae'. These cisternae are stacked over one another.

2. They are generally found in vicinity of nucleus. However, in case of secretory cells Golgi apparatus are more prominent and are located more towards the boundary of the cell from where the secretion from the cell takes place. Structurally, it is comprised of different cisternae depending on the shape, position and enzymatic activity **(Figure 1.3).**

3. The Golgi complex works in collaboration with the Rough ER. The proteins synthesized and modified in the RER are passed towards the Golgi apparatus. In the Golgi apparatus, the proteins are appropriately processed, and packaged to form 'membrane or secretory vesicles'.

4. Thus, packaging is main function of Golgi apparatus and it packages the proteins after receiving from endoplasmic reticulum. The packaged proteins are released into the extracellular fluid in the form of secretory vesicles **(Figure 1.4).**

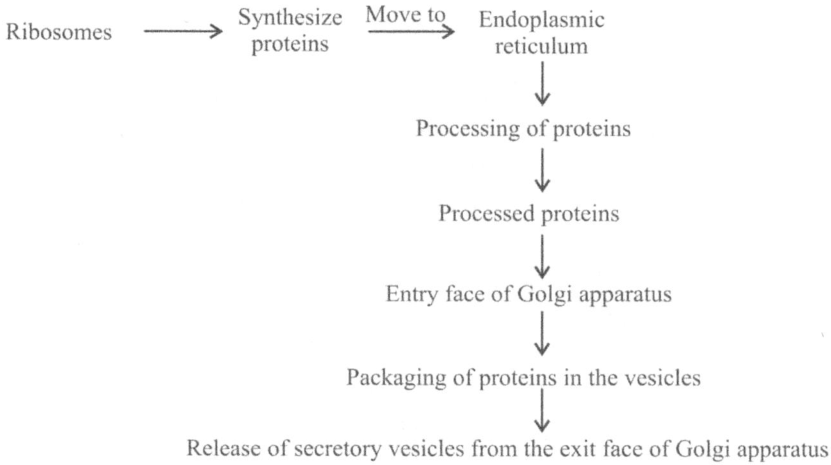

FIGURE 1.3 Key structural features of Golgi Apparatus

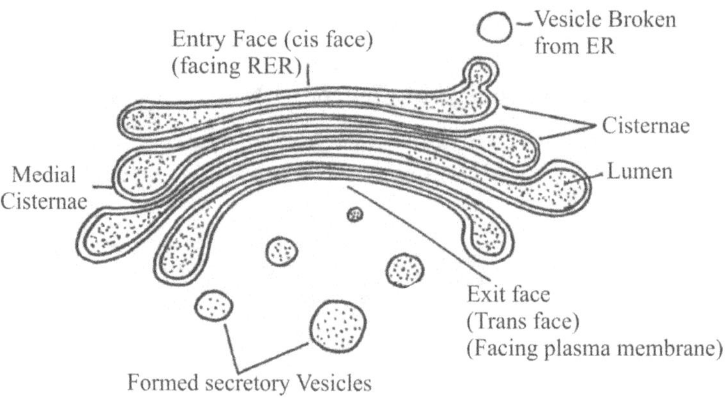

FIGURE 1.4 Golgi apparatus works in association with ribosomes and endoplasmic reticulum to form secretory vesicles

MITOCHONDRIA

1. This organelle is also referred to as the "powerhouse of the cell" because the most of the ATP (energy) required for cell to function is produced by mitochondria. In their absence, all cellular activities come to a halt due to unavailability of energy to work.

2. Their number in a cell depends on the metabolic activity of the cell. More active a cell, more is the number of mitochondria present in the cell such as in skeletal muscles and liver cells.

3. Structurally, mitochondrion has two membranes: outer membrane and inner membrane. The structure of these membranes is similar to that of lipid bilayer of plasma membrane. **(Figure 1.5)**

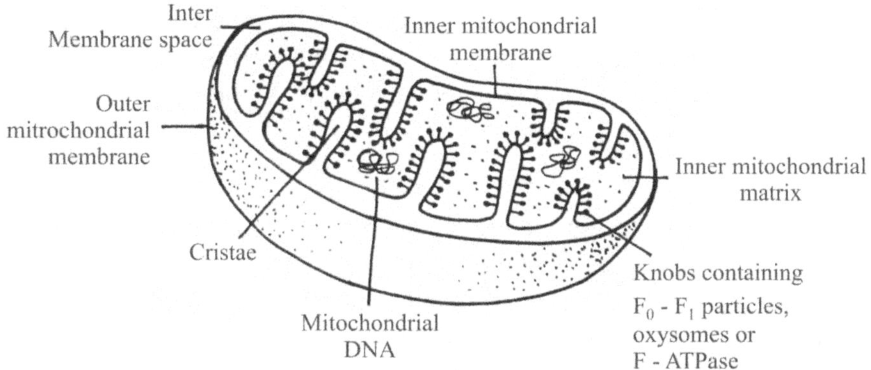

FIGURE 1.5 Ultra-structure of mitochondria showing different components.

4. The outer membrane is smooth. However, the inner membrane is folded to form finger like structures called 'cristae'. On these cristae, enzymes known as 'F_0-F_1 particles' or 'oxysomes' or 'F-ATPase' are present. These enzymes are involved in ATP synthesis.

5. The inner cavity of mitochondria is called as 'mitochondrial matrix' and is formed by inner mitochondrial membrane. The matrix contains a large amount of enzymes (dissolved in it) that are responsible for carrying out oxidative phosphorylation and ATP production.

6. Mitochondrion has its own independent genome (DNA), which shows a lot of similarity to bacterial genome. With increase in ATP demand, mitochondria can self replicate to meet the increasing demand. Therefore, it is also termed as 'semi-autonomous'.

LYSOSOMES

1. These are minute, membranous vesicles present throughout the cytosol. These are formed from the combined and coordinated actions of rough ER and Golgi complex.

2. These lysosomes contain large number of (at least 40-60) different types of digestive enzymes. These enzymes require acidic pH for optimum activity. The membrane of lysosomes prevents these powerful digestive and hydrolytic enzymes from coming in contact with the organelles. These enzymes perform digestion of
    (i)   Intracellular worn out, damaged and un-repairable cell organelles
    (ii) Food material ingested by cell
    (iii) Foreign material in the cell
    (iv) Sometimes, whole cell itself. Therefore, these are also known as 'suicidal bags of the cell'

3. Apart from intracellular digestion, these are also involved in extracellular digestion. For example, the lysosomal enzymes released from the sperm head helps in dissolving the outer membrane of the oocyte and help in fertilization.

Digestion of worn-out organelles/Cell

The worn-out organelles are engulfed by the lysosomes, where these are digested with the help of lysosomal enzymes. The digested material is returned back to the cytosol for re-use. This process of auto-digestion is termed as 'autophagy'. In this process, the worn out organelles are entrapped in an ER-derived membrane to form 'autophagosome'. This structure then fuses with the membrane of the lysosome, leading to digestion of the organelle inside the lysosome (Explained in chapter 3 necrosis and autophagy, Figure 3.2). The whole cell may also be destroyed with the help of lysosomes. This process of degradation of the entire cell is called 'autolysis'. It generally occurs in certain pathological conditions and is responsible for cell death.

PEROXISOMES

These are small sized organelles, also known as 'microbodies'. They are rich in enzymes called 'oxidases' which oxidize various organic and toxic substances. The oxidation process leads to the formation of hydrogen peroxide (H_2O_2), reactive oxygen species. Catalase enzyme present in the peroxisome neutralizes H_2O_2 to form water and protect the cell from the harmful effects of hydrogen peroxide. The peroxisomes may enlarge in size and ultimately divide to give rise to new peroxisomes. The main function of peroxisome is detoxification of harmful substances using oxidation.

PROTEASOMES

Proteasomes are minute structures and these appear like four rings placed one over the other. These are rich in large number of protein digesting enzymes termed as 'proteases'. Their major function is to degrade proteins which are not required, damaged or faulty. These proteins are disposed/digested with the help of proteases present in the proteasomes. These proteases cleave the proteins into peptides, which are further degraded into amino acids. The resulting amino acids are recycled to produce new proteins. The dysfunction of the proteasomes may cause development of various diseases such as Parkinson disease and Alzheimer's disease.

CYTOSKELETON

1. Cytoskeleton refers to structures that provide support to cell as bones provides support to body. These structures mechanically support the cell and the organelles to help maintain their shape.

2. These are mainly composed of protein filaments that form a network and are present throughout the cytosol. These protein filaments include microfilaments, intermediate filaments and microtubules.

   (i) Microfilaments

   (a) These have the smallest diameter of all three types of protein filaments. These are mostly found at the cell boundary. They are mainly made up of protein called as 'actin'. The diameter of actin microfilaments is around 7 nm.

   (b) Actin is globular proteins. These proteins assemble and form a linear filamentous structure **(Figure 1.6).**

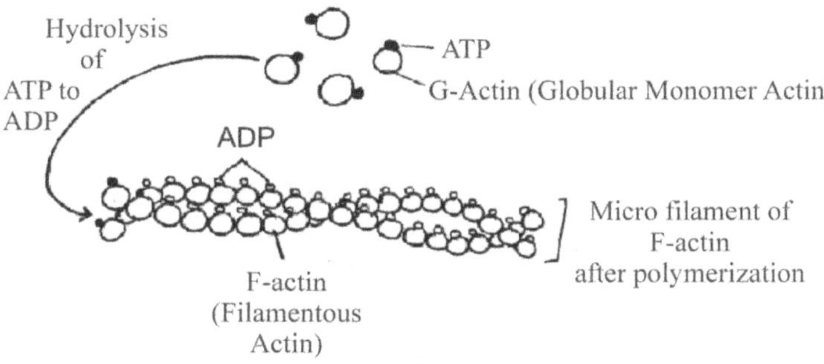

FIGURE 1.6 Structure of microfilaments made up of actin protein

   (c) Apart from providing support and shape to cell, microfilaments composed of actin also helps in movement of the cell; contraction of skeletal muscles through actin-myosin interaction, endocytosis, exocytosis and cell division.

   (ii) Intermediate filaments (IF)

   (a) These have a diameter larger than that of the microfilaments but less than that of microtubules. The diameter of these filaments is around 10 nm.

   (b) These are composed of several very strong proteins. They are mainly found in the organelles and regions of the cell, which are exposed to higher mechanical stress

   (c) These are various types and some of examples of intermediate filaments include 'keratin' that makes up hair, nails; 'desmin' that forms sarcomere in skeletal muscles; 'Glial Fibrillary Acidic Protein' (GFAP) that is found in astrocytes; 'peripherin' which is found in peripheral neurons; 'vimentin' which is widely distributed in fibroblasts, leukocytes, and endothelial cells.

(iii) Microtubules

(a) These have the largest diameter (25 nm) amongst all protein filaments. These are also the longest protein filaments.

(b) Microtubules are long, hollow cylinders and made up of α- and β-tubulin proteins. α- and β-tubulin proteins form a dimer. The dimer of α- and β-tubulin proteins polymerize to form microtubules **(Figure 1.7)**.

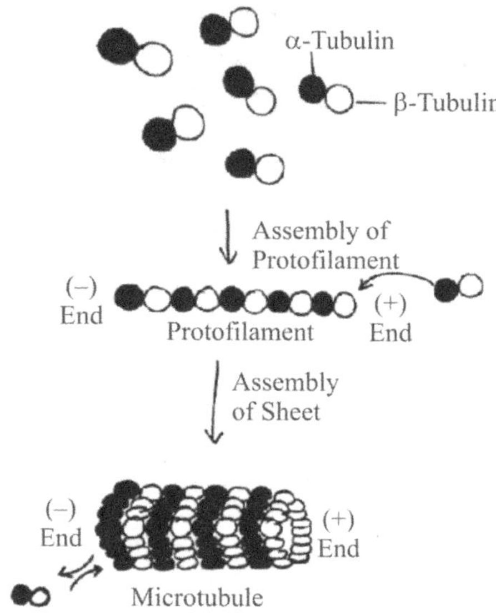

FIGURE 1.7 Structure of Microtubules made of α and β-tubulin proteins

(c) These play an important role in cell division and chromosomes move apart towards two ends through microtubules. Indeed, these are assembled in centrosome, from where they grow towards the boundary of the cell. These are the major constituents of mitotic spindles.

(d) Other functions of microtubules include maintaining the shape of the cell, movement of cell organelles, movement of cilia and flagella and movement of secretory vesicles.

NUCLEUS

1. Nucleus is the center of the cell and it controls all the vital functions of the cell. Therefore, it is one of the most prominent organelles in a cell. The genetic material of cell is present in nucleus.

2. Generally, one nucleus is present in each cell. However, cells composing skeletal muscle contain multiple nuclei, while mature RBCs do not have any.

3. Structurally, nucleus is composed of nuclear membrane, nucleoplasm, nucleolus and chromosomes **(Figure 1.8)**.

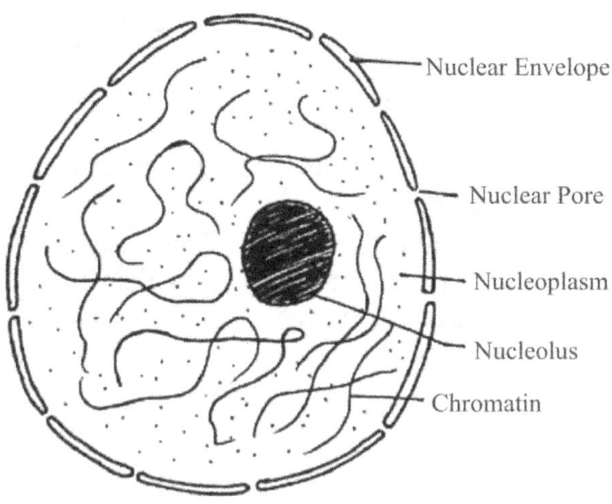

FIGURE 1.8 Structural features of nucleus

4. A nucleus is covered with a double membrane called **'nuclear envelope'** or 'nuclear membrane'. Small perforations are present in the nuclear and these are called as 'nuclear pores'. These pores regulate the movement of different substances in and out of the nucleus. Through the process of diffusion small sized molecules and ions pass through the nuclear pores. While large sized bulky molecules like proteins and RNAs are unable to pass through the small pores of the nuclear membrane by the simple process of diffusion. For their transportation, active process of transportation is used.

5. The nucleus is filled with a jelly like material called **'nucleoplasm'**, which is the site for the chemical reactions taking place inside the nucleus.

6. **'Nucleolus'** is a prominent, dark structure present in nucleus, whose major function is to produce rRNA, which in turn helps in formation of ribosomes. It is composed of proteins, deoxyribonucleic acid (DNA), and ribonucleic

acid (RNA). The cells which need more amounts of proteins have much more prominent nucleoli, for example, cells of muscles and liver.

7. **'Chromosomes'** are thread like structures present in the nucleus. These are more prominent during the process of cell division. In resting state of cell (interphase), chromatin is visualized in nucleus. Indeed, chromosomes are the condensed forms of chromatin. Chromosomes are made up of a long stretch of DNA molecule and histone proteins (explained in chapter 2 genome, Figure 2.1). Humans have 2n number of chromosomes in each cell of the body i.e., 46 chromosomes except in gametes, which contain n number of chromosomes i.e., 23. The chromosomes have specifically arranged sequence on them known as "genes". They are also known as cell's hereditary units and are responsible for transmitting the genetic information from one generation to the next. The compilation of the genetic material carrying the genetic information of an organism is known as genome. The information carried by genes is decoded by a process known as gene expression (explained in chapter 2 genome).

8. The major function of chromosomes include

 (a) These act as a carrier to transfer the genetic information from generation to generation.

 (b) Several proteins are formed from genes present on the DNA by the process known as transcription and translation. This complete process is known as gene expression.

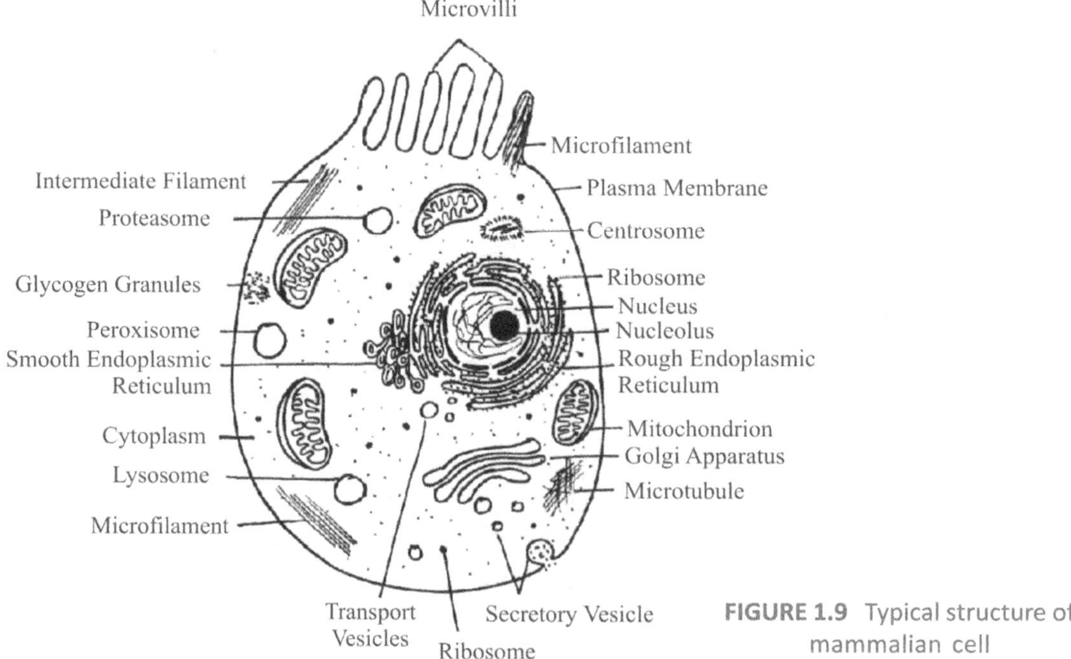

FIGURE 1.9 Typical structure of mammalian cell

TABLE 1.3 Summarized description and functions of different parts of cell

Component of cell	Description of the cell component	Functions performed
Plasma membrane	Flexible semi-permeable membrane covering the cytoplasm. Composed of phospholipids, cholesterol, glycolipids and proteins arranged in the form of fluid mosaic model.	(a) Protection of substances and organelles of the cell (b) Selective regulation of movement of substances to and from the cell (c) Site for receptors, transporters, channels, etc
Cytoplasm	Clear gel like material in between the plasma membrane and nucleus. Composed of cytosol and organelles.	Site for most of the cellular reactions
Cytosol	Intracellular fluid. Composed of different electrolytes, amino acids, glucose, ions, ATP, lipids, fatty acids, waste products and proteins suspended in 75-90% of water.	(a) Have organelles suspended in it (b) Site for many cellular reactions
Organelles	Small specialized components having characteristic structures suspended in the cytosol	Perform all the vital functions of cell
Endoplasmic reticulum	A membranous organelle containing flattened sacs, tubules and vesicles in the form of a network	
RER	Endoplasmic reticulum containing miniscule granular structures called ribosomes embedded in the outer membrane. Therefore, called rough ER.	Production and processing of various proteins
SER	Extension of RER, but lacks ribosomes on its surface. Therefore, called smooth ER.	- Synthesis of fatty acids and steroids - Detoxification of drugs or harmful substances - Storage house for Ca^{2+} ions in the form of sarcoplasmic reticulum

Table 1.3 *Contd...*

Component of cell	Description of the cell component	Functions performed
Ribosomes	Minute spherical factories for the synthesis of proteins. Made up of two subunits, a large and a small. May be attached to the surface of ER as in RER, or independently suspended in the cytosol	(a) Ribosomes on the ER for production of proteins for various processes. (b) Free or independent ribosomes for synthesis of proteins used for certain processes in the cytosol.
Golgi apparatus	Cuplike membranous organelle consisting of tubules, transport vesicles and flattened sac like structures called **cisternae.**	(a) Processing, sorting and packaging of proteins received from the ER (b) Formation of membranous vesicles to transport the modified proteins to the plasma membrane (c) Release of modified proteins into the extracellular fluid via secretory vesicles.
Mitochondria	Sausages like double membranous organelles commonly called "powerhouse of the cell". Inner membrane is folded to form finger like structures called **cristae**.	Generation of ATP via oxidative reactions of aerobic portion of cellular respiration.
Lysosomes	Minute membranous vesicles dispersed throughout the cytosol. Formed by detaching from the Golgi complex. Also called 'suicidal bags of the cell'.	(a) Digestion of foreign particles entering the cell (b) Autophagy of worn out cell organelles (c) Autolysis after death or in certain pathological conditions (d) Extracellular digestion
Peroxisomes	Structurally similar to lysosomes, but smaller in size	(a) Oxidize organic substance (b) Detoxify harmful substances (c) Degradation of hydrogen peroxide
Proteasomes	Structures resembling four rings stacked one on the other	Degradation of cytosolic proteins which are not required anymore, are damaged or faulty

Table **1.3** *Contd...*

Component of cell	Description of the cell component	Functions performed
Cytoskeleton	Protein filaments which form a network covering whole of the cytosol.	Movement of cell, provide mechanical support to cell and organelles, attachment to proteins, define and maintain shape of cell.
Nucleus	Prominent body in cell. Also known as the brain of cell.	Controls all the vital functions of the cell.
Nuclear membrane	Contains small pores called nuclear pores.	Regulate the movement of substances in and out of the nucleus
Nucleoplasm	Jelly like substance inside the nucleus	Site for chemical reactions in nucleus
Nucleolus	A prominent dark structure in the nucleus	Synthesis of rRNA
Chromosomes	Thread like structures present in the nucleus	Transfer of genetic material from one generation to other.

REVIEW QUESTIONS

TWO MARKS QUESTIONS

1. What are the functions of smooth endoplasmic reticulum?
2. What is the role of Golgi apparatus in formation of secretory vesicles?
3. Differentiate smooth and rough endoplasmic reticulum.
4. What are the difference between chromatin and chromosomes?
5. What is the role of glycoproteins on cell membrane?
6. Differentiate intrinsic and extrinsic proteins on cell membrane.
7. What are the functions of ribosomes?
8. What are the functions of mitochondria?
9. What are microtubules? Enlist any two functions of microtubules?
10. Write functions of microfilaments?

FIVE MARKS QUESTIONS

1. Explain fluid mosaic model of plasma membrane structure.
2. Explain the structure of endoplasmic reticulum, including its types and functions
3. Explain different components of nucleus with their functions.
4. What are lysosomes? What are their functions?

TEN MARKS QUESTIONS

1. What do you understand by cytoskeletal system? What are different structures that constitute cytoskeleton? Explain their structure and functions?

2. Draw and label different parts of a mammalian cell? Explain their characteristic structural features along with their functions.

MULTIPLE CHOICE QUESTIONS

---

1. Which of the following organelles is involved in steroid production?
   (a) SER   (b) Peroxisomes
   (c) Microtubules   (d) Proteasomes

2. Which of following organelles is involved in autophagy?
   (a) SER   (b) Peroxisomes
   (c) Lysosomes   (d) Proteasomes

3. Which of following is involved in antigen recognition?
   (a) Phospholipids   (b) Cholesterol
   (c) Glycoproteins   (d) Intrinsic proteins

4. Which of following is intracellular storage organelle of calcium?
   (a) SER   (b) Peroxisomes
   (c) Microtubules   (d) Proteasomes

5. Which of following organelles is involved in production of free radicals?
   (a) SER   (b) Peroxisomes
   (c) Microtubules   (d) Proteasomes

6. Actin is a constituent of following
   (a) Microtubules   (b) Microfilaments
   (c) Intermediate filaments   (d) None of above

7. The formation of secretory vesicles is a function of
   (a) Golgi Apparatus   (b) Peroxisomes
   (c) Lysosomes   (d) Proteasomes

8. F_0-F_1 particles are present in
   (a) Golgi Apparatus   (b) Mitochondria
   (c) Lysosomes   (d) Proteasomes

9. The faulty and degraded proteins are removed by
   (a) Golgi Apparatus   (b) Mitochondria
   (c) Lysosomes   (d) Proteasomes

10. DNA is present in
   (a) Mitochondria   (b) Cytoplasm
   (c) Endoplasmic reticulum   (d) Golgi apparatus

CHAPTER 2

Genome

CHAPTER OUTLINE

Genome Organization
Packaging of DNA by Histone Proteins to form Chromatin
Types of DNA depending on Reassociation Rate
Organization of Genes
Protein Coding Genes
Repetitious DNA

Gene Expression and its Regulation

SiRNA and MicroRNA

Gene Mapping
Genetic Mapping
Physical Mapping

GENOME ORGANIZATION

Genome is the genetic material of an organism and it consists of coding as well as non coding DNA. In other words, entire set of genes present in haploid state is called as genome. Accordingly, diploid organisms have two genomes (2 set of genes). The haploid human genome contains approximately 3 billion base pairs of DNA packaged into 23 chromosomes.

PACKAGING OF DNA BY HISTONE PROTEINS TO FORM CHROMATIN

In eukaryotes, DNA is packaged by histone proteins to form chromatin structure. Histones are a family of positively charged basic proteins termed H_1, H_{2A}, H_{2B}, H_3, and H_4. In turn, DNA is negatively charged, due to the phosphate groups in its phosphate-sugar backbone. Therefore, positively charged histones bind tightly with negatively charged DNA. 'Nucleosome' is the basic structural and functional unit of chromatin and one nucleosome is composed of eight histone proteins and about 146 base pairs of DNA. Two each of four histone proteins i.e. H_{2A}, H_{2B}, H_3, and H_4 combine to form a protein octamer. Over this histone octamer, 1.7 turns of DNA (146 base pairs) are wrapped to form nucleosome **(Figure 2.1)**. H_1 protein wraps about 20 base pair of DNA (linker DNA), which is usually present in between two nucleosomes. Therefore, nucleosome along with 20 base pair of linker DNA and H_1 protein form chromatosome (164 base pair DNA). Therefore, every chromosome contains hundreds of thousands of nucleosomes, and these nucleosomes are joined by the linker DNA (an average of about 20 base pairs) having H_1 protein **(Figure 2.2)**.

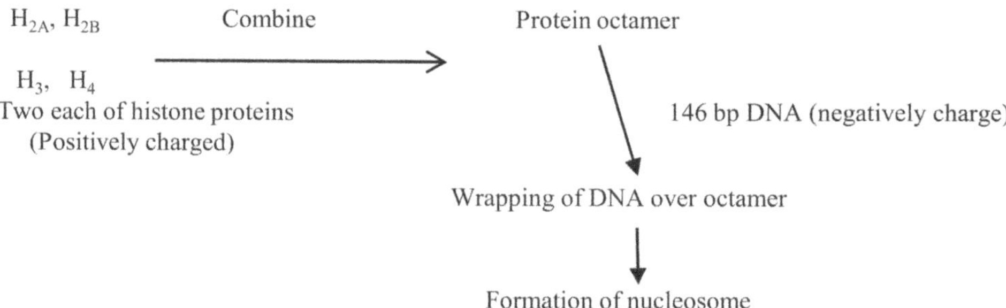

FIGURE 2.1 Formation of nucleosome using DNA and histone proteins

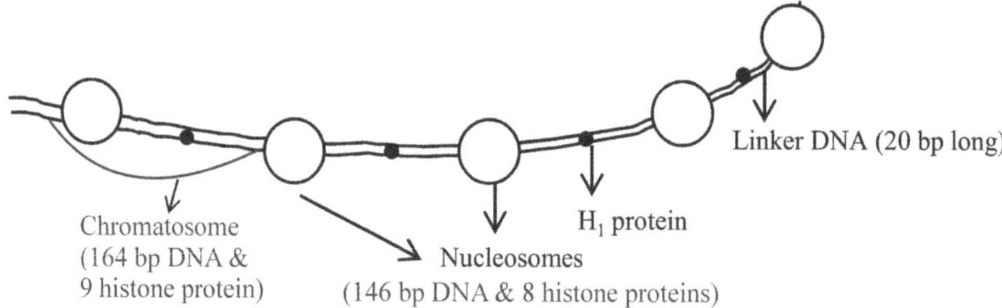

FIGURE 2.2 Joining of nucleosomes with the help of linker DNA

Inside the nucleus, chromatin exists in the form of long coils and intertwined over one another. Chromatin may exist in two forms, euchromatin and heterochromatin. Heterochromatin represents a tightly packed form of DNA and it appears darker on staining. Due to tight packing of DNA, polymerases are inaccessible and therefore, these regions do not undergo transcription. On the other hand, euchromatin represents loosely packaged form of DNA and it appears lighter on staining. Due to loose packing, polymerases can access DNA and these portions can undergo transcription **(Table 2.1)**.

TABLE 2.1 Key differences between euchromatin and heterochromatin

S. No	Euchromatin	Heterochromatin
1.	It represents loose packaging form of DNA	In this form, there is tight packaging of DNA.
2.	These regions appear light on staining	These regions appear dark on staining
3.	Polymerase can access DNA	Polymerases cannot access DNA
4.	These represent transcriptionally active form of DNA	These represent transcriptionally inactive form of DNA

TYPES OF DNA DEPENDING ON REASSOCIATION RATE

Depending on reassociation rates of denatured DNA, there are three types of DNA. Indeed to ascertain the reassociation rate, the total DNA is allowed to melt at higher temperature. The term 'melting' means separation of two strands of DNA. When two strands are completely separated from each other, the DNA is said to be 'denatured'. The process of denaturation is reversible and on lowering temperature, DNA tends to renature (reassociate) and DNA strands start forming duplex. However, the process of reassociation is not constant for whole DNA. Some portions of DNA reassociate very rapidly, some at intermediate rate and some at slow rate. Indeed, the rate of reassociation is dependent on the number of repeat sequences present in DNA. The single copy DNA with no repeat units reassociates very slowly. On the other hand, DNA with highly repetitive sequences reassociates very fast. Therefore, three types of DNA exist depending on the rate of reassociation **(Table 2.2)**.

TABLE 2.2 Types of DNA depending on reassociation rate

S. No	Types of DNA	Percentage of DNA	Characteristics
1.	DNA with slow reassociation rate	50- 60% of DNA	Single copy DNA (non-repetitious DNA) About 5% DNA codes for proteins and remaining has no known function and referred as 'spacer DNA'
2.	DNA with intermediate reassociation rate	25- 40% of DNA	DNA repeated to intermediate degree and termed as 'moderately repetitious DNA'.
3.	DNA with rapid rate of reassociation	10-15% of DNA	Highly repetitive DNA and termed as 'simple-sequence DNA'

1. **DNA with slow reassociation rate:** About 50- 60% of mammalian DNA reassociates at a slow rate and it suggests that this type of DNA is a single-copy DNA (non-repetitious DNA). However, only a small fraction of the total DNA in humans (about 5 percent) encodes for proteins or functional RNA molecules. The remainder of the single-copy DNA with no known function is referred to as 'spacer DNA'. The major function of the spacer DNA is to separate functional DNA sequences.

2. **DNA with intermediate reassociation rate:** About 25- 40% of mammalian DNA reassociates at an intermediate rate. This type of DNA has repeat sequences, which are repeated to intermediate degree. It is also termed as 'moderately repetitious DNA'.

3. **DNA with rapid rate of reassociation:** About 10-15% of mammalian DNA reassociates at a very rapid rate. This type of DNA has sequences which are highly repetitive and these are termed as 'simple-sequence DNA'.

ORGANIZATION OF GENES

There are different types of genes and these may be classified as described in **Table 2.3**.

TABLE 2.3   Classification of mammalian genes

S.No	Protein Coding Genes	Repetitious DNA		Unclassified
1.	Solitary genes	Simple-sequence DNA		Spacer DNA
2.	Duplicated Genes	Moderately repeated DNA		
		Long interspersed elements (LINES)	Short interspersed elements (SINES)	
3.	Tandemly repeated genes			

PROTEIN CODING GENES

1. **Solitary Genes:** In eukaryotes, about 25–50 percent of the protein-coding genes are represented only once in the haploid genome and thus, these genes are termed as 'solitary genes'. For example, chicken lysozyme gene is a type of solitary gene.

2. **Duplicated Genes, Gene Family and Pseudogenes:** About half of the protein-coding DNA genes in eukaryotes are duplicated genes. The DNA

that lies within 5 – 10 kb of a particular gene contains sequences that are similar, but not exact copies of that gene. These similar genes or sequences arise by duplication of an ancestral gene. Such closely placed genes with very similar (but non-identical) sequences are referred to as duplicated protein-coding genes.

A set of duplicated genes that encode proteins with similar, but non-identical amino acid sequences is called a gene family. For example, β-like globin gene family contains five functional genes designated as β, δ, A_γ, G_γ, and G_ϵ. Two identical β-like globin polypeptides combine with two identical α-globin polypeptides along with heme groups to form a hemoglobin molecule. Hemoglobins containing either the A_γ or G_γ polypeptides are expressed only during fetal life. The fetal hemoglobins having A_γ or G_γ polypeptides possess higher affinity for oxygen than adult hemoglobins.

The duplicated genes which do not code for proteins are termed as 'pseudogenes'.

3. **Tandemly Repeated Genes for rRNAs, tRNAs, and Histones:** There are multiple copies of genes present in the cell that code for rRNAs, tRNAs and histone proteins. In other words, these genes are tandemly repeated and these repeated genes encode for identical proteins or functional RNAs. It is in contrast to duplicated genes that encode for similar but non-identical proteins. These multiple copies are present in a sequence one after another, in a head-to-tail fashion, over a long stretch of DNA. The tandemly repeated rRNA, tRNA, and histone genes are required to meet the great cellular demand during active protein synthesis.

REPETITIOUS DNA

1. **Simple Sequence DNA:** In higher organisms, simple sequence consists of 5- to 10-bp long repeat sequences and such repeat sequences extend up to 10^5 base pairs in length. The long stretches of simple-sequence DNA are also referred to as 'satellite DNA'. The physiological function of simple sequence DNA is not clear yet. However, experimentally, these sequences are used in 'DNA fingerprinting' i.e. to distinguish one person from another on the basis of simple sequence DNA. Every individual is unique in terms of number of repeat units and length of repeat units. In other words, the length of repeat sequence (length of repeat unit) and number of times these sequences are repeated (number of repeat units) are different for every individual.

2. Moderately repeated DNA, or Intermediate-repeated DNA: These are classified into two types:

   (i) *LINES (long interspersed elements):* These represent repetitive DNA with repeat units of length around 7000 base pairs. In other words, about 7000 base pair long DNA sequences are repeated many a times in genome. In contrast to SINES, LINES can undergo transcription and translation to form proteins. Therefore, LINES can express proteins, which is in contrast to SINES. However, most of LINES belong to the class of transposons (discussed below).

   (ii) *SINES (short interspersed elements):* SINES represent repetitive non protein coding DNA with repeat unit of length ranging from about 500 to 700 base pairs. In other words, 500-700 long DNA sequences are repeated many a times in genome. Most of SINES belong to the class of retro transposons (discussed below).

TRANSPOSABLE ELEMENT (MOBILE UNITS)

Transposable element is a DNA sequence that can change its position within a genome leading to alteration in genetic identity and genome size. In other words, these genes tend to change their position within genome and are capable of moving from one position to another. Because of their property of moving from one portion of DNA to another, these are also called as 'jumping genes' or 'mobile elements'. These genes do not produce any known physiological function in the body and these just tend to maintain their identity in genome. Therefore, these are also called as 'selfish DNA'. These jumping genes were discovered by Barbara McClintock and she was awarded with a Nobel Prize in 1983. Transposable elements belong to two classes and DNA is transferred from donor DNA to target DNA either directly as DNA (transposons) or indirectly as RNA (retrotransposons) **(Figure 2.3).**

1. **Transposons:** These DNA elements are transferred directly as DNA from donor DNA to target DNA. Enzyme 'transposase' non-specifically binds to DNA and makes a cut to release a DNA segment. The released DNA segment is joined to target DNA.

2. **Retrotransposons:** These DNA elements are transferred indirectly through RNA. In this process, retrotransposons undergo transcription to form RNA, which is acted upon by reverse transcriptase to form DNA. The copied DNA is inserted into new site of target DNA.

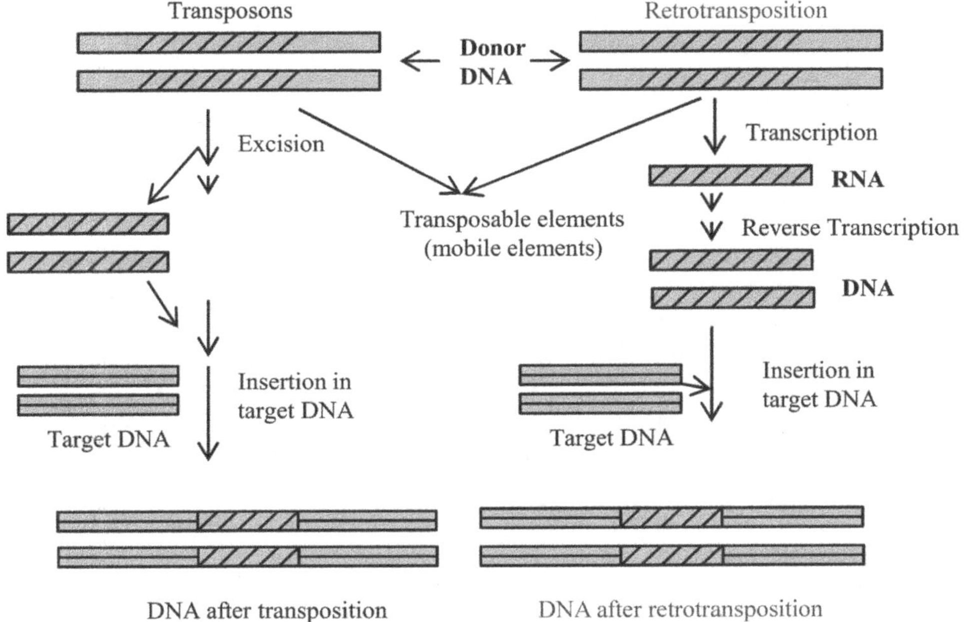

FIGURE 2.3 Two methods of transferring DNA using DNA (directly as transposons) or RNA (indirectly using retrotransposons)

GENE EXPRESSION

It is the process in which gene is used for the synthesis of proteins. Gene expresses itself by synthesizing proteins. In most of cases, gene expression refers to protein production from protein coding genes. However, it also refers to formation of functional RNA from non-protein coding genes such as transfer RNA (tRNA) or small nuclear RNA (snRNA) genes. Different steps involved in gene expression include transcription, RNA processing (splicing), translation, and posttranslational modification of a protein **(Figure 2.4)**.

1. **Transcription:** It is the process of formation of a single stranded RNA from double stranded parent DNA in nucleus with the help of an enzyme "RNA polymerase". DNA has two strands and these are termed as "template strand," and "coding strand". Template strand is used by RNA polymerase to form RNA molecule. Therefore, RNA is complementary to template strand of DNA. On the other hand, RNA molecule has sequence which is identical to "coding strand" of DNA, except that RNA has uracils in comparison to thymines in coding DNA strand. In eukaryotes, transcription also requires the presence of "promoter" and "transcription factors". There are three types of RNA polymerases in eukaryotes.

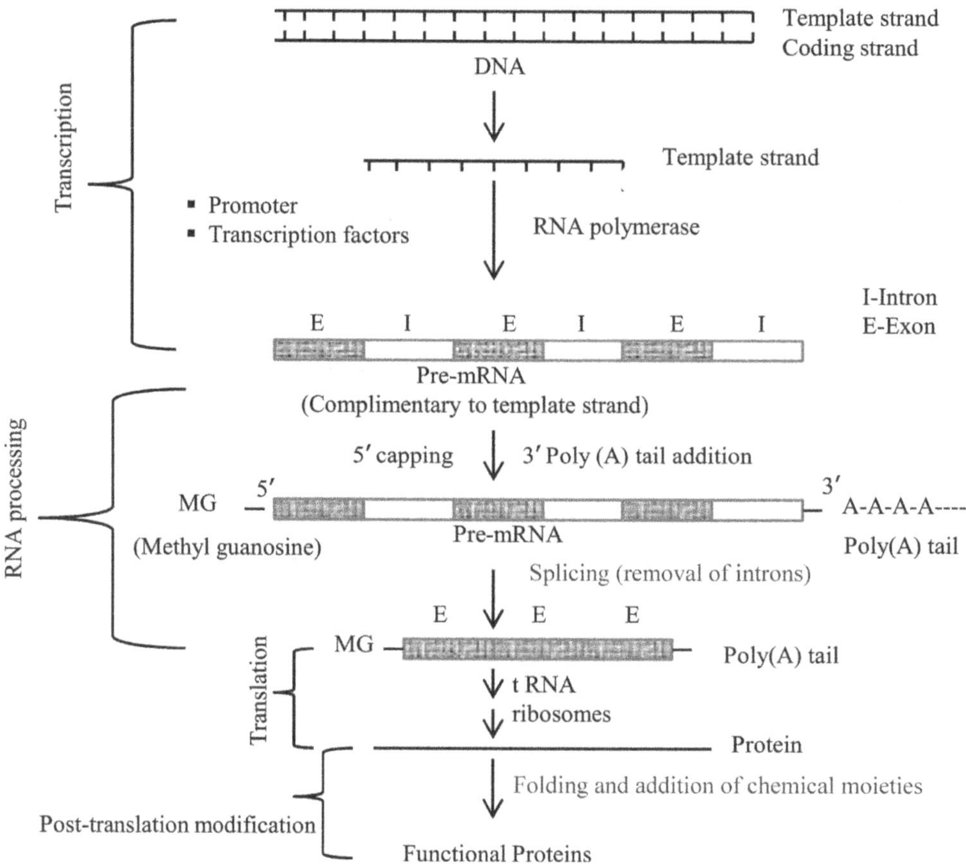

FIGURE 2.4 Different steps involved in gene expression

   (i) **RNA Polymerase I:** It is responsible for transcription of ribosomal RNA genes.

  (ii) **RNA Polymerase II:** It is responsible for transcription of all protein-coding genes and some non-coding RNAs.

 (iii) **RNA Polymerase III:** It is responsible for transcription of 5S ribosomal RNA, transfer RNA (t-RNA) genes, and some small non-coding RNAs.

2. **RNA Processing to form mature RNA:** In eukaryotes, transcription forms primary transcript of RNA (pre-mRNA), which undergoes a series of changes to form a mature mRNA.

   (i) **5' Capping:** This includes a reaction in which 7-methylguanosine is added to the 5' end of pre-mRNA. 7-methylguanosine cap protects mRNA from degradation by exonucleases.

  (ii) **3' Cleavage and Addition of Poly(A) Tail:** In this step, the pre-mRNA is cleaved at 3' end and thereafter, about 200 adenines (A) are added to form poly(A) tail. Poly(A) tail protects mRNA from degradation. 5' cap and 3' poly (A) tail are important structural characteristic features of mRNA.

(iii) RNA splicing: It constitutes a very important step in the modification of eukaryotic pre-mRNA. Eukaryotic pre-mRNAs are composed of alternating 'exons' and 'introns'. Exons refer to protein coding portions, while introns refer to non-protein coding portions. In this process, 'spliceosome' catalyzes transesterification reactions to remove introns and join neighbouring exons together. Thus, mature mRNA consists of only exons and is much shorter in length as compared to pre-mRNA which is much longer in length.

(iv) RNA Export: In this process, mature RNAs are exported from the nucleus to the cytoplasm through the nuclear pores.

3. **Translation:** It is the process of joining different amino acids to form proteins by utilizing the coding sequence of mRNA. For non-protein coding genes, formation of mature RNA is the final step of gene expression. However, for protein coding genes, synthesis of functional proteins is the final outcome of gene expression. Translation takes place over ribosomes (protein factories) in the cytoplasm. The important features of translation may be explained as below:

(i) Structural Features of mRNA: Mature mRNA consists of three regions, a 5' untranslated region (5'UTR), a protein-coding region or open reading frame (ORF), and a 3' untranslated region (3'UTR). 5'UTR and 3' UTR are non-protein coding sequences and their sequences are not used in protein synthesis.

(ii) Protein encoding Information on mRNA in the form of Codons: The coding region of mRNA has information regarding protein synthesis. This information is in the form of 'genetic code' and each triplet of nucleotides is called 'codon'. In other words, three adjacent nucleotides constitute one codon (say, AUG) and correspond to one amino acid (methionine for AUG).

(iii) Anticodon triplets in transfer RNA and transfer of amino acids to ribosomes: Corresponding to codons on mRNA, there are complementary anticodons on transfer RNA. Transfer RNAs with the complimentary anticodon (to codon of mRNA) carry amino acids and add amino acids to ribosome. Amino acids are joined together by the ribosome as per the sequence of triplets (codons) in the mRNA.

4. **Post Translational Modifications:** It refers to a series of reactions in which after translation (protein synthesis), proteins are altered/modified to make functional proteins. It may involve folding of proteins to form three dimensional structures and it may involve use of enzyme 'chaperones', which

help in attaining proper three dimensional structure. However, post-translational modifications may also involve addition of some other chemical moieties such as phosphorylation, acetylation, glycosylation etc. These modifications depend on the type of protein and are carried out in cytoplasm.

Regulation of Gene Expression

It refers to processes that control the amount and timing of protein production. Gene expression is highly regulated and is very important for the survival of organisms. Uncontrolled gene expression may lead to diseases such as cancer. Therefore, all genes are regulated and their expression is dependent on the need of organisms. For example, release and production of hormones is highly regulated. Insulin release is dependent on the amount of glucose in the body. The expression of 'cyclins' is dependent on the stage of cell cycle and whether cell has to divide or not **(discussed in chapter 6 cell cycle).** There are several terms used in relation to gene regulation:

1. **Constitutive Genes:** These genes are continuously expressed in the body. For example, eNOS (endothelial nitric oxide synthase) is constitutive gene and it synthesizes NO (nitric oxide) constitutively. In stomach, COX is constitutive enzyme and forms prostaglandins to regulate acid secretion. NSAIDS inhibit COX in stomach and may lead to peptic ulceration due to increase in acid secretion.

2. **Inducible Genes:** The expression of such genes is under the control of some environmental stimuli. For example, iNOS (inducible nitric oxide synthase) is an inducible enzyme and its expression is enhanced (NO production) only under inflammatory conditions.

There are different ways in which gene expression may be regulated **(Table 2.4):**

1. **Transcriptional Regulation:** It is one of the most important mechanisms of controlling gene expression. DNA has a number of regulatory binding sites and the process of transcription may be inhibited by binding to these regulatory sites.

    (a) The binding of RNA polymerase to DNA is an important step in transcription and inhibition of its binding is one of the mechanisms of gene regulation.

    (b) Transcriptional factors are also important in regulating transcription. The binding of inhibitory type of transcriptional factors to DNA duplex may stabilize the DNA structure and inhibit DNA opening to prevent transcription.

    (c) Epigenetic changes also constitute an important mechanism in controlling gene expression. Epigenetic refers to changes in gene

TABLE 2.4 Different mechanisms of regulating gene expression

S. No	Methods of gene regulation	Mechanisms	Examples
1.	Transcriptional Regulation	Inhibition of transcription i.e decrease in RNA synthesis from DNA	(a) Inhibition of binding of RNA polymerase to DNA (b) Binding of inhibitory transcriptional factors to DNA(c) (c) Epigenetic mechanisms
2.	mRNA regulation	Inhibition of translation or degradation of mRNA	Binding of miRNA and repressor proteins at 3' UTR region of mRNA
3.	Translational Regulation	Inhibition of Protein Synthesis	Antibiotics and Toxins
4.	Post-Translational Regulation	Protein Degradation	Ubiquitin- proteasome pathway

expression without any change in DNA sequence. It usually refers to alteration in histone proteins (packaging proteins), which changes DNA packaging. Acetylation or methylation of histone proteins are important epigenetic alterations responsible for altering gene expression. For example, acetylation of histone proteins leads to decrease in interaction between negatively charged DNA and positively charged histone proteins. Due to decrease in interaction, DNA is less folded and becomes more accessible for RNA polymerase to begin transcription. On the other hand, decrease in histone acetylation packs DNA more compactly and transcription is decreased.

2. **mRNA regulation:** As described earlier, structurally mRNA has non-coding 5'UTR and 3'UTR at either end. However, 3'UTRs of mRNAs has regulatory sequences, which may influence gene expression. 3'UTRs has binding sites for microRNAs (miRNAs) and regulatory proteins. Indeed in 3'UTR, 'microRNA response elements' (MRE) are present and miRNAs may bind to these sites to decrease translation or degrade mRNA. Furthermore, 3'-UTR also may have 'silencer regions' and different repressor proteins may bind to this region to inhibit translation **(Figure 2.5)**. The defect in miRNA dysregulation of gene expression may be important in the development of cancer, schizophrenia, bipolar disorder, major depression, Parkinson's disease and Alzheimer's disease.

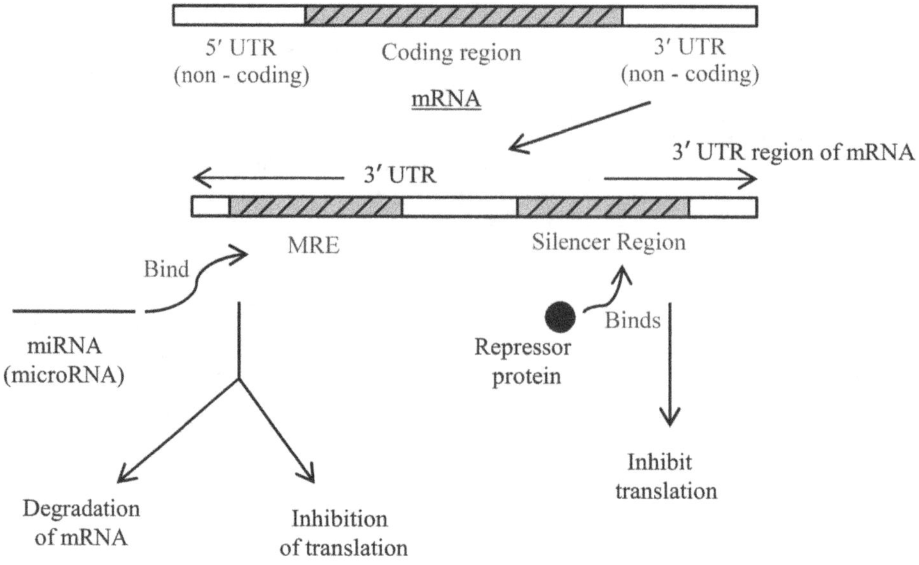

FIGURE 2.5 Regulation of gene expression through 3′UTR

3. **Translational Regulation:** It is a less common method of gene regulation as compared to transcriptional regulation. Certain toxins (ricin) and antibiotics (gentamicin, tetracyclins for killing prokaryotes) overcome gene expression by inhibiting protein translation.

4. **Protein Degradation:** Even after translation i.e. protein production, the activity of proteins may be regulated by altering the protein degradation. The proteins may be degraded by ubiquitin-proteasome pathway, which mainly degrades unneeded or damaged proteins.

Small Interfering RNAs (siRNAs)

siRNAs are 21 to 25 base pairs long, double stranded RNA molecules and produce post-transcription inhibition of RNA in a sequence specific manner. These are exogenous in contrast to miRNA, which arise from endogenous RNA. Indeed, microRNA (miRNA) and small interfering RNAs (siRNAs) are two major types of RNAi. RNA interference (RNAi) is a gene silencing method, which was first experimentally documented in 1998 in *Caenorhabditis elegans.* There are many similarities as well as dissimilarities between miRNA and siRNA.

FORMATION OF siRNA AND SILENCING OF mRNA

The different steps involved in the formation of siRNA and inhibition of RNA are illustrated below **(Figure 2.6)**:

1. Upon entry of exogenous virus or transgene in the body, double stranded RNA (dsRNA) is produced from foreign genes. The immune response responds to dsRNA by cleaving it in small interfering RNAs (siRNAs). Indeed, dsRNA is cleaved to 21- to 25- nucleotide siRNA duplexes by RNase III enzyme, Dicer.

2. Thereafter, siRNAs are unwound by an ATP-dependent enzyme called helicase and the single-stranded siRNAs combine with a protein complex to form RNA/Protein complex called as RNA-induced silencing complex (RISC).

3. The synthetic siRNAs, which may be directly administered in the body from outside, are not acted upon by RNase III, Dicer. Rather, these are directly converted to single strands by ATP-dependent helicase enzyme. It is followed by its combination with protein complex to form RISC.

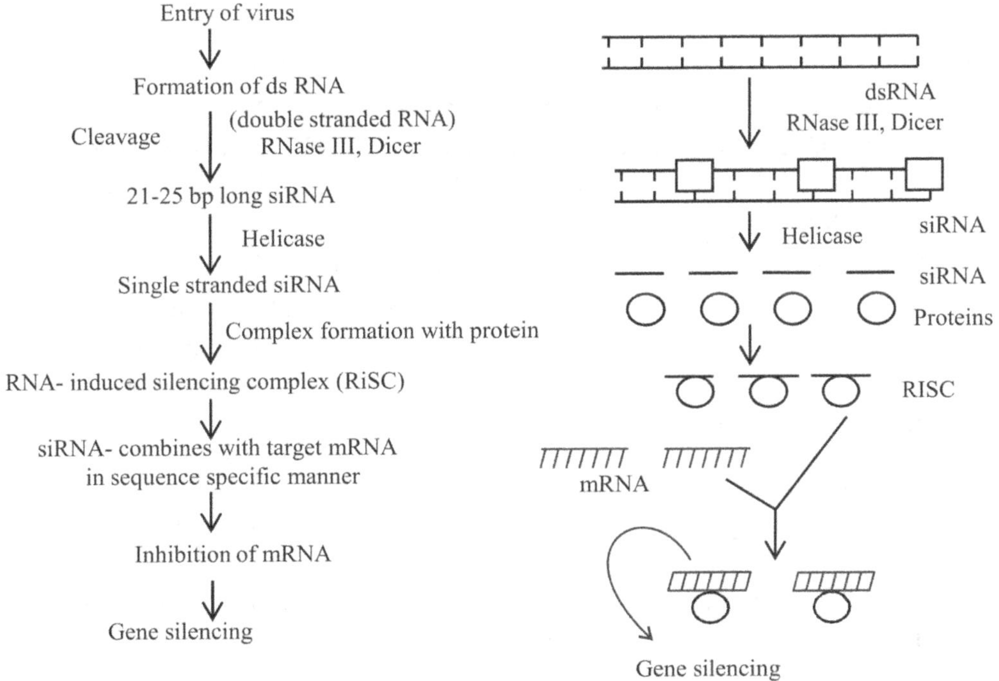

FIGURE 2.6 Formation of siRNA and gene silencing function

4. In subsequent steps, RISC degrades endogenous mRNA in a sequence specific manner. A single stranded siRNA finds complementary mRNA and binds with it in a sequence specific manner.

5. The binding of siRNA with endogenous mRNA is followed by cleavage of mRNA or inhibition of translation process. Thus, siRNA produces gene silencing by binding to target mRNA in a sequence specific manner.

MICRO RNA (miRNA)

A microRNA is a small non-coding RNA molecule, 22 nucleotides in length, and is widely distributed in plants, animals and some viruses. miRNAs are mainly located inside the cell; however, some miRNAs are also present extracellularly and these are termed as 'circulating miRNAs' or 'extracellular miRNAs'. These mainly function to silence coding RNA (RNA silencing) and thus, regulate gene expression. The human genome encodes more than 1000 miRNAs. In contrast to siRNA, miRNA arise endogenously from larger pre-mRNA.

NOMENCLATURE

There is a specific pattern of naming these microRNAs. 'miR' is used as prefix and it is followed by a dash and a number. The number indicates the order of naming. For example, miR-112 and miR-234 are two different microRNAs, and miR-112 was characterized and named prior to miR-234. Moreover, 'miR-' (R in capital letters) denotes the mature form of miRNA, while 'mir' (r in non capital letters denotes the pre-miRNA and 'MIR' (All letters in capital) refers to gene that encodes microRNA. To denote the species a three-letter prefix is added such as hsa-miR-124 indicates microRNA of human (*Homo sapiens*).

FORMATION OF MICRO RNA AND SILENCING OF mRNA

The different steps involved in synthesis of miRNA and gene silencing functions may be described as follows **(Figure 2.7)**:

1. miRNA is formed endogenously from nuclear DNA through transcription by enzyme RNA polymerase II. The polymerase enzyme leads to production

of double stranded pre-miRNA with hairpin loop. This pre-miRNA is transported from nucleus to cytoplasm, where it is acted upon by RNAase enzyme RNase III 'dicer' to cleave hair pin loop and form miRNA.

2. miRNA is converted to single stranded miRNA by helicase and later, it forms a complex with a protein called as RISC.

3. A single stranded miRNA inhibits the functioning of mRNA (gene silencing) in a sequence specific manner. In other words, miRNA are complementary to mRNA, which are to be silenced.

4. miRNAs silence the functioning of protein encoding mRNA via complementary base-pairing with mRNA molecules. The base pairing of miRNA with protein encoding mRNA may produce gene silencing either by cleaving the protein encoding mRNA or inhibiting translation of the mRNA into proteins **(Figure 2.8)**.

5. As described earlier, miRNAs may regulate gene expression by binding to 3'UTR region of mRNA. miRNAs may bind to 'microRNA response elements' of 3'UTR to decrease translation or degrade mRNA.

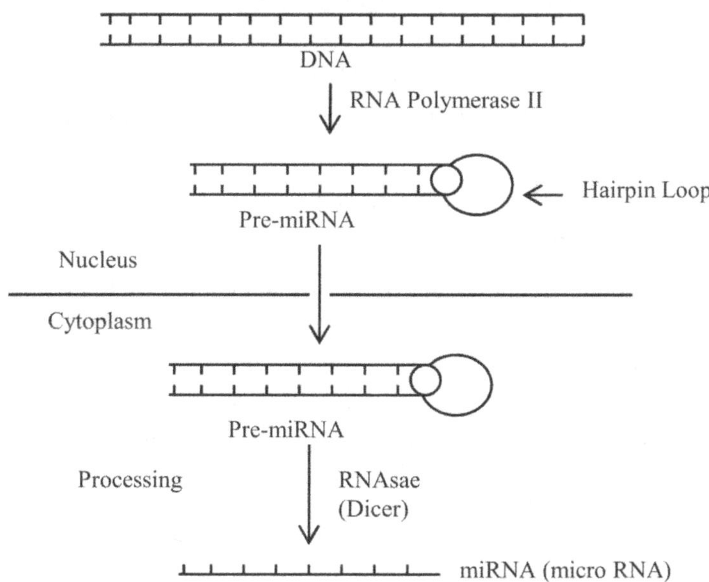

FIGURE 2.7 Steps involved in formation of miRNA

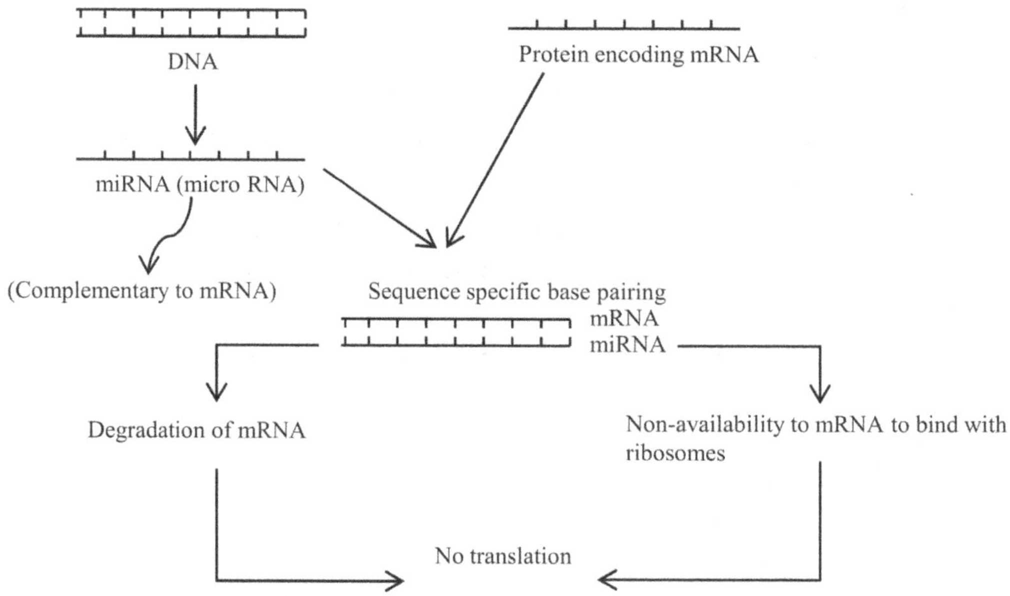

FIGURE 2.8 Mechanism of inhibition of protein encoding mRNA by miRNA

SIMILARITIES BETWEEN siRNA AND miRNA

There are some similarities between siRNA and miRNA:

1. These have approximately same size, around 20 to 25 nucleotide base pair in length

2. These are the part of the RNA interference system and both function to silence mRNA (gene silencing)

3. Both produce gene silencing by similar mechanism. Both involve the formation of RISC, which performs cleavage of target mRNA in a sequence specific manner.

4. The formation of miRNA as well as siRNA require the presence of RNase III enzyme Dicer, which produces a cut in lengthy RNA to form shorter miRNA or siRNA

DIFFERENCES BETWEEN siRNA AND miRNA

1. The major difference between these two is that miRNA arises from endogenous RNA, with hairpin loop. RNase III enzyme dicer acts over endogenous RNA to form miRNA

2. However, siRNA is exogenous in origin. Upon entry of viruses or transgene, double stranded RNA is formed, which is cut into smaller siRNA duplexes with the help of enzyme dicer.

3. siRNA are more speific in action. A single siRNA inhibit a single type of mRNA and its binding to mRNA is highly specific.

4. However, the binding of miRNA with mRNA is relatively unspecific. Therefore, a single miRNA is capable of inhibiting a large number of mRNAs.

BIOLOGICAL SIGNIFICANCE OF miRNA

Endogenous miRNAs are involved in key biological processes, including development, differentiation, apoptosis and proliferation. A decrease in miRNA may lead to excessive or uncontrolled activity of protein encoding mRNA and may lead to development of number of diseases.

1. **Diabetes Mellitus:** miRNAs play an important role in endocrine function and the changes in their expression is responsible for alteration in hormone regulation. For example, a pancreatic islet-specific miRNA, miR-375, inhibits insulin secretion in mouse pancreatic cells. Therefore, it may be suggested that an increase in miR-375 may possibly contribute in diabetes by inhibiting the release of insulin.

2. **Cancer:** Chronic lymphocytic leukemia was the first human disease that was found to be associated with miRNA deregulation. It is found that over-expression of miRNAs reduce the expression of DNA repair proteins, which leads to accumulation of damaged proteins, which ultimately results in development of cancers. It is also possible that overexpression of miRNA that down-regulate tumor suppressor genes may also contribute to tumor formation.

3. **Others:** Similarly, miRNAs have physiological as well as pathological role in cardiovascular system, urinary system and nervous system. The dysregulation of miRNA may also cause skeletal and growth defects.

POTENTIAL THERAPEUTIC USES OF siRNA

Based on the basic functions of siRNA, short synthetic interfering RNAs have been designed to inhibit the functioning of over expressing genes. The achievement of gene silencing functions by exogenous delivery of siRNA have a large number of potential therapeutic uses. For therapeutic purposes, these siRNAs are administered using viral or non-viral vectors (gene carriers). siRNA based therapeutic agents are in different stages of preclinical or clinical stages. These have been employed for the management of diseases such as dyslipidemia, chronic obstructive lung disease, hearing loss, cancer, AIDS, viral diseases, etc. Nevertheless, overcoming the systemic delivery system remains the most crucial challenges for the success of siRNA as drugs.

GENE MAPPING

It refers to mapping or localizing the position of genes on chromosomes. Mainly, there are two types of gene mapping, genetic mapping and physical mapping:

1. **Genetic Mapping:** It uses 'linkage analysis' to determine the relative position between two genes on a chromosome. A genetic map is based on the frequencies of recombination between markers (genes) during crossover of homologous chromosomes. The greater the frequency of recombination (segregation) between two genetic markers, the greater the distance between the genes. Conversely, the lower the frequency of recombination between the markers, the smaller the physical distance between them.

PURPOSE OF GENETIC MAPPING

1. It is a very important technique for medical genetics. The ultimate purpose of gene mapping is to clone genes, especially disease genes. After cloning of genes, its DNA sequence is determined followed by study of its protein product. For example: the gene related to cystic fibrosis was mapped to chromosome 7q31-q32 by linkage analysis. Later, gene was cloned and protein was analyzed to reveal that the defect of a chloride channel is mainly responsible for the disease.

2. It offers the evidence that a disease transmitted from parent to child is linked to one or more genes.

3. It also provides the information about which chromosome contains the gene and where the gene lies on that chromosome.

GENETIC/BIOCHEMICAL MARKERS

Markers are very valuable for tracking inheritance of traits (characters) from one generation to another.

1. In gene mapping, only those genes can be studied that specify some visual phenotypes such as eye color, height etc. Thus, a particular phenotype is considered as genetic marker.

2. Alternatively, those genes that specify biochemical phenotypes may also be studied. For example, blood typing is a type of biochemical parameters and is used in humans. These include the standard blood groups such as the ABO series and also the human leukocyte antigens (the HLA system).

METHODOLOGY

1. For mapping genes, family studies are done to determine whether two genes show linkage, when passed from one generation to the next. This technique in animals involves cross-breeding experiments. The first genetic map was constructed in 'fruit fly' and used genes as markers.

2. In the case of humans, the examination of family histories (pedigrees) is performed. A pedigree is a family tree/chart made of symbols and lines that represent a patient's genetic family history. It is a visual tool for documenting biological relationships in families.

3. Thus, for making a genetic map, a pedigree is established.

4. Thereafter, estimate of number of recombination frequency is made. From, recombination frequency estimate, LOD (logarithm of the odds) score is calculated.

5. The LOD score is used in linkage analysis in human populations. In pedigree analysis, LOD score is calculated. It is a statistical estimate whether two genes are likely to be located near each other on a chromosome and are therefore likely to be inherited. A LOD score of 3 or higher indicates that two genes are located close to each other on the chromosome. A LOD score of - 2.0 excludes the possibility of linkage and it means that genes are far apart.

IMPORTANT CHARACTERISTICS OF GENETIC MAP

The important points that can be deduced from gene map are:

1. In a genetic map, genes are shown in an order and distances between these genes are based on pedigree analysis. For example in **Figure 2.9**, genes A, B, C, D, E and F are placed in an order.

2. The unit of distance between genes is centiMorgans (cM). 1 cM refers to 1% chance of recombination between markers (genes).

3. The larger the distance between two genes, more is the chance of their separation or recombination. For example in **figure 2.9,** A and F are far apart and there are more chances of separation during crossing over in the process of meiosis.

4. On the other hand, smaller the distance between two genes, the lesser chances of their separation. In other words, there are very high chances that two closely placed genes are inherited together. For example, genes A and B are closely placed and there are a very few chances of their separation during crossing over.

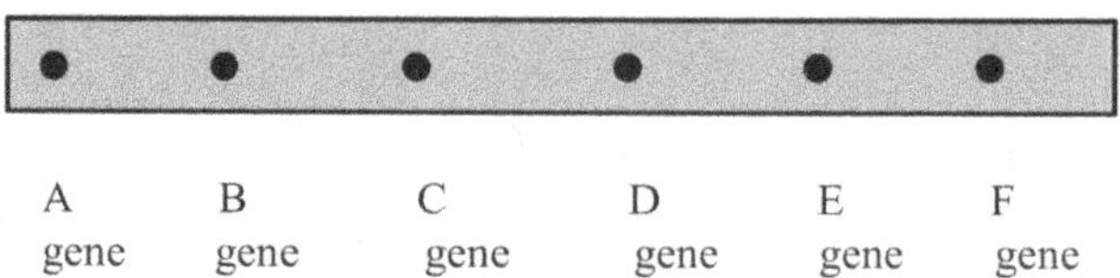

FIGURE 2.9   Genetic map showing relative location of genes on a chromosome

2. **Physical Mapping:** It uses molecular biology techniques to determine the absolute position of a gene on a chromosome. The different steps in physical mapping include:

   (i) The blood/tissue is collected from family members that carry a prominent disease/trait and from family members that do not carry disease or particular trait.

   (ii) Thereafter, DNA is isolated and closely examined to identify the unique patterns in the DNA.

   (iii) The unique patterns are identified by first cutting DNA into small pieces using restriction endonuclease enzyme or physical process by sonication.

   (iv) The DNA fragments are separated by gel electrophoresis and the pattern of DNA migration is used as its genetic fingerprint (unique pattern).

   (v) The difference in DNA pattern is identified between the family members who carry the disease and those who do not carry the disease. These unique molecular patterns in the DNA are called as 'polymorphisms', or 'markers'.

   (vi) The genetic markers are linked to a physical map by processes like 'in situ hybridization'

In situ **Hybridization:** One of the techniques for physical gene mapping is 'in situ hybridization'. In this technique, genes are localized in a tissue or cell using a labeled probe (DNA or RNA). The labeled probe has sequence which is complementary to gene to be localized on chromosomes. The probe is allowed to hybridize with a gene (to be detected) and hybridization of probe with gene is detected using a signal obtained depending on the label. In case, the target gene is not present, probe does not bind with gene and does not give any signal. Therefore, getting a positive signal after addition of probe in a tissue signifies the presence of target gene **(Figure 2.10)**.

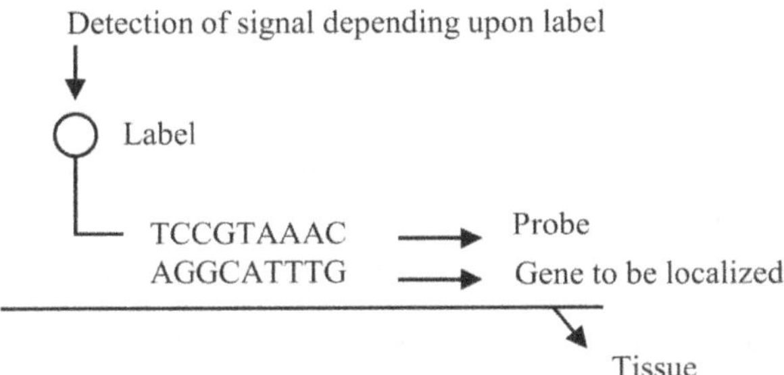

FIGURE 2.10 Basic principle of identifying gene on tissue by *in situ* hybridization in which probe binds to gene in sequence specific manner to give signal depending on label

FISH (Fluorescent *In situ* Hybridization) is a type of in situ hybridization in which probe is labeled with fluorescent dye. Therefore, fluorescence (as a signal) is obtained after successful binding of probe with target gene.

REVIEW QUESTIONS

TWO MARKS QUESTIONS

1. How may miRNA produce gene regulation by acting on 3'UTR?
2. How may gene regulation be controlled at post translational level?
3. What is miRNA?
4. What is siRNA?
5. What is gene splicing?
6. What are different steps involved in gene processing in gene expression?
7. What are epigenetic mechanisms of gene regulation?
8. What are transposons?
9. What do you understand by retro transposons?
10. What is gene mapping?
11. What are solitary genes?
12. What are duplicated genes?
13. What do you understand by pseudogenes?

14. What is linkage analysis?

15. What is in situ hybridization?

FIVE MARKS QUESTIONS

1. What are the similarities and differences in siRNA and miRNA?

2. What is gene regulation? What are different mechanisms involved in gene regulation?

3. What are different steps involved in gene expressions?

4. What do you mean by repetitive genes? What is their significance?

5. Write a note on genetic mapping? How is it different from physical mapping?

TEN MARKS QUESTIONS

1. What are siRNA? How are these formed? How these perform gene silencing functions? What are their potential therapeutic uses?

2. Write a note on gene expression and regulation of gene expression?

3. What is gene mapping? Write different methods of gene mapping?

MULTIPLE CHOICE QUESTIONS

1. Which of following is true?
   (a) MiRNA is endogenous
   (b) SiRNA is endogenous
   (c) Both miRNA and siRNA are endogenous
   (d) Both are exogenous

2. Gene splicing include
   (a) Removal of introns
   (b) Removal of exons
   (c) Removal of both introns and exons
   (d) Inhibition at 3'UTR region

3. iNOS is an
   (a) Constitutive gene   (b) Inducible gene
   (c) Housekeeping gene   (d) None of above

4. The structural features of mRNA include
   (a) 3' cap   (b)   5' poly (A) tail
   (c) Both a and b   (d)   None of above

5. Transcription involves the following
   (a) RNA polymerase   (b)   DNA polymerase
   (c) RNase III   (d)   Dicer

6. Epigenetic changes involves
   (a) Changes in DNA   (b)   Changes in RNA
   (c) Changes in histone   (d)   All the above

7. Pseudogenes are
   (a) Functional duplicated genes   (b)   Non functional duplicated genes
   (c) Single copy genes   (d)   None of above

8. Which of following is true?
   (a) Physical map tells exact locus of genes
   (b) Genetic map tell exact locus of genes
   (c) Both a and b
   (d) None of above

9. Nucleosome is composed of
   (a) Histone octamer and DNA
   (b) Histone dimer and DNA
   (c) Linker DNA and H_1 protein
   (d) Naked DNA

10. siRNA is
    (a) Exogenous   (b)   Silences RNA
    (c) Double stranded   (d)   All the above

CHAPTER 3

Necrosis and Autophagy

CHAPTER OUTLINE

Necrosis

Definitions and General Features

Characteristic Features of Necrosis

Different types of Necrosis (Morphological Patterns of Necrosis)

Morphological Changes in Nucleus during Cell Death

Autophagy

Definitions and General Features

Types of Autophagy

Macroautophagy

Microautophagy

Chaperone-Mediated Autophagy

Digestion of Cell Organelles, Endogenous substances and Exogenous Pathogens

Involvement of Genes in Autophagy

Steps Involved in Autophagy (Mechanism of Autophagy)

Blockade of Autophagy

Physiological and Pathological Role of Autophagy

NECROSIS

DEFINITIONS AND GENERAL FEATURES

It is defined as a spectrum of morphological changes that occur in irreversibly injured cell or lethally injured cell. Indeed, it is a type of cell death and is mainly characterized on morphological (gross appearance) basis. It is the most common form of cell death and it occurs in response to external stimuli. The common stimuli that may produce necrosis include hypoxia (decrease in oxygen supply) or ischemia (decrease in blood supply), infectious agents (bacteria, viruses), chemicals etc. Initially, an injury causing agent produces reversible injury. However, persistence of injury causing agent may produce irreversible injury and these irreversibly injured cells undergo necrosis. Examples include myocardial injury in myocardial infarction and cerebral injury during stroke.

CHARACTERISTIC FEATURES OF NECROSIS

The following may be regarded as characteristic features of necrosis:

1. It is the most common form of cell death in pathological conditions.
2. It is unprogrammed death of cells and living tissue.
3. The cells undergoing necrosis exhibit swelling.
4. There is recruitment of inflammatory cells (WBC) and release of cytokines, leading to initiation and propagation of inflammatory reactions in tissues undergoing necrosis.
5. There are different patterns of necrosis depending on appearance of tissue undergoing necrosis.

DIFFERENT TYPES OF NECROSIS
(MORPHOLOGICAL PATTERNS OF NECROSIS)

On the basis of appearance of necrotic cell/tissue, there are different morphological patterns of necrosis (**Table 3.1**).

TABLE 3.1 Different morphological patterns of necrosis

S. No	Type of Necrosis	Key Features	Examples
1.	Coagulative necrosis	• Preservation of the structural features of cell • Cell death occurs due to denaturation of proteins· • Invading WBC release digestive enzymes to digest the irreversibly injured cell	Hypoxic cell death e.g. myocardial infarction
2.	Liquefactive necrosis	• Digestion of dead cells to form a viscous liquid mass • Cellular framework is destroyed· • Release of lysosomal enzymes produce cell digestion	Hypoxic injury to cells of central nervous system
3.	Gangrenous necrosis	• Ischemic injury is superimposed by infection • In dry gangrene, ischemic injury is predominant • In wet gangrene, infection is predominant	Diabetic and Cigarette smokers are more susceptible to gangrene development

Table 3.1 Contd...

S. No	Type of Necrosis	Key Features	Examples
4.	Caseous necrosis	• Whitish appearance of the central necrotic area • Combination of coagulative and liquefactive necrosis	Infection by *Mycobacteria tuberculosis* or some fungi.
5.	Fibrinoid Necrosis	• Deposition of fibrin in the area of necrosis around blood vessels	Injuries to blood vessels.
6.	Fat Necrosis	• Lipase digest triglyceride esters to release fatty acids, which combine with calcium to produce white chalky appearance	Acute pancreatitis

1. **Coagulative Necrosis:** In this type of necrosis, there is preservation of the structural features of cells for few days. In this type, cell death occurs due to denaturation of both functional as well as structural proteins. Since, enzymes are also proteins; therefore, due to denaturation of enzymes, cellular proteolysis does not take place and cellular structural framework is preserved. The dead cells are invaded by large number of WBCs. The resulting WBCs release digestive enzymes including proteolytic enzymes to digest the irreversibly injured cell. This type of necrosis is a characteristic of hypoxic cell death of all tissues e.g. myocardial infarction. However, brain is the exception, which undergoes liquefactive necrosis during hypoxia.

2. **Liquefactive Necrosis:** In this type of necrosis, there is a digestion of dead cells to form a viscous liquid mass and cellular structural framework is completely destroyed. In this type, there is release of lysosomal enzymes that produce digestion of cellular components. This type of necrosis follows bacterial or fungal infections. The cells of central nervous system undergo liquefactive necrosis in response to hypoxic injury.

3. **Gangrenous Necrosis:** Gangrene is a type of necrosis, when ischemic injury is superimposed by infection. It may be 'wet' or 'dry', depending on whether the ischemic injury is predominant or infection. In dry gangrene, ischemic injury is predominant, with a minor component of infection. On the contrary, in wet gangrene, infection is predominant. Diabetic patients and cigarette smokers are more susceptible to gangrenous necrosis.

4. **Caseous Necrosis:** It is a distinctive form of necrosis and the word "caseous" is derived from ''cheesy''. It generally refers to a whitish gross appearance of the central necrotic area. It can be considered as a combination of coagulative and liquefactive necrosis and is caused by *Mycobacteria tuberculosis* or some fungi. In this type, the central necrotic portion appears like cheese (liquefactive component) and this area is surrounded by intact cell components (coagulative component).

5. **Fibrinoid Necrosis:** It is characterized by smooth muscle necrosis surrounding arterioles and other vessels. There is deposition of fibrin and other plasma protein in the area of necrosis. Fibrin is identified in light microscopy due to the eosinophilic appearance. It is caused by injuries to blood vessels.

6. **Fat Necrosis:** It mainly occurs in acute pancreatitis. During pancreatic inflammation, lipase enzyme is released into the pancreatic tissue. The lipases digest the triglyceride esters and release fatty acids. The released fatty acids combine with calcium to produce white chalky appearance (fat saponification). It is caused by direct mechanical injury or inflammation of the pancreas (acute pancreatitis).

MORPHOLOGICAL CHANGES IN NUCLEUS DURING CELL DEATH

During cell death, nuclear changes can assume one of three patterns (Table 3.2) (Figure 3.1):

(a) **Karyolysis:** Due to activation of DNAse enzyme, there is degradation of DNA or chromosomes and hence, nucleus is lightly stained with basic dye. The light staining of nucleus is also referred to as fading of basophilia of chromatin. It mainly occurs in necrotic cell death.

(b) **Pyknosis:** This type is characterized by nuclear shrinkage and DNA condenses into a solid shrunken mass and hence, nucleus is darkly stained with basic dye. The dark staining of nucleus is also referred to as an increase in basophilia of chromatin. It mainly occurs in early stage of apoptosis.

(c) **Karyorrhexis:** In this type, nucleus undergoes pyknosis followed by fragmentation of nucleus. In other words, the pyknotic nucleus undergoes fragmentation. It occurs in late stage of apoptosis.

TABLE 3.2 Different forms of nuclear changes occurring during cell death

S. No	Nuclear change	Features
1.	Karyolysis	• Activation of DNAse activity • Degradation of DNA or chromosomes • Fading of basophilia of chromatin • Occurs in necrosis
2.	Pyknosis	• Shrinkage of nuclear components • DNA condenses into a solid shrunken mass • Increase in basophilia of chromatin· • Occurs in early stage of apoptosis
3.	Karyorrhexis	• Nucleus undergoes pyknosis followed by fragmentation of nucleus • Pyknotic nucleus undergoes fragmentation • Occurs in late stage of apoptosis

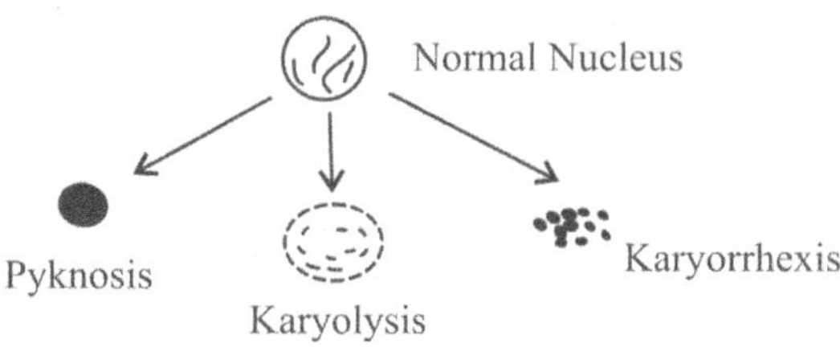

FIGURE 3.1 Morphological changes in nucleus during irreversible cell injury

AUTOPHAGY

DEFINITIONS AND GENERAL FEATURES

It refers to digestion of the body's own cellular components using lysosomes. It may also be defined as degradation of cytoplasmic components within lysosomes. Like inflammation, autophagy has dual role. Basal autophagy is required to maintain cellular homeostasis. However, excessive autophagy is detrimental and may be involved in disease progression. Hence, both physiological and pathophysiological roles of autophagy have been explored such as during starvation, cellular adaptation, intracellular protein and organelle clearance, anti-aging, elimination of microorganisms, cell death, tumor suppression, and antigen presentation during immune system activation. Apart from autophagy, there is another digestion pathway in cells, which is termed as 'ubiquitin–proteasome system'. In this system, only ubiquitinated proteins undergo proteasomal degradation.

TYPES OF AUTOPHAGY

There are three types of autophagy:

1. **Macroautophagy:** The term "autophagy" usually refers to macroautophagy. In this type, there is a formation of a double membrane bound vacuole known as 'autophagosome'. This is formed by engulfment of small part of the cytoplasm or organelles. Thereafter, autophagosome fuses with lysosomes to degrade the enclosed material. The final products including amino acids, lipids and nucleotides are released into the cytoplasm via permeases (enzymes that increase permeability) present on the lysosomal membrane **(Figure 3.2)**. These molecules participate in anabolic reactions required to maintain cellular functions.

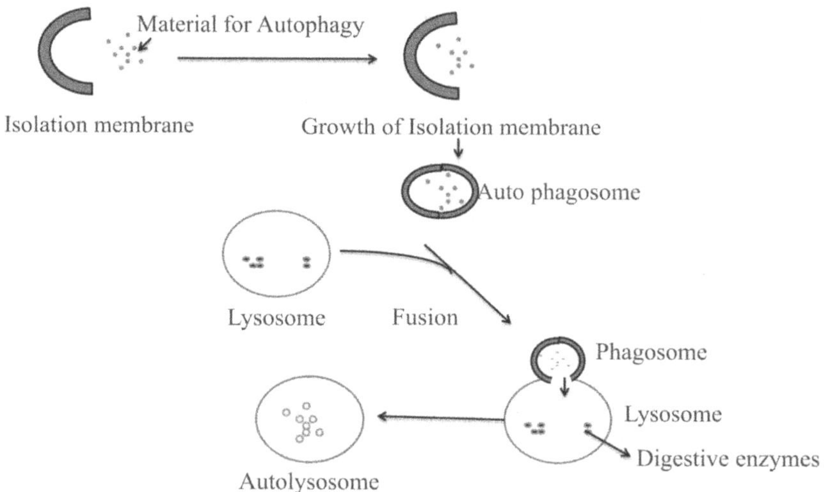

FIGURE 3.2 Different steps involved in macroautophagy and formation of autolysosomes

Macroautophagy may further be sub-classified into 'Induced Autophagy' and 'Basal Autophagy':

(a) **Basal Autophagy:** This type of autophagy is important for constitutive turnover of cytosolic components. This type of autophagy is required to keep cells free of damaged proteins and organelles because all damaged organelles are degraded by autophagy.

(b) **Induced Autophagy:** It is activated during stressful conditions such as during starvation and it helps to produce amino acids by degrading internal cellular proteins. Induced autophagy has pathophysiological role and may be involved in cell death during disease conditions.

2. **Microautophagy:** It involves direct uptake of fractions of the cytoplasm by the lysosomal membrane **(Figure 3.3)** and it is dependent on GTP hydrolysis and calcium. However, exact molecular mechanisms are unclear.

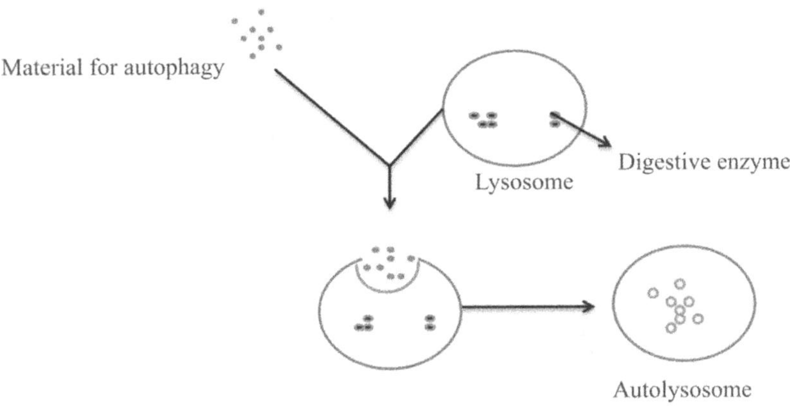

FIGURE 3.3　Different steps involved in microautophagy

3. **Chaperone-Mediated Autophagy (CMA):** Chaperones refer to those proteins that assist the folding/unfolding or assembly/disassembly of other macromolecular structures. It is a selective autophagy and is described only in mammalian cells. In this type, proteins required to be digested are delivered to lysosomes with the help of chaperons. The proteins that are to be digested contain a 'specific motif', which is recognized by chaperone, Hsc70. It is a cytosolic heat shock protein and is a member of the Hsp70 family. The molecules undergoing autophagy bind to Hsc70 and are delivered to lysosomes through lysosomal receptors (Lamp2A) **(Figure 3.4)**. Lamp refers to 'lysosomal associated membrane proteins'. Thereafter, molecules are digested inside the lysosomes.

DIGESTION OF CELL ORGANELLES, ENDOGENOUS SUBSTANCES AND EXOGENOUS PATHOGENS

Autophagy is capable of digesting different cell organelles, endogenous substances and exogenous pathogens. Depending on the type of organelle, endogenous substance or exogenous pathogen, different terms are employed. 'Mitophagy' refers to specific elimination of mitochondria, 'Ribophagy' for ribosomes, 'Pexophagy' degrades peroxisomes, 'Lipophagy' for the degradation of lipid droplets, 'Aggrephagy' degrades intracellular protein aggregates and misfolded proteins such as those observed in many neurodegenerative conditions. 'Xenophagy' denotes the degradation of intracellular pathogens such as viruses and intracellular bacteria.

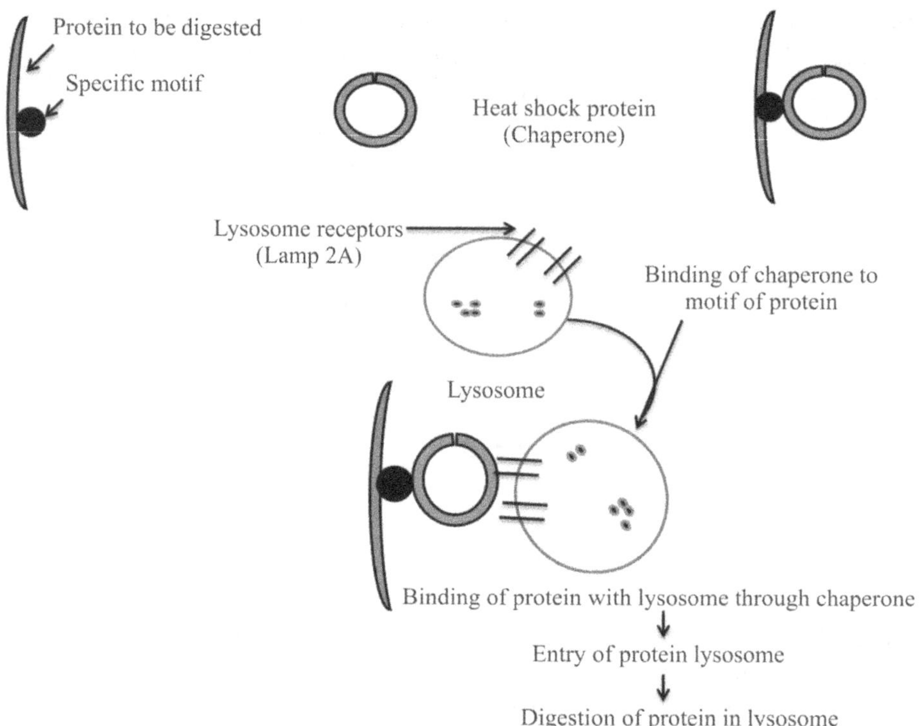

FIGURE 3.4 Different steps involved in Chaperone mediated autophagy

INVOLVEMENT OF GENES IN AUTOPHAGY

1. Autophagy is conserved from yeast to humans and is regulated by the Atg family of proteins. Atg proteins are involved in various stages of the process including induction, autophagosome formation, fusion and degradation. The role of different Atg proteins is explained in subsequent sections.

2. Beclin 1 is one of best characterized gene regulating the functions of Atg proteins. Beclin 1 was originally identified as an interaction partner of Bcl-2, an anti-apoptotic protein. However, it also controls autophagic reactions. It has been shown that during starvation, there is dissociation of Beclin 1 and Bcl-2, which may activate autophagy. Therefore, it is proposed that Bcl-2 is not only an anti-apoptotic, but also an anti-autophagic protein. Bcl-2 suppresses autophagy by inhibiting elevation of cytosolic calcium and decrease in calcium may inhibit autophagy.

STEPS INVOLVED IN AUTOPHAGY (MECHANISM OF AUTOPHAGY)

Autophagy consists of sequential steps including induction, sequestration, fusion, degradation, and amino acid/peptide generation **(Figure 3.2)**.

1. **Induction:** The most typical trigger of autophagy is nutrient starvation and lack of essential nutrient can induce autophagy. Depletion of total amino acids strongly induces autophagy in many types of cultured cells. How cells sense amino acid concentration is not fully understood. In organisms, each cell does not necessarily sense nutrient availability. Instead, the endocrine system manages autophagy regulation. Amongst different hormones, the role of insulin, growth factors has been described in regulating autophagy. Apart from starvation, other stimuli may also induce autophagy such as hypoxia, radiations, organelle damage, aggregation of abnormal proteins etc.

2. **Sequestration and Autophagosome Formation:** Autophagy is initiated by the formation of a double membrane bound vacuole known as the autophagosome. Autophagosome formation is a multistep process that consists of biogenesis of the 'isolation membrane', also termed as 'phagophore'. In the first step of autophagosome formation, phagophore or isolation membrane begins sequestering cytoplasmic constituents, including organelles. In a sequential process, there is elongation of the phagophore membrane, which fully encloses the cytoplasmic constituent and it leads to formation of autophagosome. There is a key role of the endoplasmic reticulum in the initiation of autophagy. The mitochondrial outer membrane has been proposed as another source of the isolation membrane. Furthermore, the Golgi apparatus and post-Golgi compartments containing Atg9 also contribute to the formation of the autophagosome membrane.

    Among the 31 Atg proteins, 18 Atg proteins—Atg1–10, Atg12–14, Atg16–18, Atg29, and Atg31 are involved in autophagosome formation and are called "AP-Atg proteins". These Atg proteins are hierarchically recruited at the preautophagosomal structure (PAS) to form autophagosome. It has been shown that the AP-Atg proteins depend on each other for recruitment to the PAS. Atg17 functions as a scaffold for PAS organization.

3. **Fusion of Autophagosome with Lysosomes:** In the next step, autophagosomes fuse with lysosomes to form 'autolysosomes' or 'autophagolysosomes'. Sometimes, autophagosome can merge with endosomes before fusing with the lysosomal compartment. The term 'amphisome' was coined by Per O. Seglen to describe the vacuole resulting from the fusion of the autophagosome with the endosome. Two types of fusion have been documented:

    (a) *Complete Fusion*: In this, there is a complete fusion of the autophagosome with the lysosome and two vacuoles merge with each other.

    (b) *Partial Fusion*: In second type of fusion, there is transfer of material from the autophagosome to the lysosomal compartment via a kiss-and-run fusion process. In this case, two separate vesicles are maintained and do not merge with one another.

The definition of autophagosomes, amphisomes, and autolysosomes is based on their function, not on morphology. Therefore, it is easy to distinguish these structures by electron microscopy. In such cases, the term 'autophagic vacuoles' may be used to cover all autophagic structures. The average half-life of autophagic vacuoles appears to be around 10 min.

4. **Degradation and Amino acid/Peptide generation:** The inner membrane of the autophagosome and the cytoplasm-derived materials contained in the autophagosome are degraded by lysosomal hydrolases. Following degradation of proteins, amino acids are produced. Thereafter, these amino acids are exported from lysosomes to the cytosol with the help of vacuolar permeases.

BLOCKADE OF AUTOPHAGY

The blockade of any of the process including autophagosome formation, fusion with the lysosomal compartment or impairment of lysosomal function results in an accumulation of autophagosomes. This slows down or interrupts the autophagic process. The blockade may be achieved through following:

1. **Microtubules:** Studies have confirmed the role of microtubules in fusion process of autophagosome with lysosomes. Autophagosomes move bidirectionally along microtubules. The destabilization of microtubules by vinblastine blocks autophagosome maturation and inhibits fusion between autophagic vacuoles and lysosomes.

2. **Lysosomal Membrane Proteins:** Lysosomal associated membrane proteins (Lamps) are glycosylated, lysosomal transmembrane proteins and autophagy is dependent on presence of these functional proteins. An impairment in lysosomal surface receptors (proteins) inhibits autophagy.

3. **Vacuolar ATPases (v-ATPases):** Vacuolar ATPases (v-ATPases) are surface proteins present on lysosomes and these function to maintain acidic pH in lysosomes by controlling movement of H^+ ions. Inhibition of the activity of v-ATPase by certain drugs or chemicals blocks the lysosomal pumping of H^+ and inhibits lysosomal enzymes, which are active at low pH. Therefore, inhibition of acidification in lysosomes may also prevent autophagy.

PHYSIOLOGICAL AND PATHOLOGICAL ROLE OF AUTOPHAGY

1. **Development and Differentiation:** Autophagy is essential during development and differentiation. During preimplantation period after oocyte

fertilization, there is autophagic degradation of components of oocyte cytoplasm. It is also implicated in eliminating apoptotic bodies during embryonic development. Autophagy-mediated remodeling of cytoplasm is also involved in the differentiation of erythrocytes, lymphocytes, and neural stem cells to neurons.

2. **Utilization of Degradation Products:** Under normal conditions and during very short periods of starvation, maintenance of the amino acid pool is dependent on the ubiquitin–proteasome system. However, during prolonged starvation, there is up-regulation of autophagy as an adaptive response, which provides necessary amino acids due to degradation of cytosolic proteins. These amino acids are used as an energy source after depletion of carbohydrates. Amino acids produced by autophagy may also be used to synthesize stress adaptive proteins, which are important for developing adaptation during starvation.

3. **Elimination of Damaged Organelles:** Autophagy participates in intracellular clearance of damaged, excessive or unneeded organelles. Peroxisomes induced by metabolic demand are selectively degraded by autophagy, when these are no longer needed. Similarly, damaged mitochondria are selectively eliminated by macroautophagy.

4. **Preventing Development of Neurodegenerative Diseases:** Autophagy is essential to eliminate abnormal intracellular protein aggregates and it helps in preventing the development of neurodegenerative diseases such as Huntington's, Alzheimer's and Parkinson's diseases. However, dysregulation of this process has important consequences and may lead to accumulation of protein aggregates in the brain to produce neurodegenerative diseases.

5. **Elimination of Intracellular Pathogens:** Various pathogenic bacteria, such as *Streptococcus pyogenes* and *Shigella flexneri* are sequestered by large autophagosomes and degraded following fusion with lysosomes. Another well-known pathogen persisting inside phagocytes is *Mycobacterium tuberculosis*. These bacteria inhibit phagosome maturation and survive in premature phagosomes. However, when autophagy is stimulated by starvation, rapamycin, or interferons, there is full formation of phagosomes followed by delivery of bacteria to lysosomes to produce its death.

6. **Immunity:** Autophagy is also used to present endogenous antigens on major histocompatibility complex (MHC) class II molecules, which are recognized by $CD4^+$ T cells. It also degrades endogenous antigens into peptides, which are then delivered to endoplasmic reticulum for its processing. MHC class I molecules load these peptides and move to the cell surface to be recognized by $CD8^+$ T cells.

7. **Obesity and Insulin Resistance:** Autophagy is involved in the regulation of metabolism in the peripheral tissues. Decreases in hepatic autophagy may produce obesity and insulin resistance. Animal studies have shown that restoration of Atg7 expression may decrease obesity and rescue insulin resistance.

8. **Cancer:** The role of autophagy in cancer is highly complex and dependent on cancer stage and context. Autophagy acts as a tumor suppressor in initial stages. Several of the functions of autophagy such as the elimination of defective organelles, which reduces oxidative stress and prevents DNA damage, contribute to its tumor suppressive effects. However, autophagy is required in the later stages of tumor progression to enable tumor cells to cope with metabolic stress.

REVIEW QUESTIONS

TWO MARKS QUESTIONS

1. Describe Caseous necrosis.
2. What do you understand by Liquefactive necrosis?
3. Explain fat necrosis.
4. What is pyknosis?
5. What do you understand by autophagy mediated cell death?
6. What is chaperon mediated autophagy?
7. What is the difference between basal and induced autophagy?
8. What is the difference between macro and microautophagy?
9. What is autophagosome?
10. What is the role of autophagy in cancer?

FIVE MARKS QUESTIONS

1. Explain different types of necrosis with examples.
2. Write characteristic features of necrosis.
3. What is gangrene? What are its different types? How is it different from fibrinoid and liquefactive necrosis?
4. What are the different morphological changes that may take place during cell death?
5. Explain the mechanism of autophagy.

TEN MARKS QUESTIONS

1. Define Necrosis. Mention its types. Explain the causes and pathology of each type of necrosis.
2. What is the physiological and pathological significance of autophagy?

MULTIPLE CHOICE QUESTIONS

1. Coagulative necrosis is characterized by
   (a) Digestion of cell
   (b) Influx of WBC
   (c) Preserved structural feature
   (d) Destruction of cellular framework

2. Liquefactive necrosis is characterized by
   (a) Viscous liquid mass
   (b) Destruction of cellular framework
   (c) Involvement of lysosomal enzymes
   (d) All of the above

3. Fibrinoid necrosis occurs due to injury in
   (a) Blood vessels   (b) Brain
   (c) Pancreas   (d) None of above

4. Karyolysis is a characteristic feature of
   (a) Apoptosis   (b) Necrosis
   (c) Both a and b   (d) None of above

5. Shrinkage of nuclear components takes place in
   (a) Pyknosis   (b) Karyarrhexis
   (c) Karyolysis   (d) A and B

6. Direct uptake of fractions of the cytoplasm by the lysosomal membrane is termed as
   (a) Macroautophagy
   (b) Microautophagy
   (c) Chaperon-mediated autophagy
   (d) None of above

7. Mitophagy' refers to specific elimination
   (a) Mitochondria   (b) Nucleus
   (c) Peroxisomes   (d) None of above

8. Degradation (dissociation) of Beclin 1 and Bcl-2
   - (a) Promote autophagy
   - (b) Reduce autophagy
   - (c) No effect
   - (d) Depends on the cell

9. Amphisome is formed by fusion of autophagosome with
   - (a) Lysosomes
   - (b) Endosomes
   - (c) Both a and b
   - (d) None of above

10. Autophagy may be inhibited during
    - (a) Starvation
    - (b) Microtubule disruption
    - (c) During differentiation process
    - (d) Accumulation of abnormal protein

CHAPTER 4

Apoptosis

CHAPTER OUTLINE

Definition and General Features
Morphology of Apoptosis

Early Stage

Late Stage
No Inflammation during Apoptosis
Characteristic Features of Apoptotic Cell Death
Mechanisms of Apoptosis

Extrinsic (Death Receptor) Pathway

Intrinsic (Mitochondrial) Pathway

Perforin-Granzyme System

Execution (Common) Pathway
Caspases
Laboratory Methods to Detect Apoptosis

Physiological Role of Apoptosis

Pathophysiological Role of Apoptosis

DEFINITION AND GENERAL FEATURES

The term apoptosis (a-po-toe-sis) was first used in a paper by Kerr, Wyllie, and Currie in 1972 to describe a morphologically distinct form of cell death. It is defined as 'programmed cell death', which involves genetically determined elimination of cells. It is a coordinated and often energy-dependent process that involves the activation of cysteine proteases called 'caspases'. It includes a complex cascade of events that link the initiating stimuli to the final demise of the cell. Both physiological and pathological stimuli can trigger apoptosis. Physiologically, apoptosis occurs normally during development and aging and it acts as a homeostatic mechanism to maintain the cell populations in tissues. However, it may also be activated in pathological conditions.

It is different from another type of cell death 'necrosis' (described in Chapter 3). However, it is interesting to note that apoptosis and necrosis can occur independently, sequentially, or simultaneously. It is the type of stimuli and/or degree of stimuli that determines if cells die by apoptosis or necrosis. At low doses, a variety of injurious stimuli such as heat, radiation, hypoxia and cytotoxic anticancer drugs can induce apoptosis. However, the same stimuli can result in necrosis at higher doses. Furthermore, apoptosis may be followed by necrosis and it is termed as 'apoptosis-induced necrosis'.

MORPHOLOGY OF APOPTOSIS

The morphological features of cell depend on the stage of apoptosis:

1. **Early Stage:** During the early process of apoptosis, there is cell shrinkage and pyknosis, which can be seen under light microscope. With cell shrinkage, the cells become smaller in size, cytoplasm becomes dense and the organelles are more tightly packed. Pyknosis refers to chromatin condensation (see Figure 3.1 of Chapter 3) and is the most characteristic feature of apoptosis. Under light microscope, the apoptotic cell appears as a round or oval mass with dark eosinophilic cytoplasm and dense purple nuclear chromatin.

2. **Late Stage:** As apoptosis proceeds, there is karyorrhexis i.e., fragmentation of pyknotic nucleus. The cell also undergoes fragmentation and cell fragments are divided into apoptotic bodies during a process called "budding". Apoptotic bodies consist of cytoplasm with tightly packed organelles with or without a nuclear fragment. An interesting point is that the organelle integrity is maintained even at the last stage of apoptosis and components are enclosed within an intact plasma membrane. These apoptotic bodies are subsequently phagocytosed by macrophages. Macrophages that engulf and digest apoptotic cells are called 'tingible body macrophages'.

NO INFLAMMATION DURING APOPTOSIS

It is very important to understand that there is no inflammatory reaction associated with the process of apoptosis or with the removal of apoptotic cells. This is in sharp contrast to necrosis, which is characterized by initiation and maintenance of inflammation. There are following factors that contribute to non-inflammatory process during apoptosis:

1. Apoptotic cells do not release their cellular constituents into the surrounding interstitial tissue and plasma membrane remains intact throughout the process of apoptosis

2. Apoptotic bodies are quickly phagocytosed by surrounding cells (macrophages) and prevent the initiation of inflammation

3. The engulfing tingible body macrophages do not produce inflammatory cytokines

CHARACTERISTIC FEATURES OF APOPTOTIC CELL DEATH

1. It is programmed cell death and involves genetically determined death of cells
2. It is highly coordinated and energy-dependent process
3. Both physiological and pathological stimuli can trigger apoptosis.
4. Apoptosis is initiated and executed through caspases
5. There is cell shrinkage and pyknosis in early stage of apoptosis
6. There is karyorrhexis and budding of cell in late stage of apoptosis to form apoptotic bodies, which are phagocytosed by macrophages
7. The plasma membrane remains intact throughout the process of apoptosis
8. There is no inflammatory reaction associated with the process of apoptosis

KEY DIFFERENCES BETWEEN NECROSIS AND APOPTOSIS

The key differences between necrosis and apoptosis may be summarized as follows **(Table 4.1)**:

TABLE 4.1 Key differences between necrosis and apoptosis

S. No	Necrosis	Apoptosis
1.	It is an un-programmed cell death	It is programmed cell death
2.	It is pathological in nature	It can be both physiological and pathological
3	It involves inflammatory reactions	Generally, inflammatory reactions are not present
4.	Cell swelling is the first sign of	Cell shrinkage is the first change injury in apoptosis
5.	It is energy independent process	It is energy dependent process
6.	The DNA is cut in a random manner and in gel electrophoresis, smear (due to all pieces of DNA of different sizes) is observed **(Figure 4.1)**	DNA is cut at specific points only and in gel electrophoresis, laddering is observed (due to bands of DNA of specific sizes) **(Figure 4.1)**
7.	It is characterized by karyolysis	It is characterized by pyknosis and Karyorrhexis
8.	Plasma membrane is ruptured	Plasma membrane remains intact throughout apoptosis

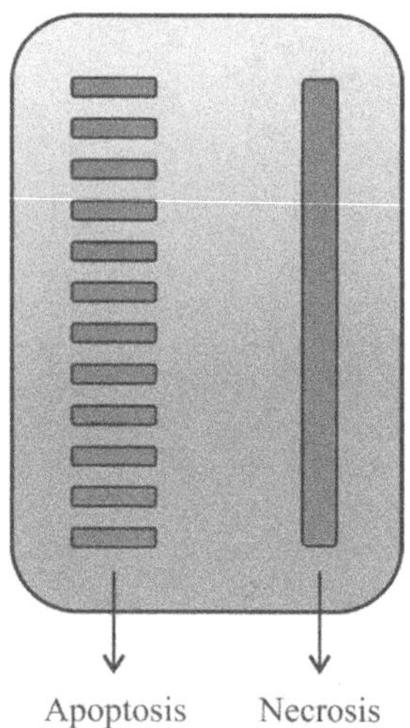

FIGURE 4.1

Appearance of DNA laddering in gel electrophoresis is a characteristic feature of apoptosis.

MECHANISMS OF APOPTOSIS

The mechanisms of apoptosis are highly complex and sophisticated, involving an energy-dependent cascade of molecular events. Cells undergo apoptosis through following steps:

1. Initiation Pathway 2. Execution Pathway

1. **Initiation Pathway:** Initiation of apoptosis involves two main apoptotic pathways: the extrinsic or death receptor pathway and the intrinsic or mitochondrial pathway. Additionally, T-cell mediated cytotoxicity involves another pathway termed as 'perforin-granzyme system'.

(a) ***Extrinsic (Death Receptor) Pathway:*** The extrinsic signaling pathways that initiate apoptosis involve 'death receptors' that are members of tumor necrosis factor (TNF) receptor super family. Ligands bind to these death receptors and signal is conveyed through these death receptors to inside the cell. Some examples of ligands and corresponding death receptors include Fas ligand (FasL)/Fas receptor (FasR), TNF-α/ TNFR1, Apo3L/ DR3, Apo2L/DR4 and Apo2L/DR5 **(R-receptors; L-Ligand, DR-Death Receptors)**. Upon ligand binding, cytoplasmic adapter proteins are recruited and bind to inside of death receptors. These adapter proteins have a 'death domain', which in turn conveys death signal. The binding of Fas ligand to Fas receptor results in the binding of the adapter protein FADD (Fas associated Death Domain) and the binding of TNF ligand to TNF receptor results in the binding of the adapter protein TRADD (TNF receptor associated Death Domain). It is followed by formation of a death-inducing signaling complex (DISC), which in turn activates procaspase-8 to form caspase-8 (initiator caspase). Once caspase-8 is activated, the initiation pathway ends and execution phase of apoptosis is triggered by activating caspase 3 (executioner caspase) **(Figure 4.2)**.

Regulation (Inhibition) of Extrinsic Pathway

(i) Death receptor-mediated apoptosis may be inhibited by a protein called 'c-FLIP', which binds to FADD and caspase-8, rendering them ineffective.

(ii) Apoptosis may also be regulated through a protein called 'Toso', which blocks Fas-induced apoptosis in T cells by inhibiting caspase-8 processing

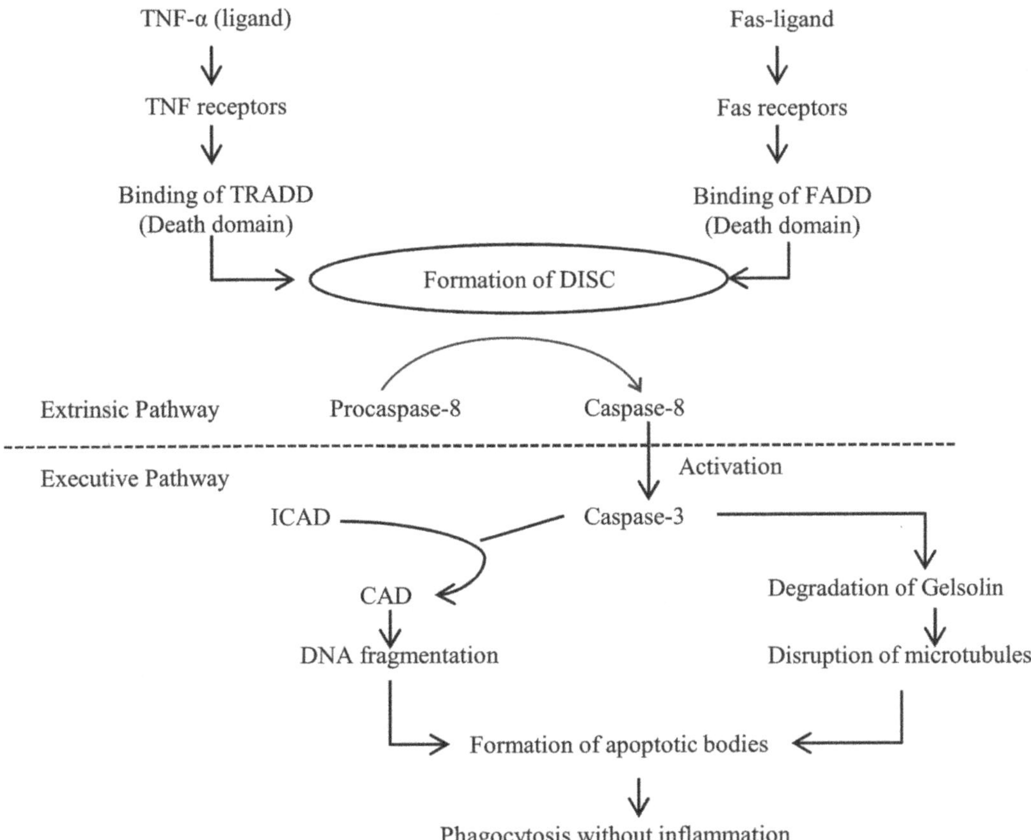

FIGURE 4.2 Extrinsic (receptor mediated) and executive pathway involved in apoptosis

(b) ***Intrinsic (Mitochondrial) Pathway***: The intrinsic signaling pathways that initiate apoptosis are non-receptor-mediated and death signals are directly transmitted from outside to mitochondria. These death signals include absence of growth factors, hormones and cytokines or exposure to radiations, toxins, hypoxia, hyperthermia, viral infections, and free radicals. All these stimuli may converge on mitochondria and may lead to opening of the mitochondrial permeability transition pore (mPTP). The opening of this pore increases the permeability of mitochondrial membrane and it is called as Mitochondrial Outer Membrane Permeabilization (MOMP). Increase in permeability leads to loss of the mitochondrial transmembrane potential and release of two main groups of pro-apoptotic proteins from mitochondria to cytosol **(Figure 4.3)**.

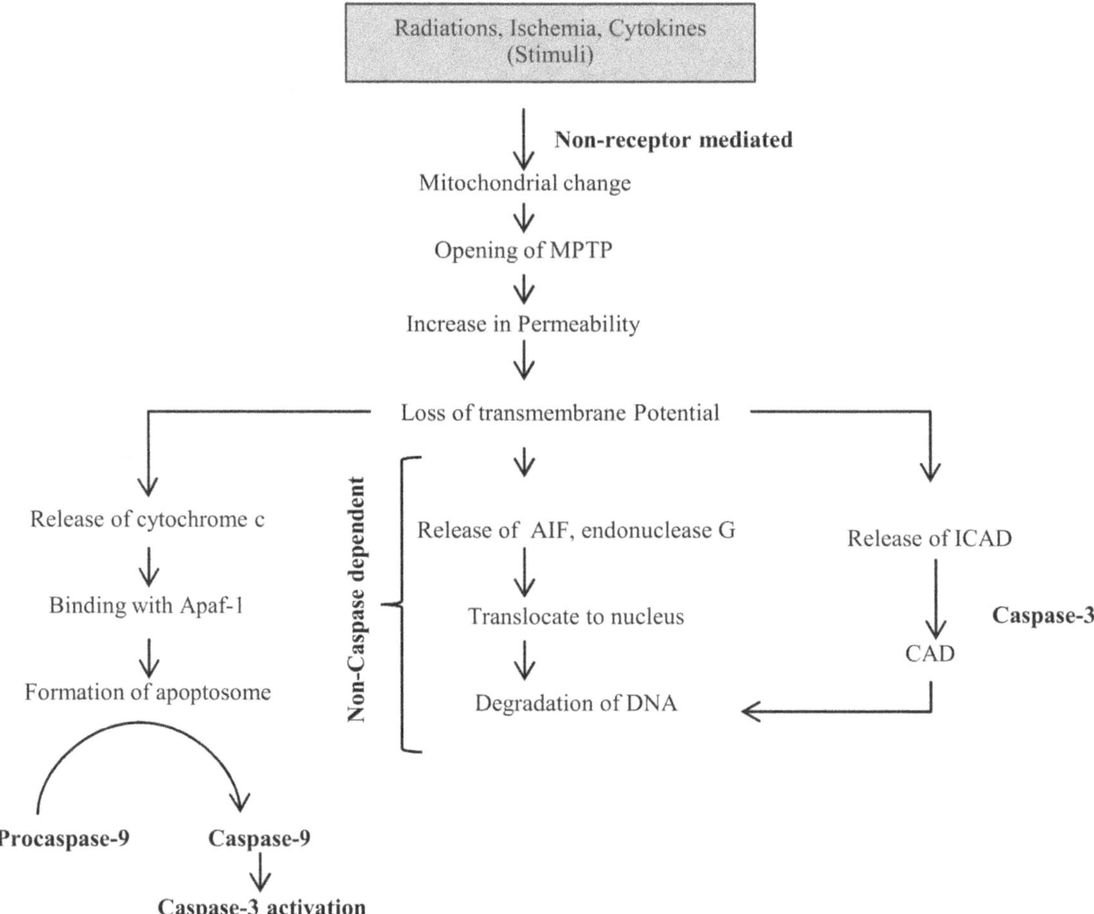

FIGURE 4.3 Intrinsic (mitochondrial) pathway involved in apoptosis

(i) ***First Group of Pro-apoptotic Proteins:*** It consists of cytochrome *c*, Smac/DIABLO, and the serine protease HtrA2/Omi. These proteins activate the caspase-dependent mitochondrial pathway. Furthermore, these proteins act much earlier in the apoptosis process. Cytochrome c binds with Apaf-1 (Apoptotic protease activating factor) to form an 'apoptosome'. This is followed by activation of procaspase-9 to form caspase-9 (initiator caspase). In turn, caspase-9 activates caspase 3 (executioner caspase) to execute apoptosis. Smac/DIABLO and HtrA2/Omi promote apoptosis by inhibiting IAP (inhibitors of apoptosis proteins) activity.

(ii) ***Second Group of Pro-apoptotic Proteins:*** The second group of pro-apoptotic proteins including AIF (Apoptosis Inducing Factor), endonuclease G and CAD (caspase activated DNAase) are released from the mitochondria. However, the release of these groups of proteins is a late event that occurs after the cell has committed to die. AIF and endonuclease G translocate to the nucleus and causes DNA fragmentation to produce condensation of chromatin in nucelus. This early form of nuclear condensation is referred to as 'stage I' condensation. AIF and endonuclease G both function in a caspase- independent manner.

CAD is also released from the mitochondria and translocates to the nucleus. Inside the nucleus, it is activated by caspase-3 and then, it leads to oligonucleosomal DNA fragmentation, which is more pronounced and advanced chromatin condensation occurs. This latter and more ronounced chromatin condensation is referred to as 'stage II' condensation.

Regulation of Intrinsic Pathway

These mitochondrial events involved in apoptosis occur through members of the Bcl-2 family of proteins. The Bcl-2 family of proteins governs mitochondrial membrane permeability and these proteins can be either pro-apoptotic or anti-apoptotic. A total of 25 genes have been identified in the Bcl-2 family. Some of the anti-apoptotic proteins include Bcl-2, Bcl-x, Bcl-XL, Bcl-XS, Bcl-w, BAG, and some of the pro-apoptotic proteins include Bcl-10, Bax, Bak, Bid, Bad, Bim, Bik, and Blk. These proteins regulate apoptosis by controlling the cytochrome *c* release from the mitochondria via alteration of mitochondrial membrane permeability. For example, when Bad (pro-apoptotic) is un-phosphorylated, it is translocated to the mitochondria to release cytochrome C. However, on its phosphorylation, it is trapped and sequestered in the cytosol and cannot move inside the mitochondria to release cytochrome C.

Puma and Noxa are also two members of the Bcl 2 family that are also involved in pro-apoptosis. These play an important role in *p53*-mediated apoptosis. It has been shown that increase in Puma leads to increase in BAX expression, which translocates to the mitochondria to release cytochrome *c* release and induce apoptosis.

(iii) Perforin-Granzyme System: The cytotoxic T lymphocytes are able to kill target cells via the extrinsic pathway and the FasL/FasR interaction is the predominant method of T lymphocytes-induced apoptosis. However, they cells also exert their cytotoxic effects on tumor cells or virus-infected cells via a novel pathway i.e., 'Perforin-Granzyme system'. It involves secretion of the transmembrane pore-forming molecule 'perforin' from T cells and perforin is attached to target cell. This is mainly a channel through which contents of cytoplasmic granules of T cells enter into target cells. The serine proteases granzyme A and granzyme B are the most important components, which are passed from T cells to target cells through perforin channel. Granzyme B activates pro-caspase-10 to form caspase 10 (initiator caspase) and activates pro-caspase 3 to form caspase 3 (executioner caspase). It may also act through mitochondrial pathway to amplify intrinsic pathway. Granzyme A is also an important enzyme in cytotoxic T cell-induced apoptosis and activates caspase independent pathways. It activates DNA degradation via DNAase NM23-H1 by cleaving the 'SET complex' and thus, releasing inhibition of NM23-H1 **(Figure 4.4)**.

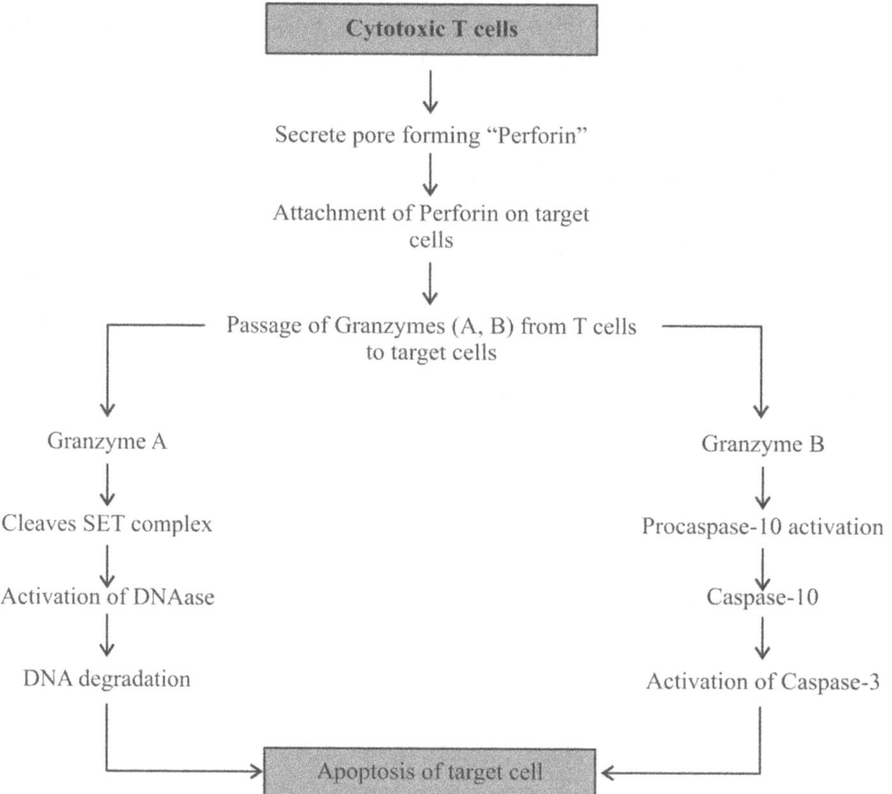

FIGURE 4.4 Perforin-Granzyme system of inducing apoptosis by cytotoxic T cells

2. **Execution (Common) Pathway:** The extrinsic, intrinsic and perforin-granzyme pathways converge at the point of the execution phase. Therefore, it is also termed as common or final pathway of apoptosis. It may further be divided into two phases:

   (a) **Activation of Executioner Caspases:** This phase is characterized by activation of execution caspases, which produce final cell death in apoptosis. Caspase-3, caspase-6, and caspase-7 function as effector or "executioner" caspases. Executioner caspases activate cytoplasmic endonuclease, which degrades nuclear material (DNA), and proteases that degrade the nuclear and cytoskeletal proteins.Caspase-3 is the most important of executioner caspase and is activated by any of the initiator caspases (caspase-8, caspase-9, or caspase-10). The mechanisms that may be involved in caspase 3 mediated apoptosis include the followings **(Figure 4.2)**:

(i) Caspase 3 specifically activates the endonuclease CAD, described earlier in intrinsic pathway. In normal cells CAD is complexed with its inhibitor, ICAD and in apoptotic cells, activated caspase-3 cleaves ICAD to release CAD. CAD specifically degrades DNA to produce chromatin condensation.

(ii) Gelsolin, an actin binding protein, has been identified as the key substrate of activated caspase-3. Gelsolin provides a site for actin polymerization and helps in formation of microtubules. Caspase-3 cleaves gelsolin and thus, there is disruption of the cytoskeleton, intracellular transport, cell division, and signal transduction.

(b) Phagocytosis of Apoptotic Bodies: Nuclear fragmentation and condensation is followed by cytoplasmic fragmentation and there is formation of large number of small sized 'apoptotic bodies'. The plasma membrane in these apoptotic bodies remains intact; however, there is movement of the normal inward-facing phosphatidylserine of the cell's lipid bilayer to outer surface of cell membrane. Externalization of phosphatidylserine on apoptotic bodies is a well-known recognition ligand for macrophages. These macrophages rapidly phagocytose apoptotic bodies without initiating inflammation.

CASPASES

Caspases are a family of proteins that are one of the main effectors of apoptosis and their activation is a hallmark of apoptosis. About 14 mammalian caspases have been identified and all caspases share a number of common features. These are widely expressed in the form of an inactive proenzyme as 'procaspases' and upon activation, procaspases are converted to 'caspase'. Caspases have proteolytic activity and are able to cleave proteins at aspartic acid residues. Once caspases are initially activated, there seems to be an irreversible commitment towards cell death. These caspases have been broadly categorized into three classes:

1. **Apoptotic Initiator Caspases:** These caspases possess long prodomains and these mediate the interaction with upstream adaptor molecules and initiate apoptosis. These include caspase-2,-8,-9 and 10.

2. **Apoptotic Effector Caspases:** These are also termed as executioner caspases. These are characterized by the presence of a short prodomain.

These are processed and activated by upstream caspases. They perform the downstream execution steps of apoptosis by cleaving multiple cellular substrates. These include caspase-3,-6 and 7.

3. **Inflammatory Caspases:** This group includes caspase-1, -4, -5, -11, -12, -13 and -14, which are involved in inflammation, instead of apoptosis.

LABORATORY METHODS TO DETECT APOPTOSIS (ASSAYS FOR APOPTOSIS)

1. **Cytomorphological Alterations:** During apoptosis, there are morphological changes in cells that may be visualized using light microscope or electron microscope.

    (i) **Light Microscopy:** The evaluation of hematoxylin and eosin-stained tissue sections with light microscopy allow the visualization of apoptotic cells. The cell is smaller in size with much darker blue colored nucleus (hematoxyllin stain) and pinkish cytoplasm (eosin stain). Moreover, tissue sections can also be stained with toluidine blue or methylene blue to reveal intensely stained apoptotic cells. This methodology depends on the nuclear and cytoplasmic condensation that occurs during apoptosis.

    (ii) **Electron Microscopy:** Transmission electron microscopy is considered the gold standard to confirm apoptosis. It allows visualization of trastructural morphological characteristics including chromatin condensation, nuclear fragmentation, presence of intact cell membrane even late inthe cell disintegration and apoptotic bodies.

2. **DNA Fragmentation:** DNA fragmentation is characteristic feature of apoptosis and it may be visualized using gel electrophoresis and TUNEL staining.

    (i) **Gel Electrophoresis:** Calcium-dependent endonucleases produce DNA breakdown, which results in formation of DNA fragments of 180 to 200 base pairs. The DNA laddering technique is used to visualize the endonuclease cleavage products of apoptosis. This assay involves extraction of DNA from a cell homogenate followed by agarose gel electrophoresis. This result in a characteristic 'DNA ladder' with each band in the ladder separated in size by approximately 180 base pairs **(Figure 4.1)**. This methodology is easy to perform and is useful for tissues and cell cultures with high numbers of apoptotic cells per tissue mass or volume.

    (ii) **TUNEL Staining:** The TUNEL (Terminal dUTP Nick End-Labeling) method is used to assay the DNA fragments by enzymatic end-labeling the DNA strand breaks. Enzyme terminal transferase adds labeled UTP to 3' ends of the DNA fragments. In apoptotic cells, DNA fragments are selectively labeled with UTP and depending on the label attached with UTP, apoptosis may be visualized by light microscopy, fluorescence microscopy or flow cytometry. It is a fast technique and can be completed within 3 hours.

3. **Membrane Alterations:** In early stage of apoptosis, there is an alteration in plasma membrane morphology. There is outward movement of the normally inward-facing phosphatidylserine of lipid bilayer. In other words, phosphatidylserine is externalized on the surface of plasma membrane. Annexin V is a recombinant phosphatidylserine-binding protein that interacts strongly with phosphatidylserine residues. To detect apoptosis, FITC-labeled Annexin V is added and its binding with phosphatidylserine can be seen using fluorescence microscopy.

4. **Other Assays:** Mitochondrial assays and cytochrome c release may also be used to detect apoptosis. Laser scanning confocal microscopy can be used to monitor mitochondrial events including mitochondrial permeability transition, depolarization of the inner mitochondrial membrane and mitochondrial redox status. Cytochrome c release from the mitochondria can be assayed using fluorescence and electron microscopy. Apoptotic or anti-apoptotic regulator proteins such as Bax, Bid, and Bcl-2 can also be detected using fluorescence and confocal microscopy. Moreover, various types of caspase activity assays may also be performed to analyze apoptosis.

PHYSIOLOGICAL ROLE OF APOPTOSIS

1. **To Maintain the Number of Cells:** The normal physiological role of apoptosis seems to be opposite to that of mitosis. Mitosis tends to maintain cell proliferation and increase the cell number. However, apoptosis tends to reduce the number of cells. Hence, these two systems keep the number of cells in a homeostasis.

2. **Developmental Process:** During development of embryo, initially there is overproduction of cells such as in the nervous system and immune system. However, this initial overproduction is then followed by the death of those cells that fail to establish functional synaptic connections or productive antigen specificities, respectively.

3. **Defense, Wound Healing and Preventing Excessive Activation of Immune System:** Apoptosis is helpful to remove pathogen-invaded cells and hence, tends to protect the body from pathogens. It is also a vital component of wound healing as it removes inflammatory cells and granulation

tissue. Dysregulation of apoptosis during wound healing can lead to pathologic forms of healing such as excessive scarring and fibrosis. Apoptosis is also required to eliminate excessively activated or auto-aggressive immune cells in the lymphoid tissues or in peripheral tissues.

4. **Aging:** An important role of apoptosis has been defined in aging process. A significant loss of cardiac and skeletal myocytes during normal *aging occurs due to apoptotic* mechanisms.

PATHOPHYSIOLOGICAL ROLE OF APOPTOSIS

It is shown that apoptosis has to be tightly regulated and dysfunction of apoptosis may lead to developmental defects, autoimmune diseases, neurodegeneration, or cancer.

1. **Cancer:** The suppression of apoptosis during carcinogenesis is thought to play a central role in the development and progression of some cancers. There are a variety of molecular mechanisms that tumor cells use to suppress apoptosis. Tumor cells can acquire resistance to apoptosis by the expression of anti-apoptotic proteins such as Bcl-2 or by the down-regulation or mutation of pro-apoptotic proteins such as Bax.

2. **Autoimmune Diseases:** The physiological role of apoptosis is to eliminate auto-aggressive immune cells from the body. However, failure to perform apoptosis may lead to activation of immune system against body organs resulting in development of autoimmune diseases.

3. **Neurodegenerative Diseases:** Excessive activation of apoptosis may be responsible for various neurodegenerative diseases such as Alzheimer's, Parkinson or Huntington's disease. For example, during Alzheimer's disease excessive deposition of amyloid β in extracellular deposits may induce apoptosis by increasing Fas ligand expressions in neurons and glia. It may also activate microglia, which would result in TNFα secretion and activation of the TNF-R1, leading to apoptosis.

4. **Ischemia-Reperfusion Injury:** Excessive apoptosis is also involved in ischemia-associated injury such as myocardial infarction and stroke. In myocardial ischemia, overexpression of BAX has been detected and therapy aimed at reducing apoptosis has shown some success in reducing the degree of tissue damage in animal studies.

REVIEW QUESTIONS

TWO MARKS QUESTIONS

1. What are the executioner caspases?
2. What are the morphological changes occurring in cell undergoing apoptosis?
3. What is the characteristic feature of DNA fragmentation during apoptosis?
4. What is the role of inflammation in apoptosis?
5. What are the nuclear changes occurring in apoptotic cell?
6. What is the role of apoptosis in cancer?
7. How may apoptosis be detected using TUNEL staining?
8. How may apoptosis be detected using Annexin V staining?
9. What is the basis of identifying apoptosis using gel electrophoresis?
10. What are the changes occurring in mitochondria during apoptosis?
11. What is the role of cytochrome c in apoptosis?
12. What is the significance of Bcl 2 family in apoptosis?

FIVE MARKS QUESTIONS

1. What are caspases? How may these be classified? Explain their role in different steps of apoptosis.
2. What do you mean by Perforin-Granzyme system in apoptosis?
3. Explain the key steps involved in extrinsic pathway of apoptosis.
4. Explain the key steps involved in intrinsic pathway of apoptosis.
5. What do you understand by execution or common pathway of apoptosis?
6. What is the physiological role of apoptosis?
7. Differentiate apoptosis and necrosis.
8. Explain the pathophysiological role of apoptosis.

TEN MARKS QUESTIONS

1. Explain the mechanism of apoptotic cell death.
2. What is apoptosis? Write its characteristic features. What are the different methods to assay apoptosis?

MULTIPLE CHOICE QUESTIONS

1. Cytochrome c is released in which of following pathway?
   - (a) Intrinsic pathway
   - (b) Extrinsic pathway
   - (c) Execution pathway
   - (d) All the pathways

2. Perforin-Granzyme system belongs to
   - (a) Initiator pathway
   - (b) Extrinsic pathway
   - (c) Execution pathway
   - (d) Common pathway

3. Caspase 3 is
   - (a) Inflammatory caspase
   - (b) Initiator caspase
   - (c) Executioner caspase
   - (d) All the above

4. Which of following is caspase dependent apoptotic protein?
   - (a) CAD
   - (b) AIF
   - (c) Endonuclease G
   - (d) None of above

5. Caspase 10 is activated in following pathway
   - (a) Intrinsic pathway
   - (b) Extrinsic pathway
   - (c) Execution pathway
   - (d) Perforin Granzyme system

6. TNF-alpha may trigger apoptosis through?
   - (a) Intrinsic pathway
   - (b) Extrinsic pathway
   - (c) Execution pathway
   - (d) Perforin Granzyme system

7. Pkynosis is a feature of
   - (a) Cell proliferation
   - (b) Necrosis
   - (c) Apoptosis
   - (d) All the above

8. Apoptotic bodies may be visualized in
   - (a) Light microscope
   - (b) Electron microscope
   - (c) TUNEL stain
   - (d) Annexin V stain

9. Bcl-10, Bax, and Bad are
    (a) Anti-apoptotic
    (b) Pro-apoptotic
    (c) No role on apoptosis
    (d) Pro and anti depending on cell type

10. Which of the following is not feature of apoptosis?
    (a) Inflammatory reactions
    (b) DNA laddering
    (c) Cell shrinkage
    (d) pathological and physiological cell death

Gene Sequencing

CHAPTER OUTLINE

Definitions and General Features
Maxam–Gilbert Sequencing
(Chemical Cleavage)

Sanger's Chain Termination Method

Differences between
Maxam-Gilbert and Sanger Method

Automated Fluorescence Sequencing

Applications of Gene Sequencing

DEFINITIONS AND GENERAL FEATURES

It refers to determining the order of nucleotides on a piece of DNA. DNA sequence is important as it governs the order of amino acids in proteins in the cell. Thus, an alteration in a DNA sequence leads to altered or non functional protein synthesis leading to development of genetic diseases. Thus, determination of DNA sequence is important to detect the mutations responsible for genetic diseases. In the mid-1970's, two methods were developed for directly sequencing DNA. These were the **Maxam-Gilbert** chemical cleavage method and the **Sanger** chain-termination method. These two methods represent the first generation of DNA sequencing methods. In later years, improvement has been done in Sanger Technique to have automated methods of gene sequencing.

MAXAM–GILBERT SEQUENCING (CHEMICAL CLEAVAGE)

It was the first widely adopted method for DNA sequencing. The main steps involved in sequencing include the following **(Figure 5.1)**:

1. In this method, DNA fragment to be sequenced is made single stranded and is labeled at one 5' end with radioactive ^{32}P ATP using a kinase reaction.

2. The labeled DNA fragment is then divided into four aliquots (portions), each of which is treated with a reagent which modifies a specific base. Thereafter, DNA is chemically cleaved by piperidine which cleaves the sugar phosphate backbone of DNA at the residue prior to the modified

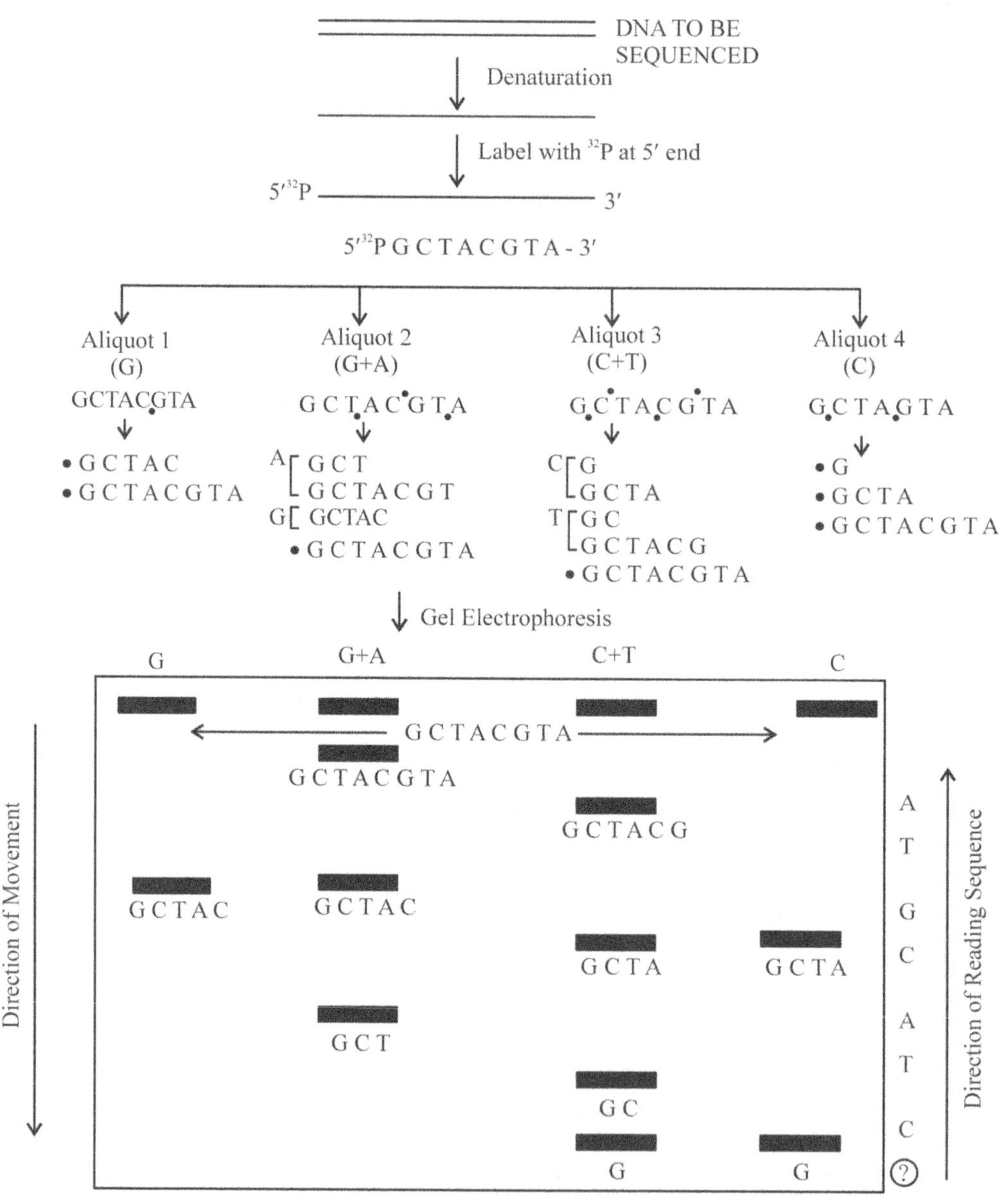

FIGURE 5.1 Maxam–Gilbert Sequencing method

base. For example, in a sequence GCTACGTA, if modification is done at G, then the cleavage points will be prior to modified G and cleavage product is GCTAC.

3. In aliquot 1, cleavage takes place at only G. In this aliquot, G residues are methylated at the N7 position by treatment with dimethyl sulfate (DMS). Piperidine is added which cleaves the phosphodiester backbone.

4. In aliquot 2, cleavage takes place at both A and G (purines). In this aliquot, formic acid is added which causes depurination. The piperidine is added to cleave the backbone.

5. In aliquot 3, cleavage takes place at C and T. In this case, treatment is done with hydrazine followed by piperidine.

6. In aliquot 4, cleavage takes place at C. In this case, treatment is done with hydrazine in the presence of 1.5 M NaCl, which protects cleavage at position T. It is followed by treatment with piperidine to cleave backbone.

7. Thereafter, DNA fragments are separated using gel electrophoresis and detection is done using autoradiography.

8. The sequence of DNA is determined using the pattern of bands obtained on gel electrophoresis.

POINTS RELATED TO DELINEATING THE SEQUENCE

1. The total number of lanes on the gel will determine the number of base pair in a sequence. For example, in **Figure 5.1**, there are eight lanes on the gel and it tells that the number of base pair is also eight.

2. The presence of band in a gel indicates the presence of the base pair. The bands which are common to G and G +A tell the presence of G. However, the bands exclusively present in G + A show the presence of A at that position.

3. There will be whole GCTACGTA band in every section.

4. The first base pair remains unknown.

5. The sequence has to be read in the opposite direction of movement of separated bands.

LIMITATIONS

However, it is not used widely these days and it has been replaced by next-generation sequencing methods.

1. Its major limitation is that it is a very tedious method.

2. It involves measurement of radioactivity. It also involves usage of hydrazine, which is a known neurotoxin. Therefore, it may not be used routinely.

3. It is difficult to scale up and cannot be used if DNA has more than 500bp.

4. Automation is not possible.

SANGER'S CHAIN TERMINATION METHOD

This is the most popular protocol for DNA sequencing. It is adaptable and scalable to large DNA sequencing too. Modern DNA sequencing methods uses the principles of the Sanger technique. Ribose has a hydroxyl group on both the 2' and the 3' carbons, whereas deoxyribose has one hydroxyl group on the 3' carbon. However, in dideoxyribose, the hydroxyl group is missing from both the 2' and the 3' carbons. Thus, the incorporation of specific dideoxynucleotides (with dideoxyribose sugar) results in chain termination and more nucleotides cannot be added to growing strand of DNA. Due to absence of hydroxyl group at 3' position, a phosphodiester bond cannot be formed and there is chain termination **(Figure 5.2)**. The steps involved in this technique include the followings **(Figure 5.3)**:

1. DNA to be sequenced is made single stranded and region to be sequenced is flanked by known sequence at 3'.

2. Four types of deoxynucleotide triphosphates (dNTPs) i.e, dATP, dGTP, dCTP, dTTP are used. Four dideoxynucleotide triphosphates (ddNTPs) i.e, ddATP,

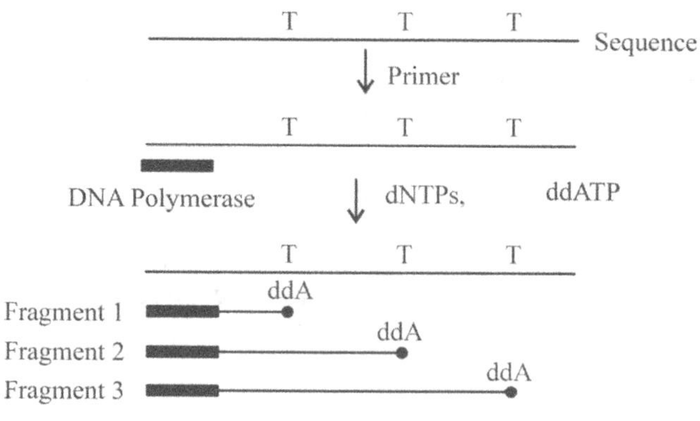

FIGURE 5.2 The different possible fragments formed due to chain termination in Sanger Method

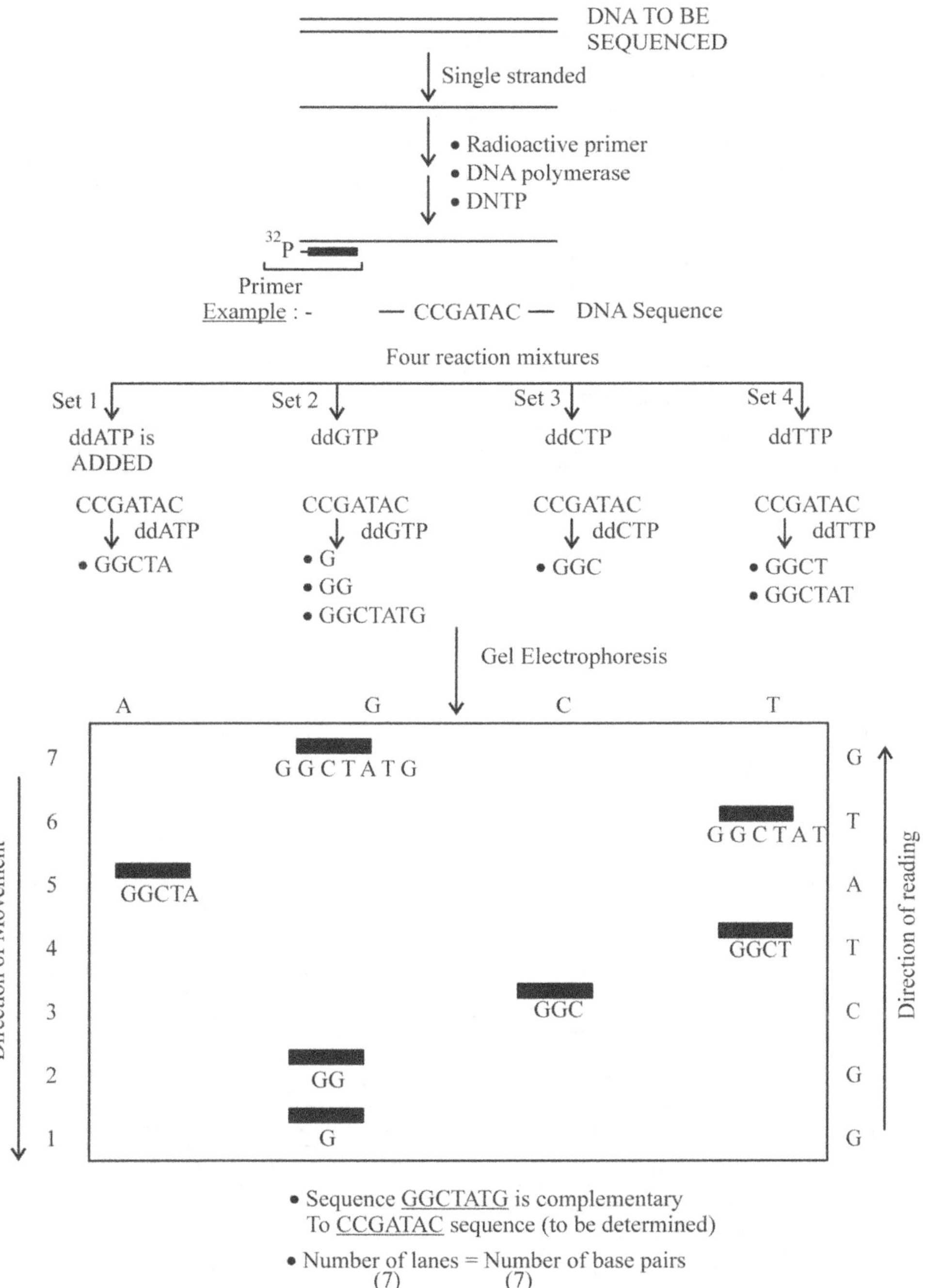

FIGURE 5.3 Sanger Method of DNA sequencing using chain termination

ddGTP, ddCTP, ddTTP are also used. Dideoxynucleotides resemble normal nucleotides, but lack the normal -OH group.

3. Four separate set of DNA sample (to be sequenced), primer, dNTP and DNA polymerase are taken. In first set ddATP is added, in second set ddGTP is added, in third set ddCTP is added and in fourth set ddTTP is added.

4. Using DNA polymerase, partial copies of DNA fragments are obtained. The full   DNA is not formed because the addition of ddNTP leads to chain termination.

5. In first set, all possible fragments of different lengths ending in ddATP are produced; in second set, all possible fragments of different lengths ending in ddGTP are produced; in third set, all possible fragments of different lengths ending in ddCTP are produced; in fourth set, all possible fragments of different lengths ending in ddTTP are produced.

DIFFERENCES BETWEEN MAXAM-GILBERT AND SANGER METHOD

The two methods of DNA sequences may be differentiated on the following basis **(Table 5.1):**

TABLE 5.1 Key differences between gene sequencing methods of Maxam-Gilbert and Sanger methods

S. No	Maxam-Gilbert Method	Sanger Method
1.	It is based on chemical cleavage of DNA sequence	It is based on synthesis of complimentary strand of DNA, which is to be sequenced
2.	Different DNA fragments are produced due to chemical cleavage	Different DNA fragments are produced due to chain termination
3.	DNA is labeled with ^{32}P	Primer is labeled with ^{32}P
4.	It is chemical method	It is enzymatic method
5.	It requires extensive DNA purification	It needs less DNA purification
6.	It cannot be automated	The process can be modified to make it automated
7.	It is not used nowadays	The modified forms are very widely used
8.	Scale up is not possible and it cannot determine DNA sequence of large DNA fragments	Scale up is possible and large DNA sequences can be determined.

AUTOMATED FLUORESCENCE SEQUENCING

There has been a significant advancement in DNA sequencing using fluorescence-labeled dideoxy-terminators. In 1986, Leroy Hood and colleagues reported a DNA sequencing method in which the radioactive labels were replaced by fluorescent labels. This is a modification of Sanger method. The modifications include:

1. In this method, only a single set of reaction mixture is used in which DNA to be sequenced, DNA primers, dNTP, DNA polymerase and ddNTP (ddATP, ddGTP, ddCTP, ddTTP) are added. It is in contrast to Sanger method, where four reaction mixtures were used.

2. In Sanger method, primers are radiolabeled. In this method, ddNTP are labeled with fluorescence dyes.

3. In this method, gel is replaced replaced by polymer filled capillary tubes.

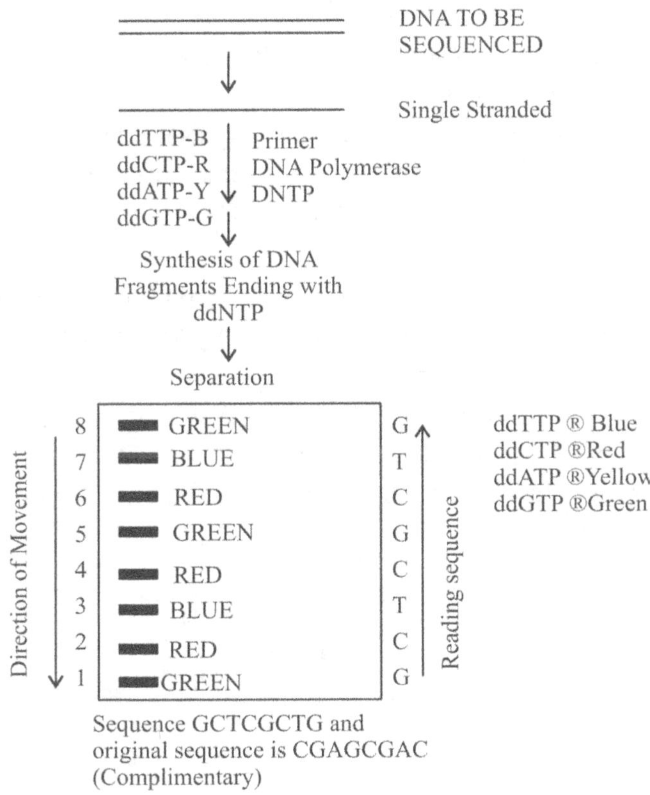

FIGURE 5.4 Automated Fluorescence method of DNA sequencing

4. The process is automated. A single gel lane has different bands of nucleotides and these bands have a distinct fluorescence. The readout process is done by laser scanner and recorded by computer.

5. Let's assume ddATP is labeled with yellow fluorescence dye, ddGTP with green, ddCTP with red, ddTTP with blue. Therefore, band with fragments ending with ddTTP has blue fluorescence, bands with ddATP have yellow fluorescence, bands with ddGTP have green and bands with ddCTP have red fluorescence. Based on the color of band, the nucleotide sequence can be determined. In this case, the sequence obtained is 'GCTCGTG' and it complimentary sequence i.e. 'CGAGCAC' is the sequence of given DNA **(Figure 5.4)**.

APPLICATIONS OF GENE SEQUENCING

1. **Disease Diagnosis:** In medical science, DNA sequence may be used to identify the genetic diseases. The sequence genes from patients may be used to determine the risk of genetic diseases.

2. **Molecular biology:** Gene sequencing is very useful to study genomes and the proteins encoded by those genes. Information from gene sequencing may be used to identify genes, phenotypes, changes in genes and along with changes in phenotype.

3. **Evolution:** It has been successfully used in evolutionary biology to study the relationship between different organisms and how these have been evolved.

4. **Forensic:** Each individual is unique because of its DNA. Therefore, DNA sequence may be used to identify a particular individual in forensic cases. Moreover, DNA sequencing has been used to match DNA sequences in paternity testing.

REVIEW QUESTIONS

TWO MARKS QUESTIONS

1. What is gene sequencing?
2. What is the use of gene sequencing in medical science?

3. What are the limitations of Maxam-Gilbert method of sequencing?
4. What are the modifications done in Sanger method to obtain new methods of sequencing?
5. What is principle of Sanger Technique?

FIVE MARKS QUESTIONS

1. What are the differences between Maxam-Gilbert and Sanger method of sequencing?
2. Explain Automated Fluorescence Sequencing method?
3. How Sanger technique is used to identify DNA sequences?
4. What is Maxam-Gilbert method of identifying DNA sequence?
5. What are the applications of gene sequencing?

TEN MARKS QUESTIONS

1. Write note on Sanger technique of DNA sequencing along with modifications to have Automated Fluorescence Sequencing method?

MULTIPLE CHOICE QUESTIONS

---

1. The following method of sequencing is based on DNA synthesis
    (a) Sanger method
    (b) Automated Fluorescence method
    (c) Maxam-Gilbert Method
    (d) a and b

2. In which of following methods, labeling is done with radioactive ^{32}P
    (a) Sanger method
    (b) Maxam-Gilbert Method
    (c) Automated Fluorescence method
    (d) A and B

3. In which of following methods, four reaction mixtures are used
    (a) Sanger method
    (b) Maxam-Gilbert Method
    (c) Automated Fluorescence method
    (d) A and B

4. Which of following is based on chemical cleavage?
   (a) Sanger method
   (b) Maxam-Gilbert Method
   (c) Automated Fluorescence method
   (d) None of above

5. Which of following is enzymatic method?
   (a) Sanger method
   (b) Maxam-Gilbert Method
   (c) Automated Fluorescence method
   (d) None

CHAPTER 6

Cell Cycle and Regulation

CHAPTER OUTLINE

Definitions and General Features

Stages of Cell Cycle

Interphase

M Phase (Mitotic Segregation)

Cell Cycle Control

Cyclins

Cyclin-Dependent Kinases

Cyclin-Dependent Kinase Inhibitors

DEFINITIONS AND GENERAL FEATURES

Cell cycle consists of a series of coordinated events which lead to cell division. In this process, nucleus is divided followed by division of cytoplasm and there is formation of two daughter cells. The cell division takes places following zygote formation, which increases the number of cells in the body. The cell division continues to take place in adults too e.g. formation of blood cells takes place continuously. This type of cell division is termed as 'mitosis', which takes place in somatic cells (non gonadal cells). In this type, the genetic matter remains same i.e., diploid (2n) cell divides to form diploid (2n) cells. Therefore, this type of cell division is termed as 'equatorial division'. It is in contrast to another cell division, which is termed as 'meiosis'. It takes place in gonadal cells and leads to formation of sperms and eggs. This type of division is termed as 'reductional division' because genetic matter is halved. From diploid (2n) gonadal cells, haploid (n) gametes are produced. However, the following section mainly focuses on mitosis and its regulation with cyclins, cyclin-dependent kinases (CDK) and CDK inhibitors.

STAGES OF CELL CYCLE

Cell cycle is a series of highly regulated steps that governs cell proliferation. The cell cycle may be mainly divided into two phases, interphase and M phase.

A. Interphase

Interphase (earlier termed as resting phase) is the period in which cell prepares itself for cell division. There is a growth of cell and there is an increase in cell size due to increase in protein synthesis. DNA replication also takes place. In this phase, chromatin is visible, which appears as long intertwining threads coiled in nucleus. The typical chromosome is visible during M phase, which is due to condensation of chromatin. Interphase is further divided in three phases, G_1, S and G_2 phases **(Figure 6.1)**:

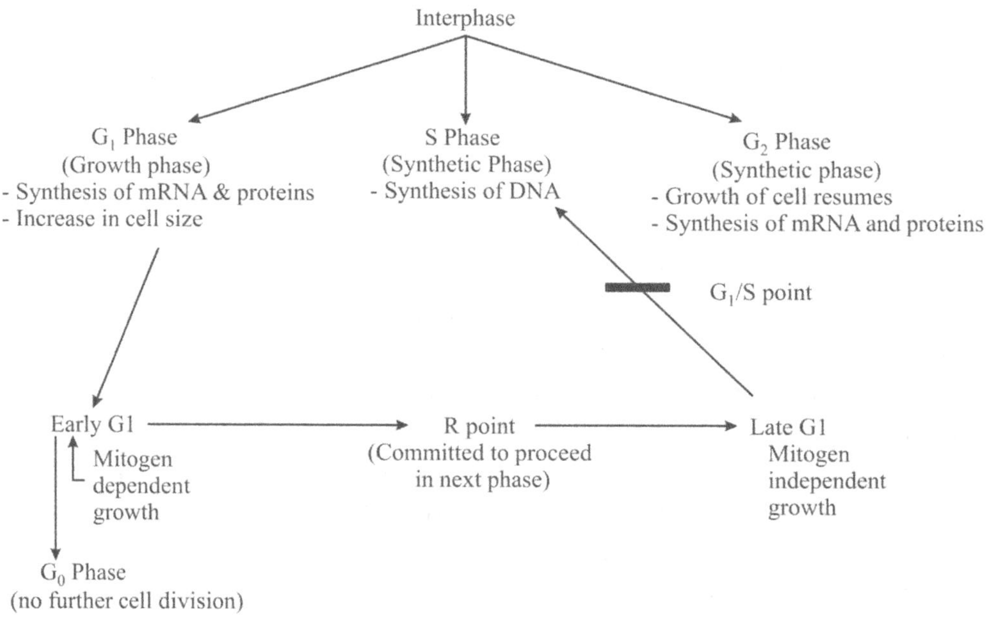

FIGURE 6.1 Different phases in interphase

I. G_1 Phase (First Gap period)

In this phase, the cell synthesizes mRNA and proteins required for cell division. Thus, there is enlargement in cell size. This phase ends and the cell moves into the S phase. This phase is particularly important in the cell cycle because it determines whether a cell commits to divide (enters in S phase) or exits the cell cycle (G_0) and becomes non-dividing cell. This gap phase is further divided into an early and a late stage, which is separated by the restriction (R) point.

1. **Early G_1 stage (Mitogen-Dependent):** This is the first phase and it starts after the completion of previous cell division (mitosis). It requires extrinsic growth factors (mitogens), which provide the stimulatory signal to proceed forward.

2. **G_0 phase (Quiescence):** Sometimes, cells exit the cell cycle and enter into the G_0 phase. In phase, cells remain in stationary phase and these have reduced metabolic activity. The cells do not proceed for cell division.

3. **Restriction (R) Point:** If cell does not enter in G_0 phase, then cell proceeds to this phase. This is called as 'point of no return', where the cell is committed to progress to the next phase and prepares itself for cell division. Hyperphosphorylation of **RB** by CDK4/cyclin D is important in passing through the R point.

4. **Late G_1 stage (Mitogen-Independent):** In this phase, there is no requirement of mitogen signal to proceed.

5. **G_1/S Checkpoint:** It is an important checkpoint and cell passes from G_1 to S phase through this checkpoint. During this transition phase, DNA integrity (damage) is checked before DNA replication proceeds in S phase. In case of DNA damage, DNA repair pathways or apoptosis is activated. The DNA repair pathways tend to repair the damaged DNA. Failure to repair the DNA damage leads to activation of apoptosis and non-repairable cell undergoes death.

II. S phase (Synthesis)

This phase is characterized by DNA replication and occurs between G_1 and G_2 phase. The DNA content is duplicated so that DNA can be distributed equally into daughter cells. During DNA synthesis, enzyme 'helicase' unwinds the DNA double helix, and the enzyme 'DNA polymerase' adds nucleotides to DNA single strand according to complementary base pairing rule to form another DNA strand.

III. G_2 phase

This is called as second gap phase. In this phase, there is rapid cell growth and protein synthesis to prepare cell for cell division. Indeed, the processes (protein synthesis) of G_1 resume in G_2 phase. G_2 phase ends with the onset of prophase. At the end of G_2 phase, cell enters in M phase through G_2/M checkpoint. At this check point, replicated DNA is checked before cell division (mitosis).

B. M Phase (Mitotic Segregation)

In this phase, the cell undergoes mitosis and cell divides. The chromosomes and cytoplasm are divided into two daughter cells. This phase is further divided into prophase, metaphase, anaphase, and telophase **(Figure 6.2)**.

1. **Prophase:** This phase starts after G2 of interphase, in which the chromatin start condensing into chromosomes and mitotic spindle formation is initiated.

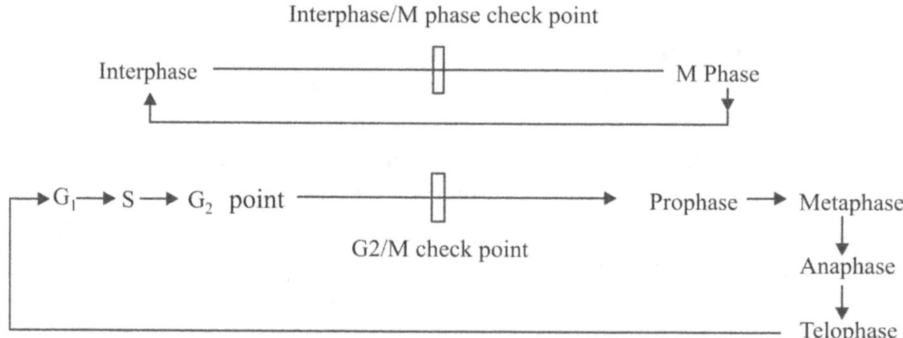

FIGURE 6.2 Different phases in cell cycle

This process is called chromosome condensation. The loosely packed genetic matter of interphase i.e., chromatin undergo condensation to form shorter chromosomes. In this stage, chromosomes are long, thin and thread-like and each chromosome has two chromatids, which are joined at a place called centromere.

2. **Metaphase:** In this phase, the nuclear envelope is disintegrated and microtubules enter in the nuclear space. Chromosomes are further condensed and become shorter in size. Typical structure of chromosomes is visible during metaphase. Microtubules attach to chromosomes and mitotic spindle is formed. The chromosomes are aligned along the metaphase plate or equatorial plane.

3. **Anaphase:** There is division of centomere and sister chromatids are separated. The shortening of microtubules pulls sister chromatids to move to opposite ends of the cell. The microtubules push against each other, causing the cell to elongate.

4. **Telophase:** It may also be termed as reversal of prophase. The chromatids reach to the ends of cell and a new nuclear envelope is formed. The new nuclear envelope surrounds the separated daughter chromosomes and the nucleolus reappears. Mitotic spindle (microtubules) is dissolved.

CELL CYCLE CONTROL

Cell cycle is controlled by cyclins, cyclin-dependent kinases (CDKs) and cyclin-dependent kinase inhibitors (CDKIs) **(Figure 6.3)**. These proteins and enzymes function in association with one another to control cell cycle.

1. **Cyclins:** These are a family of proteins that control the progression of cells through the cell cycle by activating cyclin-dependent kinase (CDK) enzymes.

Cyclins were originally named because their concentration varies in a cyclical fashion during the cell cycle. At least 13 mammalian cyclins have been identified. These have different structures and functions. However, they have a homologous region of about 100 amino acids called the 'cyclin box' and this region of cyclin is responsible for its binding with CDK. Depending on the functions, cyclins are classified in two classes:

(i) *G_1/S cyclins*: These control the cell cycle in G_1, S and at the G_1/S Checkpoint (transition). These include cyclin A, cyclin D and cyclin E. The levels of cyclin A are increased in the nucleus during S phase and it is involved in initiation and completion of DNA replication. During S phase, cyclin A associates with CDK2 to promote DNA replication. The synthesis of cyclin D is initiated during G_1 and drives the G_1/S phase transition. It interacts with four CDKs: CDK2, 4, 5, and 6. CDK4 binds with cyclin D to phosphorylate RB, which allows progression through the R point. Cyclin E binds to CDK2, which is required for the transition from G_1 to S phase of the cell cycle.

(ii) *G_2/M cyclins*: These control the cell cycle at the G_2/M checkpoint (transition). The levels of these cyclins are increased during G_2 and reduced at the end of the M-phase. For example, cyclin B regulates progression from G_2 to M phase. It is a mitotic cyclin and it binds to CDK1. The activity of the cyclin B-CDK complex rises in the cell cycle until mitosis is over. The complex of CDK and cyclin B is also called as 'maturation promoting factor' or 'mitosis promoting factor'.

2. **Cyclin-dependent kinases (CDKs):** CDKs are a family of protein kinases and these regulate the cell cycle. It binds a regulatory protein called a cyclin. Without cyclin, CDK has little kinase activity and only the cyclin-CDK complex is an active kinase. CDKs phosphorylate their substrates on serines and threonines, so these are also called as 'serine-threonine kinases'. These CDKs interact with specific cyclins as described in **Table 6.1.**

TABLE 6.1 Different types of cyclins and CDKs along with their peak rise time in different phases

S. No	Phase	Cyclin	CDK
1.	G_0	C	CDK3
2.	G_1	D,E	CDK2,-4,-6
3.	S	A,E	CDK2
4.	G_2	A	CDK1,CDK2
5.	M	B	CDK1

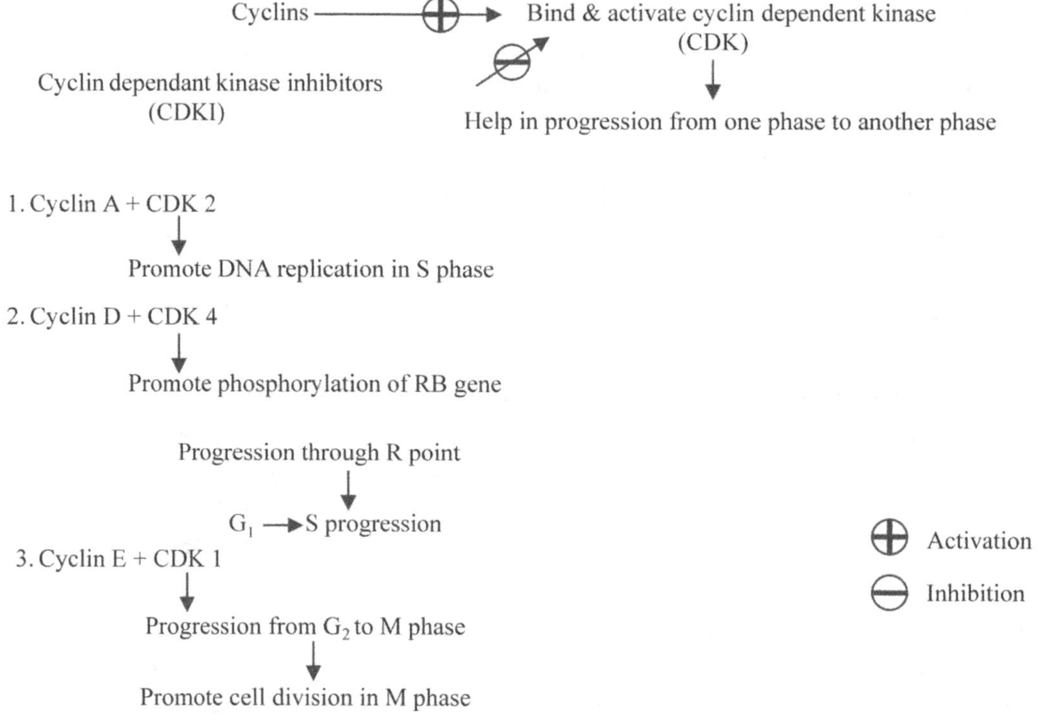

FIGURE 6.3 Role of cyclin and CDK in cell cycle regulation

3. Cyclin-Dependent Kinase Inhibitors (CDKIs): These proteins inhibit CDK and function as tumor suppressor proteins by inhibiting the proliferation of cells. In contrast, cyclins and CDK increase cell proliferation and excessive activation may promote tumor growth. CDK inhibitors promote cell cycle arrest at the G_1 phase. Some of these CDK inhibitors include p16 (CDK2A), which is a tumor suppressor protein and is encoded by CDKN2A gene. It regulates cell cycle by decelerating cells progression from G_1 phase to S phase, and therefore, acts as a tumor suppressor. CDK inhibitors that inhibit CDKs are described in **Table 6.2.**

TABLE 6.2 Different CDK inhibitors and CDKs

S. No	CDK inhibitor	Gene	CDK
1.	p16	CDKN2A	CDK 4,6
2.	p15	CDKN2B	CDK4
3.	p18	CDKN2C	CDK 4,6
4.	p19	CDKN2D	CDK 4,6
5.	p21	CDKN1A	Cyclin E_1/CDK 2
6.	p27	CDKN1B	Cyclin D3/CDK 4

REVIEW QUESTIONS

TWO MARKS QUESTIONS

1. What do you understand by cyclins?
2. What is the role of cyclin dependent kinase inhibitors in cell proliferation?
3. What is the major difference in G and S phase?
4. What do you understand by G_0 phase?
5. What are G_1/S and G_2/M check points?
6. What is Restriction point?
7. What are the characteristic features of metaphase?
8. What is the difference between chromatin and chromosomes?
9. What are cyclin dependent kinases?
10. What are the different phases of interphase?

FIVE MARKS QUESTIONS

1. How is cell cycle regulated?
2. What are the features of interphase? Elaborate different phases.
3. What is M phase? Elaborate different phases?

TEN MARKS QUESTIONS

1. What is the role of cyclins and associated proteins in controlling proliferation of cells?
2. What are the different phases in cell cycle?

MULTIPLE CHOICE QUESTIONS

1. Which of following is mitogen dependent phase?
   (a) G_0 (b) Early G_1
   (c) Late G_1 (d) All the above
2. The point of no return is also termed as
   (a) G_0 (b) G_1
   (c) R phase   (d) None of above

3. Chromosomes are best visualized in
   - (a) Metaphase
   - (b) Anaphase
   - (c) Telophase
   - (d) Interphase

4. Cell in non-dividing stage exists in
   - (a) G_0
   - (b) Early G_1
   - (c) Late G_1
   - (d) None of above

5. DNA replication takes place in following phase:
   - (a) G_0
   - (b) Early G_1
   - (c) Late G_1
   - (d) S phase

6. Cyclin A is involved in
   - (a) G_0
   - (b) Early G_1
   - (c) Late G_1
   - (d) S phase

7. p16 and p15 are
   - (a) Cyclins
   - (b) CDK
   - (c) CDK inhibitors
   - (d) None of above

8. The binding of cyclin with CDK leads to
   - (a) Activation of CDK
   - (b) Inhibition of CDK
   - (c) Depends on reactants
   - (d) No influence

9. Which of following is tumor suppressor?
   - (a) Cyclins
   - (b) CDK
   - (c) CDK inhibitors
   - (d) None of above

10. Chromatin is present in
    - (a) Interphase
    - (b) Telophase
    - (c) Metaphase
    - (d) Anaphase

Genomic and Proteomic Tools

7. Recombinant DNA Technology 95

8. Gel Electropgoresis 125

9. Gene Therapy 143

10. Polymerase Chain Reaction 165

11. ELISA and Micro Array Technique 179

12. Western Blotting 199

CHAPTER 7

Recombinant DNA Technology

CHAPTER OUTLINE

Definition and General Features

Different Steps of Recombinant DNA Technology

Isolation/Extraction of Target DNA/RNA

Selection Of Cloning Vector

Plasmids

Cutting DNA By Restriction Endonucleases

Joining the Segments by Ligases

Transformation

Selection

Application of Recombinant DNA Technology

DEFINITION AND GENERAL FEATURES

It is their process of combining two different DNA components (target DNA and vector) to form a chimeric or recombinant DNA followed by its propagation and amplification in a living cell (host) in an industrial setup for commercial goods (protein pharmaceuticals) **(Figure 7.1)**. It is also referred to as "gene cloning" or "molecular cloning". 'Cloning' refers to process of producing identical copies. Since in this process chimeric or recombinant DNA is amplified in a host cell and identical copies of that chimeric DNA is formed, therefore, it is called "gene cloning".

DIFFERENT STEPS OF RECOMBINANT DNA TECHNOLOGY

Following are the steps involved in the recombinant DNA technology **(Figure 7.1)**:

  (a) Isolation/extraction of target DNA/RNA

  (b) Selection of cloning vector

  (c) Cutting two DNA components with restriction endonucleases

  (d) Joining two DNA segments by ligase to form chimeric DNA

(e) Transformation, i.e., transfer of chimeric DNA to host cell (Bacterial cell)

(f) Selection of transformed cells

(g) Propagation and amplification of selected cells

(h) Obtaining the desired protein pharmaceutical products

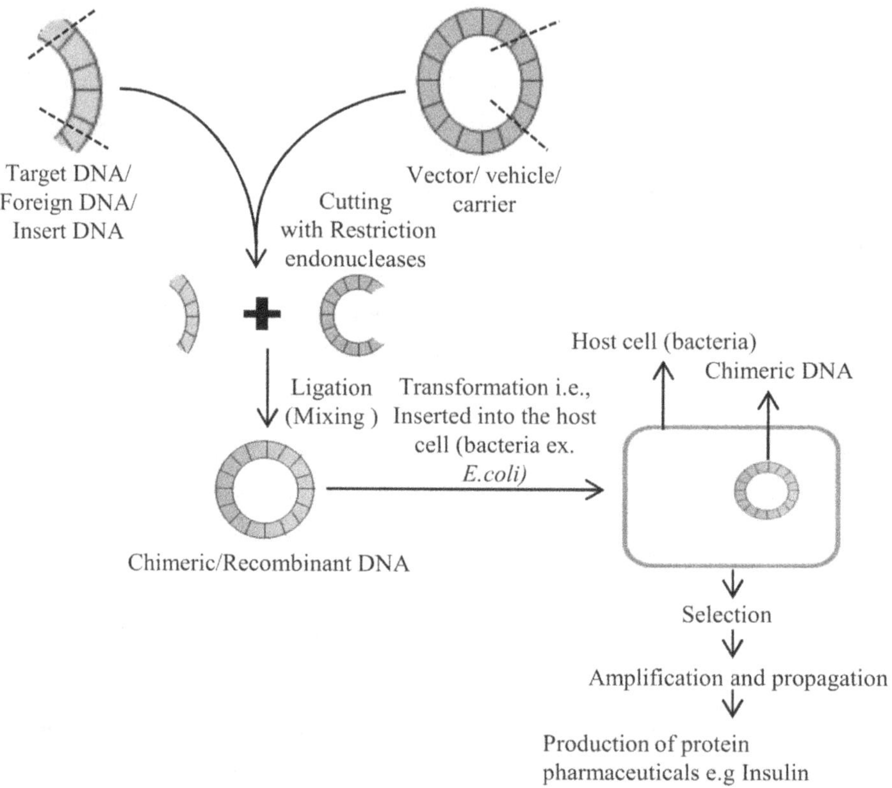

FIGURE 7.1 Different steps involved in recombinant DNA technology

ISOLATION/EXTRACTION OF TARGET DNA/RNA

The target DNA is a DNA portion for which recombinant DNA process is carried out. For example, if recombinant DNA technology is carried out for insulin production, then insulin gene is termed as target DNA. It is also referred to as "foreign DNA", "insert DNA" or "cloned DNA". In this step, the target DNA/RNA is isolated from a tissue/organ and the choice of organ depends on type of protein pharmaceutical to be produced. For example, if the purpose is to produce insulin, the DNA is isolated from pancreas.

Choice between DNA and mRNA: Although both DNA and mRNA may be used as target gene, yet RNA is preferred over DNA. The reason is that DNA has both exons (coding portion) and introns (non-coding portion) **(unit I chapter 2)**. Therefore, if DNA is to be used, then non-useful portions i.e., introns are also incorporated, which makes DNA a relatively lengthy molecule. On the other hand, mRNA is formed from DNA (transcription) and during the process the introns are removed by splicing. Accordingly, mRNA contains only exons and therefore, it is much shorter in length. Using reverse transcriptase enzyme, mRNA is converted to double stranded cDNA (complimentary DNA). cDNA is much shorter in length as compared to DNA due to absence of introns **(Figure 7.2)**.

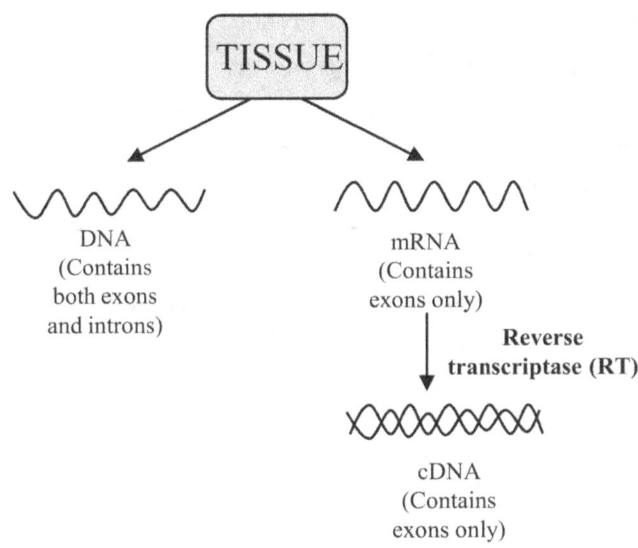

FIGURE 7.2 Isolation of DNA/mRNA from tissue

Therefore, the shorter length of DNA is preferred because the process of transformation is more efficient for shorter molecules.

SELECTION OF CLONING VECTOR

Vector refers to a carrier and cloning vector is a DNA molecule, which acts as a carrier for 'target DNA'.

Desirable properties of a vector:

1. ***Optimal Size:*** Depending on the size of target DNA (to be carried), cloning vectors of different carrying capacities are employed. For example, plasmids

are employed as cloning vectors for target DNA of size less than 10 kb. For larger sized DNA, other vectors are employed, such as, cosmids or bacteriophages.

2. ***Presence of appropriate selection marker gene:*** Two or more selection marker genes should be present in vector for selecting the desired chimeric DNA (discussed in 'selection' paragraph). Mostly, these marker genes encode for antibiotic resistance.

3. ***Presence of restriction endonuclease site:*** The vector should have DNA sequences, which are identified and selectively cut by restriction endonuclease enzyme.

4. ***Presence of Restriction endonuclease site in the marker gene***: It means that there should be DNA sequences within marker gene region, so that restriction endonuclease enzyme can produce a cut in 'marker gene' region.

5. ***Origin of Replication (ORI):*** Origin of replication should be present in vectors. Due to presence of ORI gene, the vectors are capable of self replication, which is essential for propagation and amplification.

Types of cloning vectors: There are different types of cloning vectors that are used in the process of recombinant DNA technology and some of commonly employed vectors include:

1. ***Plasmids:*** These are very commonly employed and these can carry up to 10 kb of target DNA. For example, PUC cloning vectors and pBR322 cloning vectors.

2. **Bacteriophage:** These refer to viruses that infect bacteria. Scientists have employed these bacteriophages to carry target DNA in host cells (bacteria). These have relatively larger carrying capacity, up to 20 kb of DNA. For example, bacteriophage M13 vectors, Lambda Phage Vector

3. ***Cosmids***: These have carrying capacity up to 40 kb of DNA. These are artificially created vectors with the properties of both plasmids and bacteriophages. Indeed, it is a plasmid with 'cos sites' of lambda bacteriophage (Cosmid = cos sites + plasmid). Cosmids can be used to make gene libraries.

4. ***Phagemid Vectors***: These are novel hybrid vectors made up of plasmids and M13 vectors. The term phagemids is derived from 'phage' from M13 and 'mid' from plasmid.

5. ***Bacterial artificial chromosomes (BAC):*** These have large carrying capacity, 150–350 kbp and these are used to sequence the genome of organisms in genome projects.

6. *Yeast artificial chromosomes (YAC):* These are genetically engineered chromosomes of yeast, with very large carrying capacity around 100–1000 kb. These are mainly used for sequencing genome of organisms such as in Human Genome Project.

PLASMIDS

These are extra-chromosomal units, self replicating and autonomous elements present in the bacterial cell. These replicate independent of main chromosomal DNA of bacteria. They are the circular duplex DNA, which can be isolated from bacteria. Depending upon the number of copies of plasmids, these may be 'single copy plasmids' or 'multi-copy plasmids'. Bacteria with single cell plasmids have one plasmid per cell. On the other hand, bacteria with multi-copy plasmids have more than one plasmid per cell (10-100 copies). Copy number refers to number of copies of plasmid in a cell. High copy number refers to the multi-copy plasmids, which produce up to 1000 copies of plasmid per cell. These are under relaxed replication control; therefore, these accumulate in large number. Due to increase in their number, the yield of protein pharmaceuticals is increased and these high copy number plasmids are preferred as cloning vectors.

Naturally occurring plasmids do not possess all the desirable features of cloning vector (as discussed in **Desirable properties of a vector**). Therefore, scientists have created different artificial plasmids by modifying the sequences of natural plasmids. In recombinant DNA technology, artificially made plasmids are employed and these include pBR 322, pBR 325, pBR 327, pUC 18/19, pUC 12/13, etc.

1. **pBR Vectors:** pBR stands for p for Plasmid; BR for Bolivar and Rodriguez (name of the scientists). These are commonly used vectors. These have low copy number around 25 copies/cell; thus employment of vectors leads to low yield. These are of following types:

   pBR 322: It has 4361 base pairs and two marker genes i.e., tetracycline resistant and ampicillin resistant genes are present. The restriction endonuclease produces a cut in the DNA sequence present in the marker genes, and the function of the marker gene is inactivated. It has ORI (Origin of Replication), which provides self replicating functions. It also has ROP (Repressor of primer) which represses ORI and limits plasmid replication. Due to the presence of ROP gene, there is low copy number in pBR vectors **(Figure 7.3).**

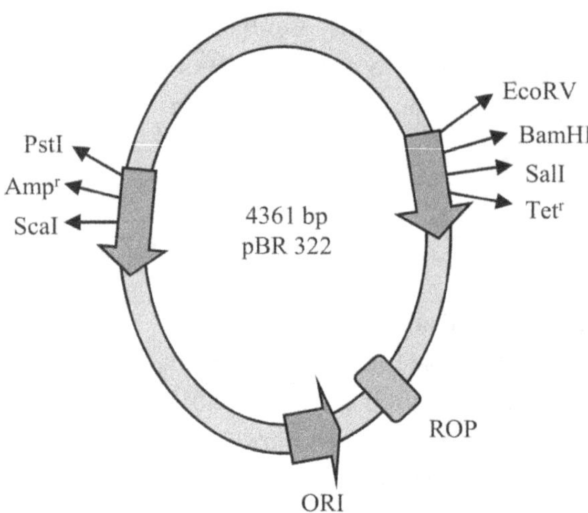

FIGURE 7.3 Plasmid Bolivar Rodriguez 322; ORI: Origin of Replication; ROP: Repressor of primer; EcoRV, BamHI, SalI, ScaI, PstI: Restriction endonucleases; Tet^r: Tetracycline resistant gene; Amp^r: Ampicillin resistant gene

pBR 325: It is a variant of pBR 322 vector. It has an extra marker gene, chloramphenicol resistance gene and this marker gene has DNA sequences, which are recognized by EcoRI (most common type of restriction endonuclease).

pBR 327: This plasmid has also been derived from pBR 322. It is smaller in size with deletion of 1427-2516 segments. Due to smaller size, the process of transformation (entry of recombinant DNA in host bacterial cell) becomes very efficient. Its main feature is that apart from prokaryotic cells as the host cells; it may be used in eukaryotic cells also, and it shows good expression.

2. **pUC vectors:** *pUC* stands for p for **P**lasmid, UC for **U**niversity of **C**alifornia. Nowadays, pBR vectors are replaced by more efficient and improved pUC vectors. The following are the salient features of pUC vectors **(Figure 7.4)**:

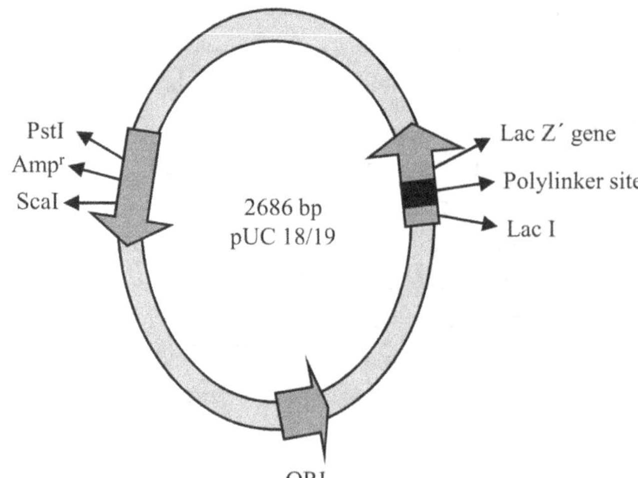

FIGURE 7.4 Structure of pUC 18/19

(i)   Their size is smaller than pBR vector, approximately 2700 base pairs.

(ii) The copy number of pUC is high i.e., 500-700 copies per cell. Due to high copy number, the yield of protein pharmaceuticals is around 3-4 µg/ml with pUC vectors in comparison to 0.23 µg/ml with pBR.

(iii) They have the 'polylinker site', which is a DNA segment with sequences recognized by more than 11 restriction endonucleases.

(iv) These possess two marker genes, ampicillin resistant gene and Lac Z′ gene Lac Z′ gene expresses to produce the α-peptide of the enzyme β-galactosidase (containing 1021 amino acids). This enzyme has β-peptide (1-92 amino acids) at the $-NH_2$ end and ω fragment at the $-$COOH end. Lac I gene is responsible for the production of repressor. which blocks the expression of Lac Z′ gene in normal resting conditions.

(v)   These vectors are made in pairs. For example, pUC 18/19; pUC 8/9; pUC 12/13. pUC 18/19 and pUC 8/9 have same polylinker site; however, the orientation of polylinker site is opposite in these two vectors.

Advantages of pUC over pBR

(i)   Smaller size, therefore, it is easy to transform into the host cell

(ii) Presence of polylinker site, so that the range of restriction endonucleases that may be used is increased

(iii) Colorimetric selection in pUC vector (due to presence of Lac Z' gene, **discussed in selection paragraph**) is another advantage in contrast to positive-negative selection in pBR vectors.

(iv) Due to high copy number of pUC, the yield is higher.

3. DNA Cutting: It is required that two different molecules (target DNA and cloning vector) are cut, so that these two different DNA molecules can be joined to form chimeric/recombinant DNA. DNA cutting may be done by two methods:

(i)   ***Random cutting methods:*** In these methods, DNA is cut randomly to produce different sets of DNA. However, it is not useful for recombinant DNA technology. The methods include sonication, high speed stirring, or passage through narrow bore syringe.

(ii) ***Specific cutting methods:*** In these methods, specific cuts are produced in the DNA. Nucleases are mostly used to produce specific cut in DNA. These are the enzymes, which cleave the nucleic acid by hydrolyzing phosphodiester bond. Nucleases are of two types: exonucleases and endonucleases. Exonucleases produce cut from the ends (sides) of the DNA, while endonucleases produce cut within (inside) the DNA **(Figure 7.5)**.

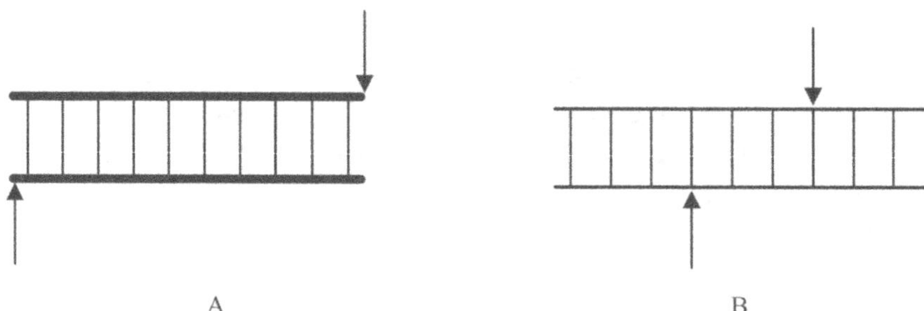

FIGURE 7.5 Cutting of DNA by exonucleases (A) and endonucleases (B).

RESTRICTION ENDONUCLEASES

These enzymes produce the cut within the DNA at specific site, which results in production of same set of DNA fragments. Restriction refers that the enzymatic activity (cutting) is restricted to certain portions. Indeed, the recombinant DNA technology became feasible only after the discovery of restriction endonucleases.

ISOLATION OF RESTRICTION ENDONUCLEASES FROM BACTERIA

Restriction endonucleases are isolated from bacteria. In bacteria, they play an important physiological role, wherein, they protect the bacteria from incoming virus. These enzymes cut DNA of infecting virus and protect bacteria. However, the bacteria's own DNA is not affected by these enzymes because the bacterial DNA is methylated. Methylated DNA provides self protection from the action of restriction endonucleases.

5′-G A A T T C-3′
3′-C T T A A G-5′

FIGURE 7.6 Palindrome sequence

Cutting a Palindrome Sequence: The special property of these enzymes is that they recognize and cut in the palindrome sequence. A palindrome sequence is a DNA sequence that is same when read in same polarity from either end. For example, the DNA sequence is same, when read from 5' to 3' from either end; or 3' to 5' from either end **(Figure 7.6)**.

Nomenclature of restriction endonucleases: The naming of the restriction endonucleases follows a specific pattern and it depends on the bacteria from which enzyme has been isolated. For example, EcoRI is one of most commonly employed restriction endonuclease. 'E' denotes genus i.e., *Escherichia;* 'co' stands for *Coli* which is the species, 'R' denotes the strain, which is optional and the roman numerical 'I' represents the order of characterization from the same microorganism (means first, second or third enzyme isolated from same microorganism) **(Figure 7.7).**

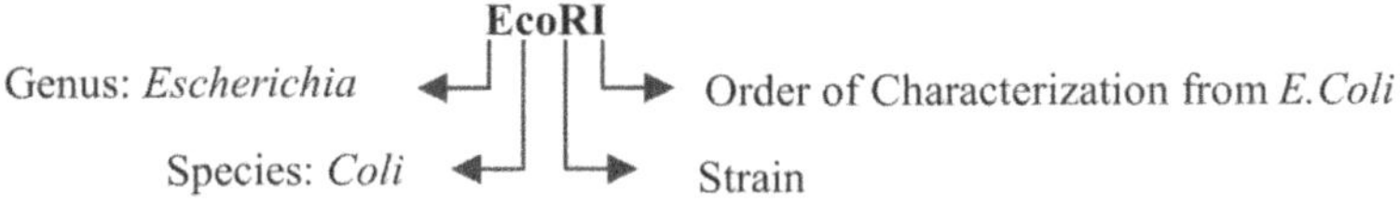

FIGURE 7.7 Nomenclature of restriction endonuclease, EcoRI

Restriction Enzymes produce two types of cuts: Restriction endonuclease may either produce sticky ends or blunt ends.

1. ***Sticky ends/ protruding ends/ cohesive ends:*** These types of nucleotide fragments have one strand extending beyond the other strand. The extending part is known as the sticky end. Such types are easy to ligate since they easily base pair with other sticky end. This feature makes them the preferred type of cuts. Two types of extensions may be produced (5′ phosphate or 3' hydroxyl) depending on the endonuclease.

   (i)   5′ phosphate extension: This type of sticky end is more common. The most commonly used restriction endonuclease produce this type of extension **(Figures 7.8, 7.9, 7.10).**

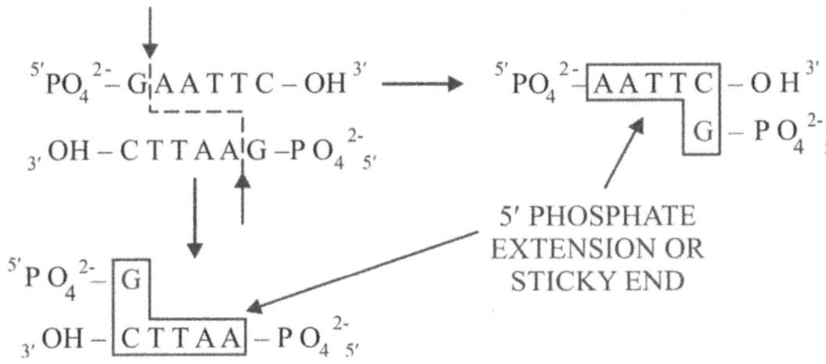

FIGURE 7.8 Cutting pattern of EcoRI obtained from *Escherichia coli* to produce sticky ends with 5′phosphate extension.

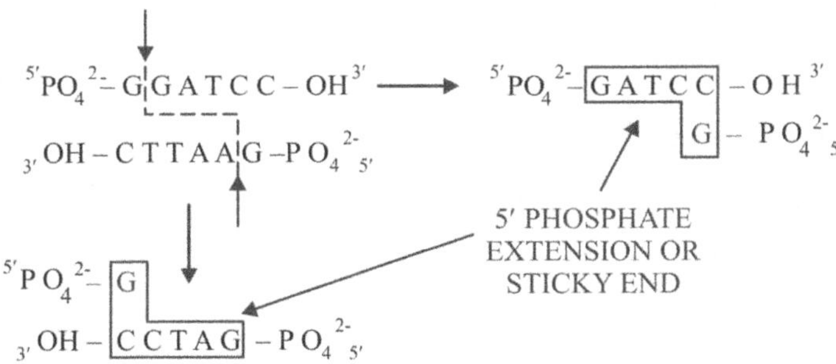

FIGURE 7.9 Cutting pattern of BamHI obtained from *Bacillus amyloliquefaciens* to produce sticky ends with phosphate extension

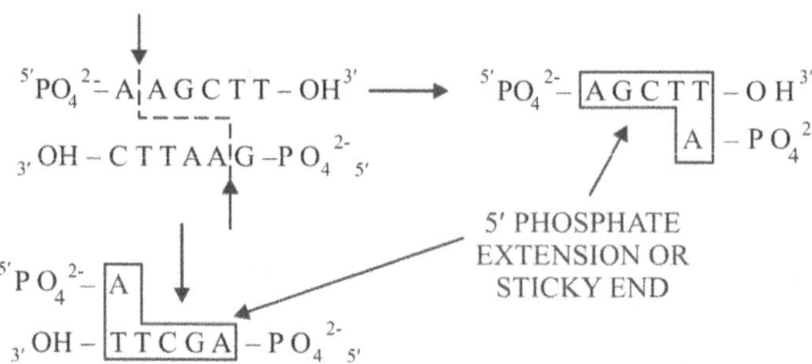

FIGURE 7.10 Cutting pattern of Hind III obtained from *Hemophilus influenza* to produce sticky ends with phosphate extension

(ii)   3′ hydroxyl extension: In this type of cutting, the sticky ends are produced ending with 3′ hydroxyl group **(Figure 7.11)**.

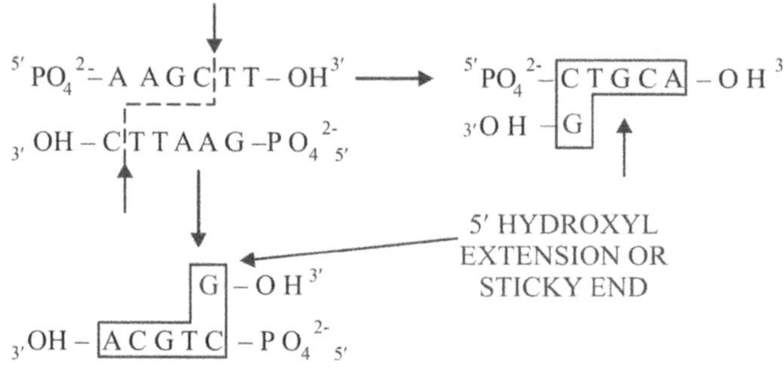

FIGURE 7.11 Cutting pattern of Pst I obtained from *Providencia stuortii* to produce sticky ends with 3' OH extension.

2. **Blunt ends:** These types of ends are difficult to join. Certain restriction endonucleases produce symmetrical cut to produce stable blunt ends **(Figure 7.12)**. For joining blunt ends, high concentration of ligases, linkers, adaptors or homopolymer tailing is used.

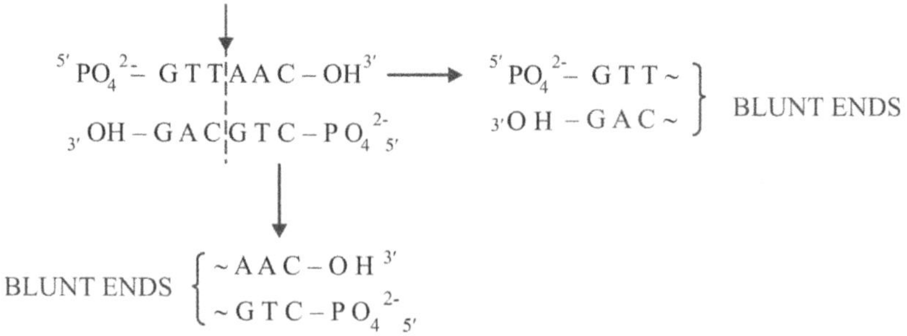

FIGURE 7.12 Cutting pattern of Hpa I, obtained from *Haemophilus parainfluenzae*

Types of Restriction endonucleases: Restriction endonucleases are mainly of three types, type I, type II and type III.

1. *Type I:* The following are the characteristic features of type I enzymes

   These are large and multimeric enzymes. Multimeric enzymes have multiple and non-identical subunits.

   (i)   The enzyme possesses endonuclease and methylase activity on different subunits.

   (ii)   Magnesium ion (Mg^{2+}), ATP, and SAM (S-adenosyl methionine) are required for the action of these enzymes.

   (iii) They recognize a particular sequence. The cut is produced 100-1000 base pairs downstream the recognition site. It means these enzymes show a specific recognition ability, but relatively non-specific cutting.

   (iv)   The cleavage is ATP dependent.

   (v)   Example of such type are EcoB, EcoK

2. *Type II:* The following are the characteristic features of type II enzymes

   (i)   These are relatively smaller in size.

   (ii)   These are either monomeric or have identical subunits in multimeric form.

   (iii) Methylase and endonuclease activities are not the part of a single enzyme complex.

   (iv) Mg^{2+} is the co-factor required for the endonuclease activity

   (v)   SAM is required for the methylase activity

   (vi)   These recognize a particular sequence and produce a cut within that recognized sequence. Therefore, these are highly specific enzymes. For example, EcoRI, BamHI, etc.

   (vii) Type II restriction endonuclease are of further six types:

   (a)   II P – These are the most commonly used enzymes. These recognize 4, 6, 8 base pair long palindrome sequence.

   (b)   II W – These recognize 5, 7 base pair palindrome sequence.

   (c)   II N – Interrupted palindrome sequence are recognized by these types of restriction endonucleases

   (d)   II S – They cleave 1-20 base pairs away from the recognition site

   (e)   II T – They produce asymmetric cutting

   (f)   II U – Unknown

3. *Type III:* The following are the characteristic features of type II enzymes

   (i)   These are large multimeric enzymes and have the endonuclease and methylase activities on the same enzyme complex.

(ii) These are specific in recognizing nucleotide sequence. However, these produce cuts 25-27 base pairs away from the recognition site.

(iii) Example: EcoP1, EcoP15, HinfIII

Other characteristics of Restriction Endonucleases

1. *Isoschizomers:* These are those restriction endonucleases that produce cut in the same recognition sequence, but at different locations. For example, XmaI and SmaI are isoschizomers **(Figure 7.13)**.

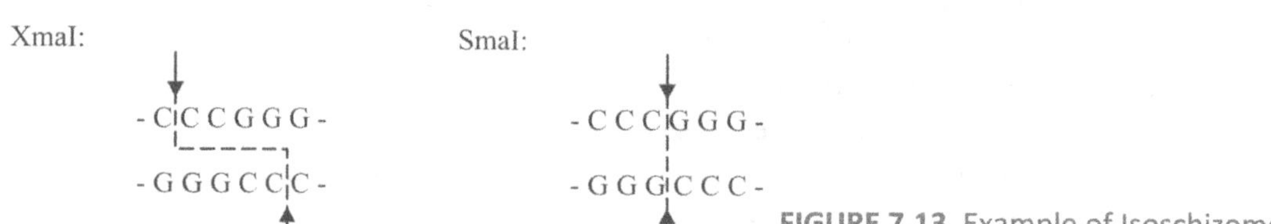

FIGURE 7.13 Example of Isoschizomers

2. *Isocaudamers:* These are those restriction endonucleases that produce cut in different recognition site, but produce same nucleotide extension sequence. For example, BamHI and Sau3AI produce $^{5'}$-G A T C-$^{3'}$ overhang or extension.

3. *Star activity:* When restriction endonucleases do not act in optimal conditions (such as in different buffer solution), then these enzymes may show non-specific cutting. In that condition, enzyme is said to exhibit star activity and it is represented by star. For example, EcoRI* means that EcoRI acts in non-optimal conditions and hence, its cutting pattern is non-specific.

4. *Storage of Restriction endonuclease:* The optimal temperature for storing restriction endonuclease is -20°C.

5. *Units:* One unit of a restriction endonuclease refers to the amount of restriction endonuclease required to completely digest 1μg of DNA in 60 min under appropriate conditions.

JOINING THE DNA SEGMENTS BY LIGASES

Ligase is an enzyme which forms phosphodiester bond between 3'-OH and 5'-PO_4^{2-} ends of DNA fragments cleaved by restriction endonucleases. Therefore, it is used to join target DNA with cloning vector to form a recombinant DNA. It is a single polypeptide with a mass of 68 kDa. For executing ligase action, it requires ATP and Mg^{2+} as co-factors. Usually, sticky ends are joined by T_4 DNA ligase. However, it also joins blunt ends at higher concentration.

Physiological Role of DNA Ligase

DNA ligase is present in almost all cells in organisms. Physiologically, ligases perform two main functions:

1. These ligate the 'nicks' produced in the sugar-phosphate backbone of double stranded DNA **(Figure 7.14)**.

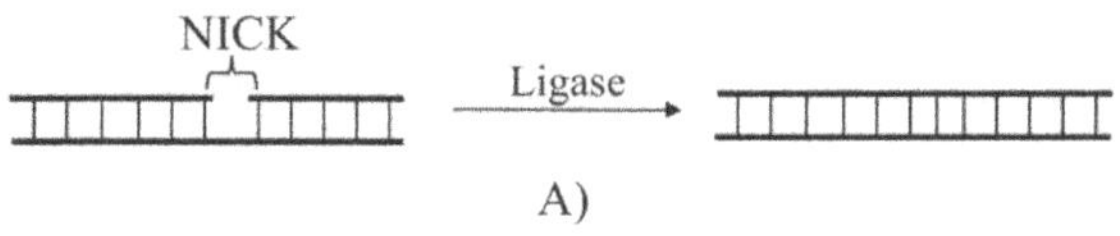

NICK

Ligase

A)

FIGURE 7.14 Joining of nick and forming a phosphodiester bond between hydroxyl and phosphate group

2. These join the DNA segments (Okazaki fragments) in "lagging strand" during DNA replication.

Source of Ligases: DNA ligase is obtained from followings:

1. The most common source of ligase is bacteria. The most commonly used ligase in recombinant DNA technology is T_4 DNA ligase. It is isolated from *E. coli*, which is infected with bacteriophage T_4.

2. However, recombinant DNA technology is also employed to obtain T_4 DNA ligase (protein product).

3. Other ligases used in recombinant DNA technology include *E. coli* DNA ligase. However, its efficacy is less as compared to T_4 DNA ligase.

Factors affecting the rate of ligation: There are some factors that may affect rate of ligation between cloning vector and target DNA. These include:

1. *Temperature:* Ligation requires optimum temperature and ligation rate is optimum at 37°C.

2. *Concentration of reactants (DNA fragments):* There needs to be an optimum ratio of cloning vector vs target (insert) DNA in terms of their weights and size.

$$\text{Vector-target DNA ratio} = \frac{W_v}{S_v} : \frac{W_i}{S_i}$$

W_v = weights of vector; W_i = weight of target DNA (in ng)

S_v = size of vector; S_i = size of target insert (in kb)

3. *Nature of ends of DNA:* Sticky ends are easy to ligate than blunt ends. Therefore, more amount of ligase is required to ligate the blunt ends in comparison to sticky ends. Blunt ends produced by restriction endonuclease such as SmaI are difficult to ligate due to lesser area available for the formation of bonds between the fragments. Therefore, special methods are

used for joining blunt ends including linkers, adapters and homopolymer tailing.

Self Ligation (Recircularization of Vector) and Prevention using Alkaline Phosphatase In recombinant DNA technology, self ligation of the cleaved fragments of cloning vector can lead to recircularization of vector (plasmid) **(Figure 3.15)**. In this situation, target DNA is unable to ligate with cloning vector and efficiency of the process is diminished. To prevent the self ligation, alkaline phosphatase is used in recombinant DNA technology. The most common alkaline phosphatase used is calf intestinal phosphatase (CIP).

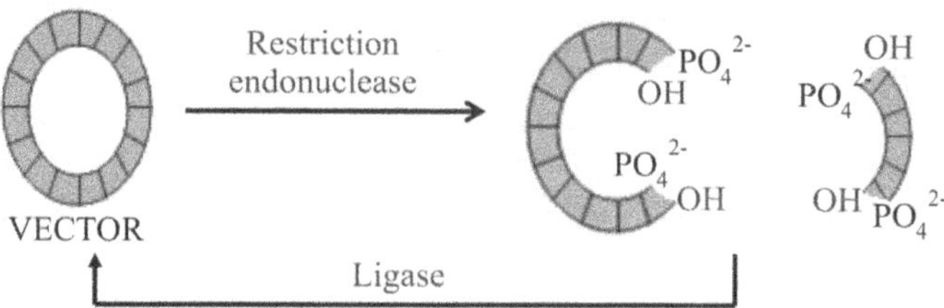

FIGURE 7.15 Recircularization of cleaved fragments of plasmid

To prevent recircularization, cloning vector is treated with alkaline phosphatase. It removes 5′-phosphate groups on vector on both strands, replacing them by hydroxyl group. As a result of this replacement, self ligation between fragments of vector cannot take place, thus, preventing the recircularization of the plasmid **(Figure 3.16)**. Thereafter, 'insert DNA' is mixed with cloning vector in the presence of ligase. The phosphodiester bond formation will take place due to presence of phosphate groups on insert DNA. However, instead of usual four bonds, only two bonds are formed and two nicks remain in chimeric construct. Even with presence of two nicks, such chimeric construct is stable at 37°C, because two DNA fragments are held together by hundreds and thousands of base pairing **(Figure 3.17)**. Moreover, once these chimeric construct enter in host cells (after transformation), the nicks are sealed after replication.

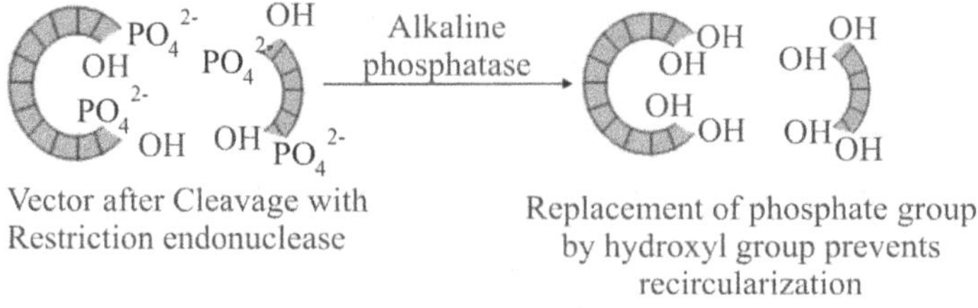

FIGURE 7.16 Alkaline phosphatase removes phosphates groups from vector and prevents recircularization

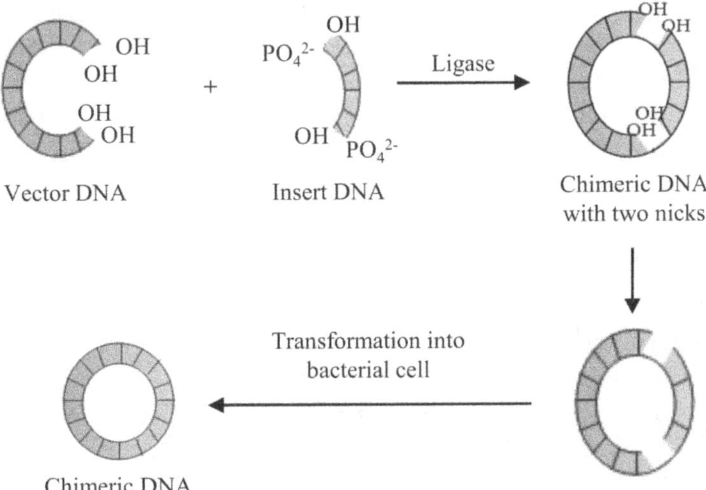

FIGURE 7.17 Joining of vector (without any phosphate group) with target DNA (with phosphate groups) to form stable chimeric DNA construct with two nicks

TRANSFER OF CHIMERIC DNA TO HOST CELL (TRANFORMATION)

After the formation of recombinant DNA, the next step is to transfer it into living cell (host cell) for its amplification. Most often, the host cell is bacteria and recombinant DNA is transferred to bacteria and the process of passage of DNA into bacterial cell is called as transformation. Transformation was discovered in 1928 by Fred Griffith and it is defined as the heritable change in the properties of bacteria due to uptake of naked DNA. On the other hand, transduction is defined as bacteriophage mediated transfer of DNA from one bacterium to another. It means viruses help in transferring DNA from one bacterium to another bacterium in transduction. The efficacy of transformation is assessed by measuring following two parameters:

1. **Transformation frequency:** It is the ratio of transformed cells to total number of treated cells.
2. **Transformation efficiency:** It refers to total number of transformed cells per unit amount of DNA added.

Methods Employed for Tranformation: Competence is the ability of bacteria to take up DNA. Natural competence of bacteria is very low and bacteria do not take DNA naturally. Therefore, competence is induced artificially so that bacteria can take up DNA and can be transformed. The process of transformation is directly dependent on the size of chimeric/recombinant DNA. The process is more efficient for small sized DNA and becomes inefficient as the size of DNA increases.

1. **Cold CaCl₂ method:** The mixture of *E. coli* (host cell) and recombinant DNA is treated with ice cold $CaCl_2$ and then exposed to high temperature (42°C) for approximately 120 seconds. Thereafter, enough of growth media is added and incubated for 30-60 minutes to allow the bacteria to recover and express DNA. Depending upon the conditions, approximately 10^4-10^9 transformants per microgram of DNA are obtained. Higher efficiency is observed with low level of DNA. As the concentration of DNA is increased, the transformation efficiency decreases.

Proposed mechanisms of DNA uptake

(i) Divalent cations (calcium ions) may shield negative charge on DNA (PO_4^2) and on the outer side of membrane, which is made up of phospholipids and lipopolysaccharides. The shielding of negative charge on DNA and membrane allow these two to come closer.

(ii) Low temperature and divalent cations may cause crystallization in regions of membrane. This makes the channels accessible for DNA uptake.

(iii) Reorganization of lipopolysaccharides may also lead to opening of channels.

2. **Electroporation:** It is standard and versatile method of transformation. It involves electric field-mediated membrane permeabilization. In this method, uptake of DNA is induced by subjecting bacteria to high voltage electric field. *E. coli* and DNA mixture (approximately 50 microliters) is taken in a chamber fitted with electrodes. A single pulse of electric field of 25 microfarads; 2.5 KV; 200 ohms is applied for 4.6 millisecond **(Figure 7.18)**. This procedure has an efficiency of 10^6 per microgram of DNA for large plasmids of approximately 136 Kilobase pairs and 10^9 per microgram of DNA for smaller plasmids of approximately 3 Kilobase pairs.

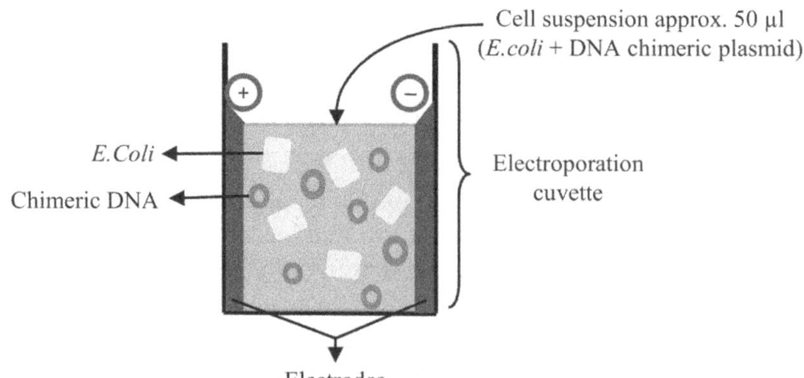

FIGURE 7.18 Procedure of carrying electroporation

Proposed mechanisms of DNA uptake: High voltage electric field causes alignment of charged molecules on the cell membrane. This alignment may lead to creation of pores and DNA may enter inside the bacteria through these pores. In other words, application of electric field leads to creation of transient pores in the membrane. However, the movement of molecules through these pores is not direction specific i.e., the materials may also come out of the cell, which may lead to cell death on applying long duration electric field.

3. **Conjugation:** It is a natural system of transmitting plasmid from one strain to another and has been employed to transfer the chimeric DNA from a donor cell to recipient cell. However, this transfer of chimeric DNA depends on presence of genes in plasmid, which encode conjugative function i.e., ability to transfer the genetic material. The plasmids used for recombinant research such as pBR and pUC vectors lack the conjugative function. Therefore, the process of conjugation employs three types of cells:

   (i)   ***Helper cells***: They possess conjugative and mobilization functions in their plasmid. Therefore, they are used to transfer the conjugative property to the cells containing the non-conjugate plasmid i.e., those lacking conjugative property. They also possess tetracycline resistant gene. These cells do not show any growth on the minimal media.

   (ii) ***Donor cells***: These cells possess mobilizable plasmid, but lack conjugative property. These plasmids are the ones containing the chimeric DNA. The plasmid of donor cells also contain Kanamycin resistant gene. Similar to helper cells, donor cells also do not grow on minimal media. These cells receive the conjugative property from the helper cells, which confers the donor cells the ability to transfer the chimeric DNA to the recipient cell. Donor cells are used when the recipient cell is not readily transformed, for example, Pseudomonas putida.

   (iii) ***Recipient cells:*** These cells lack in both conjugative and mobilizable property. Moreover, they are also deprived of any resistant gene. However, unlike helper and donor cells, recipient cells can grow on minimal media. For example: Pseudomonas putida.

Since the helper cell has the ability to conjugate and transfer its genetic material, helper cell is conjugated with the donor cell. This transfers the plasmid possessing the conjugative property to the donor cell which contains non-conjugate plasmid (chimeric DNA). The donor cell is therefore enabled to transfer its plasmid to the recipient cell (Pseudomonas putida). Therefore, this is also known as tripartite mating. All the three cells are then grown in complete media without any antibiotics. The grown cells are then transferred to a minimal media containing Kanamycin. This results in death of helper and donor cells since they lack Kanamycin resistant gene, while the recipient cells survive due to presence of Kanamycin resistant gene in their plasmid (chimeric DNA) **(Figure 7.19).**

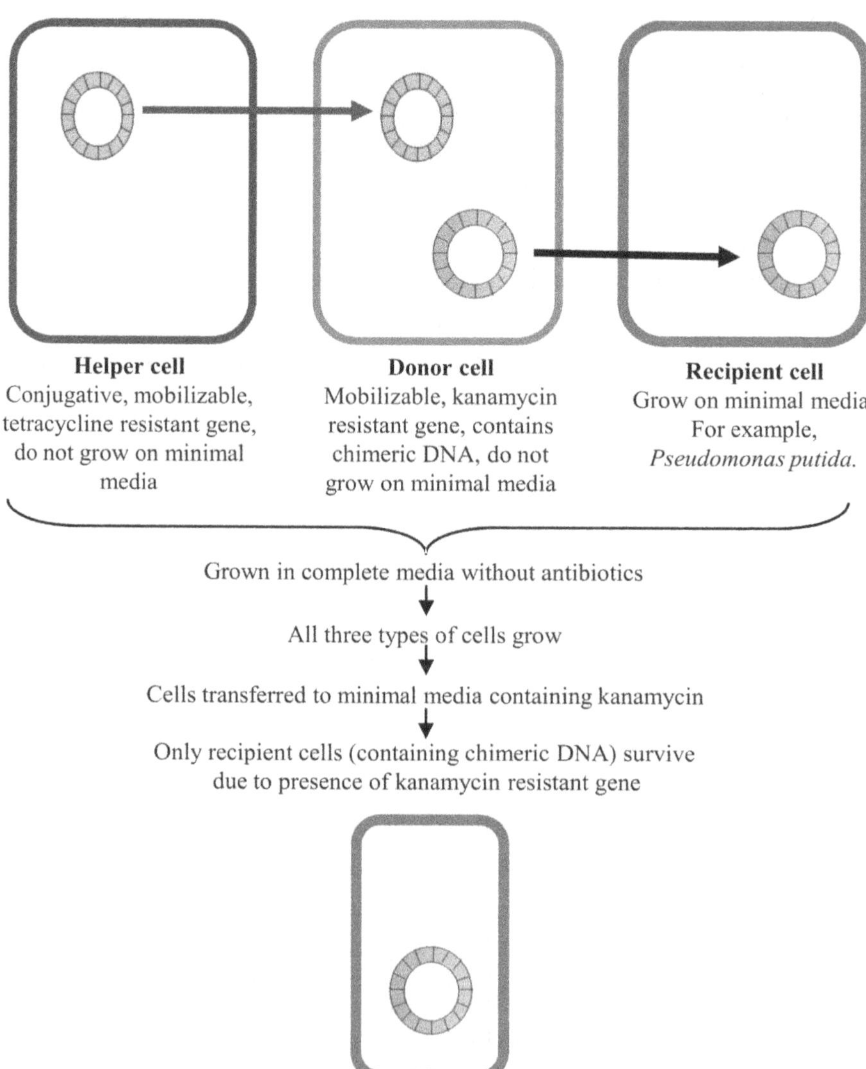

FIGURE 7.19 Conjugation method of transformation

SELECTION OF HOST CELL WITH DESIRED RECOMBINANT DNA

Following transformation, selection of host cell in which desired recombinant DNA has entered is done. After transformation, there three different possibilities arise:

(i)   No transformation takes place i.e., recombinant DNA does not enter the host cell. These types of cells are not selected.

(ii) Transformation takes place; however, recircularized vector (plasmid) enters the host cell. These types of cells are also not selected.

(iii) Transformation takes place and chimeric/recombinant DNA enters the cell. These types of cells are selected.

Depending on the type of marker genes present on cloning vectors, the different selection procedures are selected. For pBR vectors, positive negative selection procedure is used. However for pUC, colorimetric selection method is used.

Selection of host cell with pBR vector based recombinant DNA: The following are the salient points related to selection of host cells following transformation with pBR based recombinant DNA.

Addition of Target DNA in vector disrupts functioning of one of marker genes: These plasmids contain two marker genes i.e., ampicillin resistant and tetracycline resistant genes. Addition of target DNA in any one of marker gene sequence leads to loss of antibiotic resistance gene. For example, addition of target DNA in sequence of tetracycline resistant gene leads to loss of tetracycline resistance. However, ampicillin resistant gene remains intact. In certain cases, the production of chimeric DNA may fail leading to formation of recircularized plasmid, which has intact ampicillin and tetracycline resistant gene **(Figure 7.20)**.

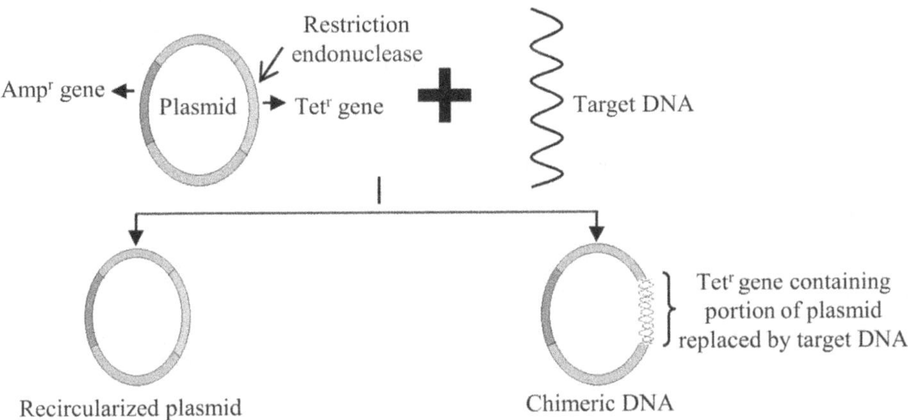

FIGURE 7.20 Addition of target gene disrupts tet^r gene functioning in chimeric DNA. However, in recircularized plasmid, tet^r gene remains functional.

Three types of Host cells after transformation : After transformation, three may be different types of host cells **(Figure 7.21)**:

1. No transformation takes place and cells are Amp^s as well as Tet^s. S stands for sensitive.

2. Transformation with recircularized plasmid takes place. The cells are Amp^R as well as Tet^R. R refers to resistance.

3. Transformation with chimeric DNA. The cells are Amp^R as well as Tet^S.

Method of selection: Host cells with pBR vectors-based chimeric DNA are selected using positive-negative selection procedure. In this procedure, some cells are allowed to grow (positive selection) and others are inhibited from growth (negative selection). The following steps are involved in selection procedure **(Figure 7.21)**:

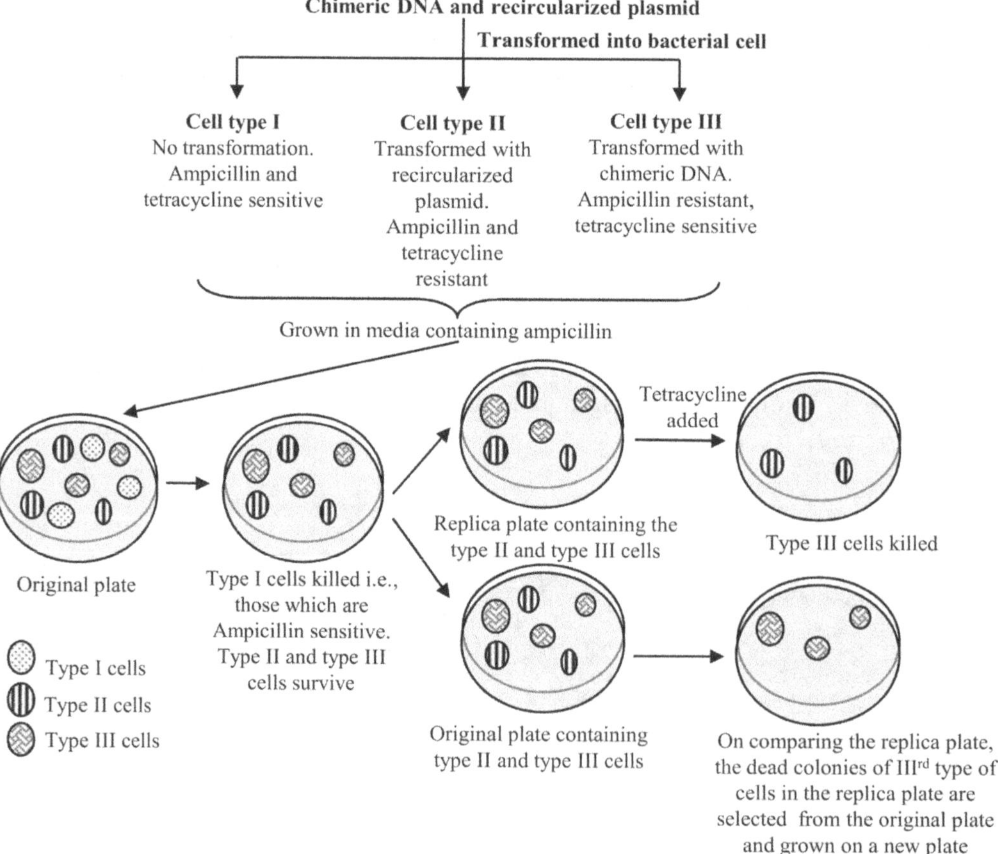

FIGURE 7.21 Possibility of three types of colonies after transformation followed by positive negative selection.

(i)   All types of cells are grown on a culture media with no antibiotic.

(ii) In a growth media, ampicillin is added which kills the cells lacking ampicillin resistant genes. In other words, cells with no transformation (cells with first possibility) are killed.

(iii) At this point, the replica of this plate (original) is made. Both original and replica plates are identical and have two types of cells (cells with second and third possibility).

(iv) The replica plate is treated with tetracycline, which kills the cells lacking tetracycline resistant gene. In other words, cells transformed with chimeric DNA are killed (cells with third possibility). Cells transformed with recircularized plasmid (cells with second possibility) remain and grow in culture media.

(v)   The comparison of original and replica plate is made. The purpose is to select the cells from original plate corresponding to killed cells in replica plate. The cells killed in replica plate are to be selected. Therefore, these are selected from original plate by comparing with replica plate.

Selection of host cell with pUC vector based recombinant DNA: The following are the salient points related to selection of host cells following transformation with pUC-based recombinant DNA.

Addition of Target DNA in vector disrupts functioning of one of marker genes: pUC vectors have two marker genes i.e., ampicillin resistant gene and Lac Z' gene. Addition of target DNA in Lac Z' region leads to loss of its functioning. However, ampicillin resistant gene remains intact; therefore, recombinant DNA has only ampicillin resistance gene without Lac Z' gene. In case of recircularized plasmid, there is intact ampicillin resistance gene and Lac Z' gene **(Figure 7.22)**.

Three types of Host cells after transformation: After transformation, there are three types of host cells **(Figure 7.23)**:

1. No transformation has taken place and the cell lacks ampicillin resistant gene and Lac Z' gene.

2. Transformation has taken place with recircularized plasmid. The host cells have both ampicillin resistant and Lac Z' gene.

3. Transformation has taken place with chimeric DNA and the cells have ampicillin resistant gene, but Lac Z' gene is non-functional.

Method of selection

The host cells following transformation with pUC based recombinant DNA are selected by colorimetric method. The different steps are:

(i)   All types of cells are grown in culture media

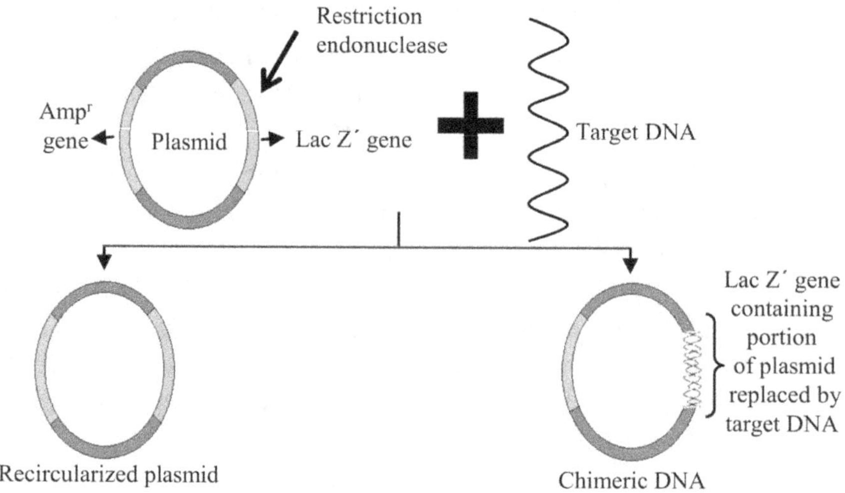

FIGURE 7.22 Addition of target gene disrupts Lac Z′ gene functioning in chimeric DNA. However, in recircularized plasmid, Lac Z′ gene remains functional.

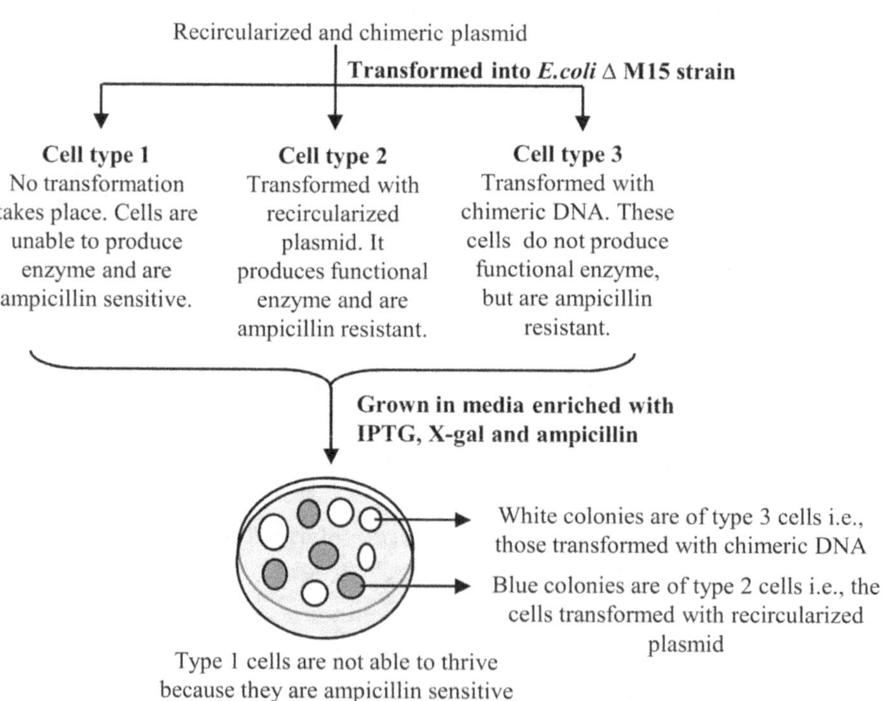

FIGURE 7.23 Three types of cells formed following transformation and selection of desired cells by colorimetric method.

(ii) Ampicillin is added in growth media, which kills the cells lacking ampicillin resistant genes. In other words, cells with no transformation (cells with first possibility) are killed.

(iii) Thereafter, IPTG (isopropyl thiogalactoside) and X-Gal (5-Bromo-4-chloro-3-indolyl-β-D-galactoside) are added in culture media. The cells having functional Lac Z' genes (cells with second possibility) start producing α-peptide of galactosidase enzyme in the presence of IPTG, which acts as inducer. The production of α-peptide results in formation of active galactosidase. Galactosidase acts on X-Gal (substrate) and forms blue colored product **(Figure 7.24)**. Thus, cells with functional Lac Z' gene (recircularized plasmid) appear blue.

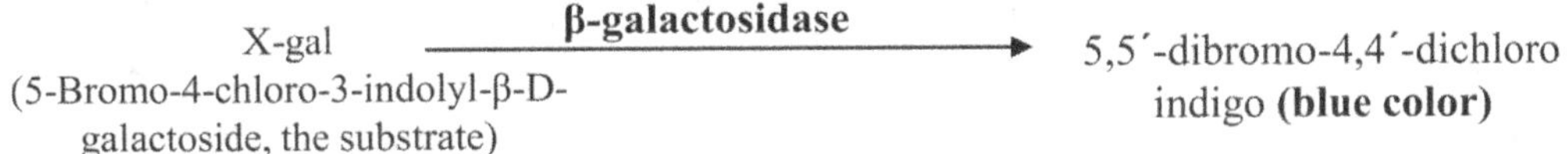

FIGURE 7.24 Conversion of X-Gal to blue colored product in the presence of beta-galactosidase

(iv) On the other hand, cells with non-functional Lac Z' genes (recombinant DNA) do not form active galactosidase enzyme and no blue colored product is formed. Thus, colorless colonies are selected amongst blue colonies.

ALPHA-COMPLEMENTATION

It refers to a process used for selection of the bacterial cells with successful transformation of pUC vectors in them. *E. coli* HM15 strain (host cell) is used for transformation of pUC vector. The pUC vector contains Lac Z' gene, which produces β-peptide of the α-galactosidase enzyme; while *E. coli* HM15 produces inactive galactosidase due to absence of α-peptide at its $-NH_2$ end. Successful transformation of pUC vector into *E. coli* enables the production of active β-galactosidase in *E. coli*. To ensure successful production of â-galactosidase, *E. coli* with β-complimenting vector is grown in IPTG, the inducer of Lac Z' gene. IPTG inactivates the repressor produced by Lac I, enabling the expression of Lac Z' gene, thus, initiating the production of α-peptide. This results in formation of active galactosidase. Addition of X-Gal (5-Bromo-4-chloro-3-indolyl-α-D-galactoside) to these cells grown in IPTG enriched media produces blue colored and white colored colonies depending on the presence or absence of α-galactosidase enzyme, respectively. This color is the result of conversion of X-Gal to 5-Bromo-4-chloro-3-indolyl in the presence of galactosidase. Furthermore, oxidation of 5-Bromo-4-chloro-3-indolyl in air leads to formation of a blue dye, 5, 5′-dibromo-4,4′-dichloro indigo. Therefore, blue stained colonies are a result of transformation of vectors with functional Lac Z′ gene in the bacterial cell; and white colonies indicate failure of transformation of the vector into the bacterial cell or transformation of the vector after being treated with restriction endonucleases specific to the polylinker site so as to recombine a new DNA segment of interest to produce the recombinant DNA **(Figure 7.25)**.

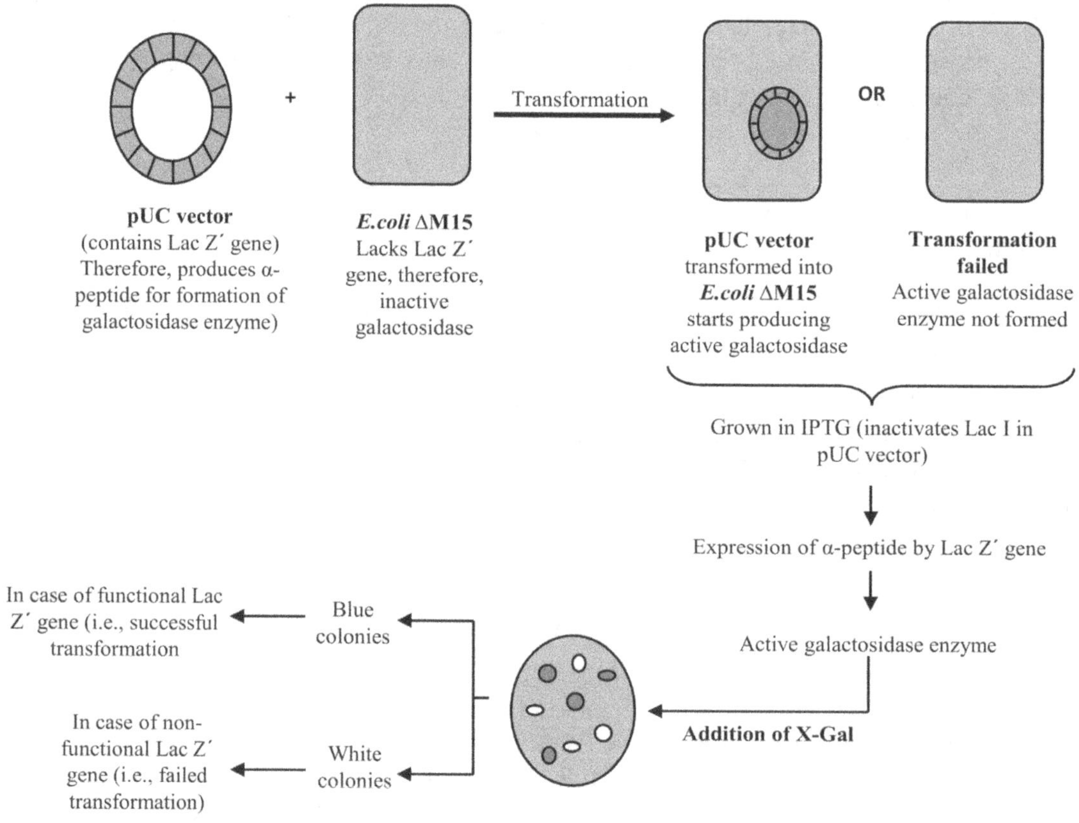

FIGURE 7.25 Alpha-complementation in selection of pUC based chimeric DNA.

APPLICATIONS OF RECOMBINANT DNA TECHNOLOGY

1. **Production of Protein Pharmaceuticals (Therapeutic Proteins):** The major application of this technology has been in the area of therapeutic protein production. 'Human insulin' was the therapeutic product obtained using recombinant DNA technology. Thereafter, a lot of other therapeutic proteins have been synthesized and these include human growth hormone,

tissue plasminogen activator, erythropoietin, active Protein C, Clotting Factor VIII, interferons and Deoxyribonuclease I (DNase I) **(Table 7.1)**

TABLE 7.1 List of therapeutic products produced using recombinant DNA technology

S. No	Products	Therapeutic Uses
1.	Insulin	Diabetes Mellitus
2.	Human Growth Hormone	Dwarfism
3.	Tissue Plasminogen Activators	Myocardial infarction, pulmonary embolism to dissolve clot
4.	Interferon	Treatment of viral diseases and cancer
5.	DNAse	In Cystic fibrosis to decrease the viscosity of mucus
6.	Erythropoietin	Renal failure associated anemia
7.	Clotting Factor VIII	Hemophilia A

2. **Transgenic Animals:** These are the animals whose genetic makeup is altered permanently (in heritable manner). These animals are made by inserting or removing target gene from the organisms.

   (i) **Disease Models:** These animals are extensively employed as 'Disease Models' to evaluate the efficacy of new drugs. In these animals, gene alteration is done to induce diseases such as hypertension, Alzheimer disease, diabetes mellitus and atherosclerosis etc. Such diseased animals are used as disease models to explore the effectiveness of new drugs.

   (ii) **Production of Protein Supplements and pharmaceuticals from Milk-producing transgenic animals:** A number of protein products including insulin, growth hormone, and blood anti-clotting factors may be obtained from the milk of transgenic cows, sheep, or goats. These animals made may be used as protein factories by adding our gene of interest in these animals.

   (iii) **Xenotransplantation:** This refers to transplantation of organs from animals to humans as there is shortage of human donors. Transgenic pigs may provide the alternative to human as organ donors. However, organ transplantation rejection is the major hurdle. Research is underway to remove the pig proteins and replace with human proteins to avoid transplantation rejection.

   (iv) **Non-medical uses:** Apart from medical uses, these animals are extensively used in agriculture and related fields. Farmers use these animals for increased milk production, high growth and disease resistance.

3. **Transgenic Plants:** Similar to transgenic animals, these are the plants whose genetic makeup is altered in a heritable manner. These plants are made to have more resistance to biotic stresses (insects, viruses, fungi and bacteria); abiotic stresses (heat, chilling, freezing, drought, salinity, ozone, intense light); have improved crop yield, shelf life (fruits and flowers), quality and nutrition. Moreover, these transgenic plants may also be used as bioreactors to yield protein pharmaceuticals, vaccines, and biodegradable plastics.

4. **Humanized and Human Monoclonal Antibodies:** The monoclonal antibodies produced by 'Hybridoma technology' produce immunogenic response because antibodies produced by B cells are obtained from mice. In order to reduce immunogenicity, humanized antibodies and human antibodies are produced using recombinant DNA technology. The protein sequences in antibodies are modified to increase their similarity to human antibodies. For example, omalizumab is humanized monoclonal antibody used for bronchial asthma.

5. **Gene Therapy:** It is the type of therapy in which exogenous gene is added or over expressing gene is silenced to cure the disease. The details of the gene therapy are explained in **gene therapy chapter.**

6. **Recombinant Vaccines:** A vaccine is a biological preparation which provides active immunity against disease. Recombinant DNA technology has been used to prepare vaccines. The vaccine prepared using recombinant DNA technology is called recombinant vaccine. These are of two types, DNA vaccines and protein subunit vaccines. In DNA vaccines, a synthetic DNA is injected to produces antigen, which evokes or activates immune response. In subunit vaccines, the synthetic peptides that represent fraction of the pathogenic organism are injected to activate an immune response. For example, Hepatitis B vaccine is recombinant vaccines and is used to prevent hepatitis B.

REVIEW QUESTIONS

TWO MARKS QUESTIONS

1. What is recombinant DNA technology?

2. What is application of alkaline phosphatase in recombinant DNA technology?

3. What are the advantages of pUC vectors over pBR vectors?

4. What do you understand by electroporation method of transformation?

5. What are restriction endonucleases? What is its significance in recombinant DNA technology?

6. What is palindrome sequence? Give example showing cutting in palindrome with suitable restriction endonuclease.

7. What do you understand by alpha-complementation?

8. What are the characteristic features of pUC vectors?

9. What is copy number? How is it regulated? What is the advantage of high copy number?

10. What is ligase? What is its role in recombinant DNA technology?

11. What is pBR? Explain its key features.

12. What is cDNA? What is its advantage over DNA in recombinant DNA technology?

FIVE MARKS QUESTIONS

1. Write a note on applications of recombinant DNA technology?

2. What are restriction endonucleases? What are its different types with special reference to type II enzymes?

3. What is transformation? What are different methods employed for transformation in recombinant DNA technology?

4. How are pUC based chimeric DNA selected in host cells?

5. What are cloning vectors? What are ideal characteristics of such vectors? What are the factors that affect the choice of vectors?

TEN MARKS QUESTIONS

1. Explain different steps involved in recombinant DNA technology?

2. What are plasmids? What is their role as cloning vectors in recombinant DNA technology? What are main types of plasmids employed in recombinant DNA technology?

3. Write applications of recombinant DNA technology.

MULTIPLE CHOICE QUESTIONS

1. Which is not present in pUC vectors?
   - (a) ORI
   - (b) RoP
   - (c) Lac Z' gene
   - (d) Antibiotic resistance marker gene

2. Which is not true for pBR?
   - (a) High copy number
   - (b) Widely used
   - (c) Named after scientists
   - (d) Self replicating

3. In electroporation, DNA moves inside the cell due to
   - (a) Neutralization of charged ions
   - (b) Creation of pores
   - (c) Removal of components hindering permeability
   - (d) All the above

4. Alkaline phosphatase in used to
   - (a) Prevent recircularizaion of plasmid
   - (b) Remove phosphate groups from plasmid
   - (c) Recombinant DNA technology
   - (d) All the above

5. Which is true for T4 Ligase
   - (a) Isolated from E Coli
   - (b) Prepared by recombinant DNA technology
   - (c) Both a and b
   - (d) Isolated from T4 ligase

6. In pUc based selection procedure, colonies with chimeric DNA are
   - (a) Blue in color
   - (b) Colorless
   - (c) Yellow color
   - (d) None of above

7. In recombinant DNA technology, which ends are preferred
   - (a) Sticky ends
   - (b) Blunt ends
   - (c) Both a and b
   - (d) None of above

8. What type of restriction endonucleases are preferred
   - (a) Type I
   - (b) Type II
   - (c) Type III
   - (d) Type IV

9. Which of following enzyme acts on palindrome sequence
   - (a) Type I
   - (b) Type II
   - (c) Type III
   - (d) Type IV

10. Which of the following is not application of recombinant DNA technology?
   - (a) Production of protein products
   - (b) Transgenic animals
   - (c) Gene therapy
   - (d) Western blotting

Gel Electrophoresis

CHAPTER OUTLINE

Introduction and General Features

Basic Concepts in Electrophoresis

GELS
Agarose Gel
Polyacrylamide Gels

Horizontal vs Vertical

Electrophoretic System

Sample Preparation

Buffer Systems
Ornstein and Davis Model of Discontinuous

Buffer System
SDS–PAGE (Discontinuous Buffer system)

Detection Methods
Detection of Nucleic acids (DNA or RNA)
Detection of Proteins

Isolation of Nucleic Acids or Proteins from Electrophoresis Gel
Passive Diffusion
Electroelution
Continuous Elution

INTRODUCTION AND GENERAL FEATURES

The word 'electrophoresis' has been derived from Greek word and it means 'carried by electricity'. Electrophoresis may be defined as migration of charged particles under the influence of electric field. Gel electrophoresis is described as a technique used to separate charged biomolecules like DNA, RNA and proteins in a gel on the basis of their charge, size, and shape. The technique is easy to perform and reliable results may be expected with minimum of practice. Electrophoresis is performed in free solution, while gel electrophoresis is performed in semi-solid gel. Gel provides an anti-convection media, which offers many advantages. For example, in free solution, the separated molecules can again mix up. However, in a gel the separated molecules remain separated as there is no possibility of mixing of those separated molecules.

There are a number of techniques available for separation of proteins and nucleic acids, based on their chemical and physical properties. The presence of charge on these molecules is much exploited in separation techniques such as in gel electrophoresis; isoelectric focusing and ion exchange chromatography.

However, gel electrophoresis is one of the most common methods available for separation of proteins and nucleic acid.

BASIC CONCEPTS IN ELECTROPHORESIS

Whenever an electric field is applied, a charged molecule experiences a force, F.

$$F = qE \qquad \qquad .....(8.1)$$

Where, q = charge on the molecule; E=electric field (Volt/cm)

As soon as a charged molecule begins to move under the influence of electric field, a frictional drag or force (F′) comes into play. F′ is directly proportional to migration speed of ion.

$$F' \, \alpha \, v$$
$$F' = fv \qquad \qquad .....(8.2)$$

Where, v = migration velocity; f = frictional coefficient, it depends on the size and shape of macromolecules (ions)

Under steady state conditions,

$$F = F'$$

So, $qE = fv$ (From Eq 8.1 and 8.2)

$$\text{Or} \quad E = \frac{fv}{q} \qquad \qquad .....(8.3)$$

Electrophoretic mobility (μ) of a molecule is defined as steady state velocity per unit electric field **(Equation 8.4)**. Units of $\mu = cm^2/v\text{-}sec$

$$\mu = \frac{v}{E} \qquad \qquad .....(8.4)$$

Putting **equation 8.3** in the above equation

$$\mu = \frac{v}{fv} \times q = \frac{q}{f} \qquad \qquad .....(8.5)$$

From **equation 8.5**, it may be deduced that electrophoretic mobility depends on charge and frictional coefficient. As written above, frictional coefficient (f) depends on the size and shape of molecule. Therefore, electrophoretic mobility of molecules depends on three factors, charge of molecule, size of molecule and shape of molecule. The basis of separation of molecules in gel electrophoresis is difference in electrophoretic mobility of those molecules. The goal of electrophoresis is to separate different molecules due to their different electrophoretic mobility.

GELS

Gels are intermediate between solids and liquids. These are three-dimensional networks of constituent polymers. As gel forms, individual components combine into fibers that aggregate into bundles to form random meshwork. In between the bundles, there are open spaces called 'pores' or sieves. Hence, gels may be defined as "3 dimensional sieves that limit the motion of migrating molecules". The major advantage of using gels is that they enhance separation due to sieving action. During electrophoresis, molecules move between 'buffer filled pores' of gel. The molecules have to squeeze through the small pores of gels and this process in dependent on size and shape of molecules. The dense regions of gel (other than pore portion) act as barrier and molecules cannot pass through those dense regions. The movement of molecules is ultimately dependent on electric field and charge of molecule. Thus, gel electrophoresis is separation of charged molecules under the influence of electric field and in turn depends on size, shape and charge of molecule. Gels are the most useful support media for carrying out electrophoresis and agarose and polyacrylamide gels are of real importance.

AGAROSE GEL

The salient features of agarose gel may be discussed as below:

1. **Structure of Agrose gel:** It is a neutral, linear polysaccharide purified from agar-agar of red algae. It consists of D-galactose and 3,6-anhydro-L-galactose linked in alternating fashion by glycosidic bonds **(Figure 8.1)**.

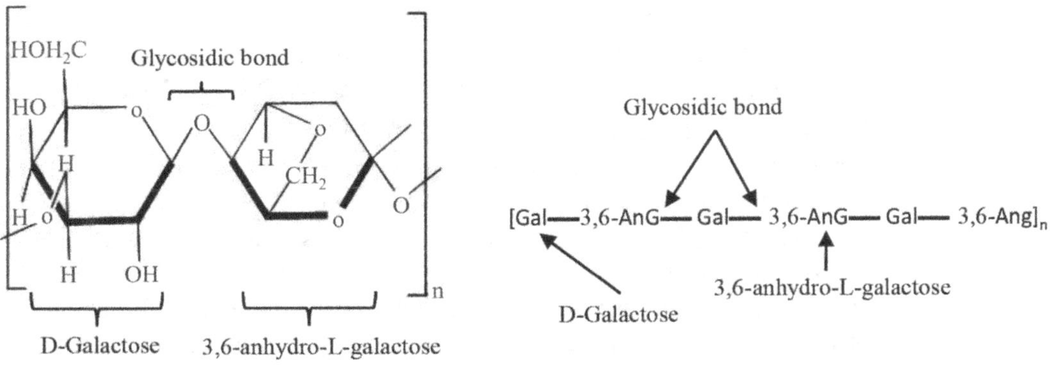

FIGURE 8.1 Structure of Agarose gel, n represents number of repeat units.

2. **Method of preparation of Gel:** Agarose is soluble in hot water and when a hot solution of agarose is cooled, a matrix (gel) is formed. The cross linking of agarose polymer chains occurs by hydrogen bonds. The formation of gel is reversible and gel can again be converted to solution form by heating. Commercially, agarose is available as a dry white powder and it is dispersed in buffered ionic solutions followed by heating until it is completely dissolved. At about 50°C, molten agarose is poured into 'casting tray' in which gelation (solidification) takes place **(Figure 8.2)**.

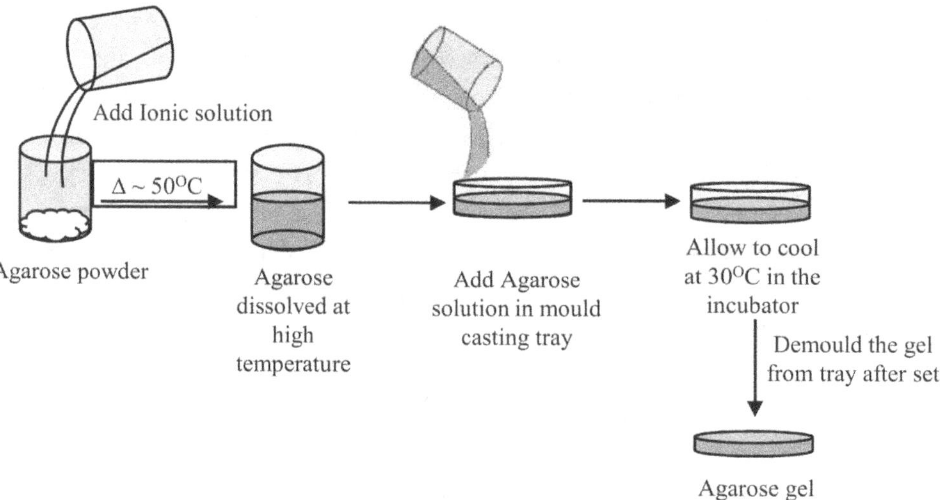

FIGURE 8.2 Procedure of setting the Agarose gel

3. **Concentration of Agarose Gel:** The concentration of agarose gel is chosen on the basis of material to be separated. Most often, the range is between 0.5-2.0% w/v **(Table 8.1)** and 1.5% w/v solution of agarose gel is mostly used. As the concentration of agarose increases, the pore size of gel decreases and hence, mobility of molecules in a gel decreases. Thus, higher concentration may be used for separating smaller DNA molecules.

4. **Separation of Proteins or Nucleic Acids:** Agarose is mainly used for the separation of nucleic acid such as DNA or RNA. The pores of agarose gels are larger than that of polyacrylamide gel. Proteins larger than 500 kDa in size and DNA larger than about 2000 base pairs can be separated in agarose gel. The pores of agarose gel are larger, and proteins are of smaller size, therefore, agarose gel cannot be used to separate normally occurring protein fragments. Indeed, agarose is a non-sieving matrix for proteins and there is increased diffusion of proteins in large agarose pores. However, it may be used for separation of proteins when combined with some other separation techniques such as 'isoelectric focusing' (agarose IEF) or when the separating protein molecules are very large in size.

TABLE 8.1 Agarose concentration used to separate DNA

S.No.	% agarose (g/ml)	Double stranded DNA size (kb)	Double stranded DNA that migrates with dye	
			Bromophenol (Tracking dye)	Xylene cyanole (Tracking dye)
1	0.3	60-5.0	-	-
2	0.6	20-1.0	0.7-1.2	9.0-10.0
3	0.7	10-0.8	0.6-0.8	6.0-7.0
4	0.9	7-0.5	0.3-0.4	3.0-4.0
5	1.2	6-0.4	0.18-0.21	1.4-1.9
6	1.5	4-0.2	0.12-0.14	0.8-1.4
7	2.0	3-0.1	<0.1	0.8-0.9

5. **Factors Affecting Mobility of DNA in Agarose gel:** The mobility of DNA in agarose gel depends on:

   (i) *Molecular size of DNA*: Mobility is inversely proportional to molecular weight. Higher is the molecular weight, lower is the mobility. Indeed, DNA travels at a rate inversely proportional to $\log_{10}$ of DNA's molecular weight.

$$\text{Mobility } \alpha \ 1/\log_{10} \text{ mol. Weight}$$

   (ii) *Agarose Concentration:* Agarose concentration determines the pore size; therefore, higher is the concentration, smaller is the pore size and slower is the mobility.

   (iii) *Conformation of DNA*: The DNA fragment with compact conformation has fast mobility. On the other hand, a linear DNA fragment moves with lesser speed.

   (iv) *Applied current:* The higher is the applied current, the faster is the movement of the DNA through the gel. However, the values of voltage or current cannot be exceeded beyond a limit because at high voltage melting of the gel may take place, due to production of heat. Moreover, very high applied current (>5-8 V/cm) also decreases the resolution.

6. **Gel Artifacts:** There are different reasons for gel artifacts:

   (i) *Overloading of sample*: If the amount of DNA that is put in gel is very high, then instead of sharp bands, broad smear will be obtained. The overloaded DNA will not migrate to longer distance in comparison to DNA samples loaded at low concentration.

   (ii) *Edge effect:* The DNA samples do not migrate at same rate, when put in different parts of the same gel. The DNA sample loaded in the centre of gel moves at a faster rate as compared to DNA sample loaded at edges. So, overall it leads to 'smiling of bands' **(Figure 8.3)**.

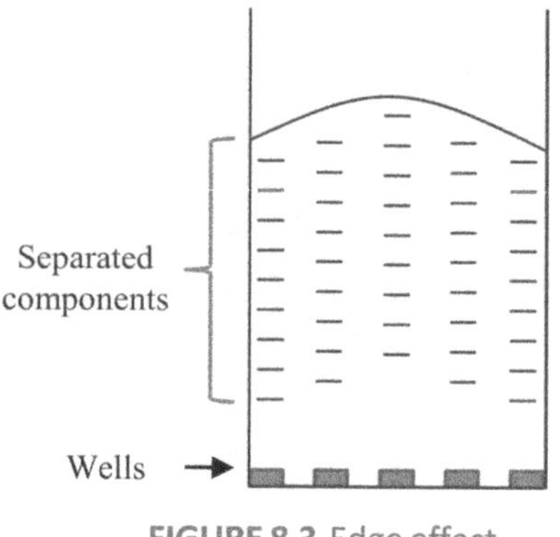

FIGURE 8.3 Edge effect

(iii)   Overheating: The gel artifact may also occur due to overheating, when a very strong electric field is applied. The edges of gel are in contact with buffer and dissipate heat more quickly than the centre of gel. Thus, the center of gel is overheated than corners. This leads to decrease in viscosity of gel in centre and DNA moves at a faster rate in the centre.

(iv)   Salt effect: For DNA fragments, an increase in salt concentration may affect DNA mobility up to 15%. An increase in ionic concentration decreases the DNA mobility. The presence of extra ions in a sample may shield the charges on DNA fragment and hence, net charge on DNA is reduced, leading to decrease in its mobility.

POLYACRYLAMIDE GELS

The use of polyacrylamide gel in electrophoresis is termed as PAGE (Polyacrylamide Gel Electrophoresis). The salient features of polyacrylamide gel may discussed as below:

1. **Structure of Gel:** This gel is made by co-polymerization of acrylamide and N, N′- methylene bisacrylamide. The polymerized units of acrylamide are cross-linked using bifunctional N, N′- methylene bisacrylamide as co-

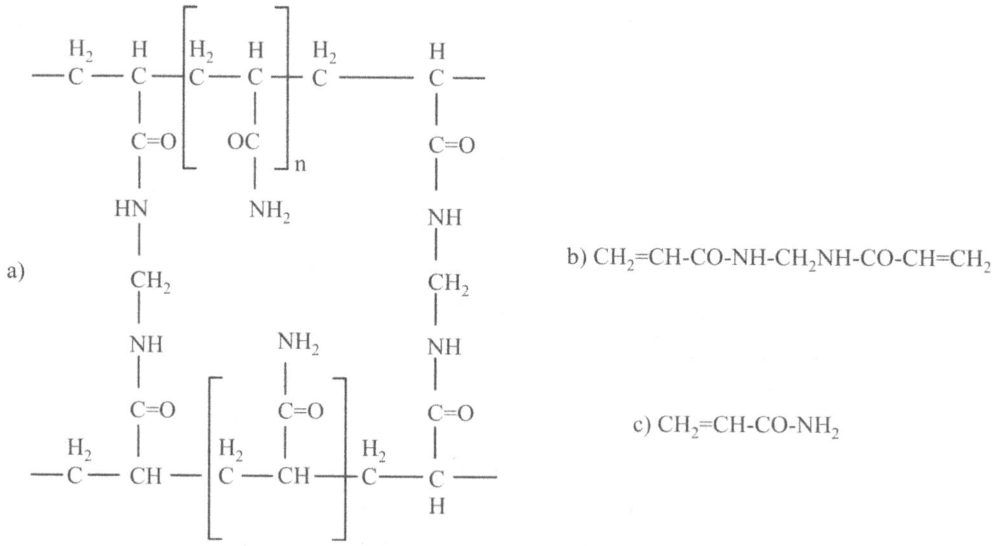

b) $CH_2=CH-CO-NH-CH_2NH-CO-CH=CH_2$

c) $CH_2=CH-CO-NH_2$

FIGURE 8.4 Structure of (a) N,N′methylene bis acrylamide, (b) acrylamide and (c) polyacrylamide

monomer or cross linkers. These cross linkers covalently link adjacent polyacrylamide chains **(Figure 8.4)**. Gels are unstable outside the pH range of 4-6. The sharpness of band decreases in old gels. Therefore, for high resolution studies, gels should be prepared fresh before use.

2. **Free radical mediated polymerization reaction:** The formation of polyacrylamide gel is free radical mediated reaction. Ammonium persulphate acts as an initiator and it provides free radicals; tetramethylethylenediamine (TEMED) acts as an accelerator. TEMED causes decomposition of ammonium persulphate and liberates two sulphate (SO_4^{2-}) free radicals. The free radicals initiate polymerization and the rate of polymerization depends upon net concentration of monomers and free radicals, temperature and purity of reagents. Any compound that acts as a free radical trap stops the polymerization. Oxygen is the most abundant radical trap, so proper degassing should be done to remove oxygen.

3. **Concentration of Gels and its relation with Pore Size:** The concentration of polyacrylamide gels is expressed by pair of values of %T **(Equation 8.6)** and % C **(Equation 8.7)**. %T is the weight percentage of total monomer including cross-linker (g/100 ml). % C is the proportion of cross-linker as a percentage of total monomer

$$\%T = \frac{(A+B)100}{V}\% \qquad\qquad .....(8.6)$$

$$\%C = \frac{B \times 100}{A+B}\% \qquad\qquad .....(8.7)$$

A = amount of acrylamide; B = amount of bisacrylamide; V = volume of buffer added

When % T is increased at fixed low cross linker concentration, the number of chain increases and pore size decreases. However, pore size is biphasic function of % C. With an increase in %C, with constant %T, the pore size decreases. But, increase in % C (beyond 5%), the pore size increases due to linking of cross linker with each other. For proteins, 30% T and 2.7% C and for nucleic acids, 30% T and 3.3% C are preferred.

HORIZONTAL VS VERTICAL ELECTROPHORETIC SYSTEM

Gel electrophoresis may be performed with gel positioned either vertically or horizontally. In vertical electrophoresis, with the sample migrates in a downward direction and it is most common way to run PAGE and is well suited for blotting. In this case, gel is contained in cassette of glass or plastic. The upper and lower parts of cassette are open and in contact with electrolyte (buffer) solution. The sample is loaded on the top of gel in the sample application wells. In horizontal electrophoresis, gel is layered on horizontal plate **(Figure 8.5)**.

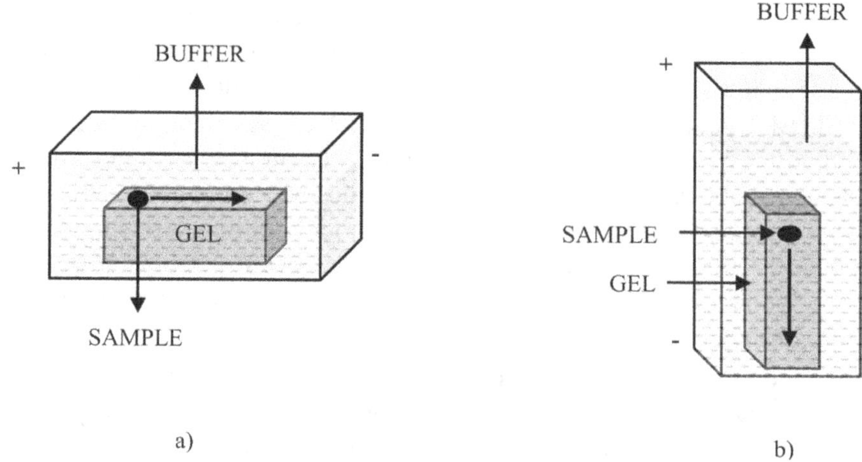

FIGURE 8.5 Representation of horizontal (a) and vertical (b) systems of gel electrophoresis

SAMPLE PREPARATION

1. **Use of detergents:** The DNA or proteins may be analyzed or separated in gel electrophoresis, when they are in solution form. If sample is difficult to dissolve, agents like detergents or urea may be necessary. However, unlike chromatography, where insoluble material may ruin the column, the presence of particles in electrophoretic sample does not interfere much with separation. Detergent such as sodium dodecyl sulphate (SDS) is added to the protein sample in order to reduce the protein-protein interaction and denature them. The use of SDS in PAGE is called as SDS-PAGE (discussed later). Several other denaturants have also been used in the process including urea, which breaks H-bonds holding the two helical strands of DNA together. This results in formation of single stranded DNA, which is important for molecular weight determination. Other denaturants used in sample preparations include, formamide and mercaptoethanol, etc.

2. **Tracking Dye:** Bromophenol blue is the most commonly employed tracking dye. It is used to visualize the sample migration in a gel.

3. Glycerol or High Concentration Sucrose: Along with detergents and tracking dye, glycerol or high concentration solution of sucrose (40%) is also added in a sample. Addition of glycerol makes the sample heavier and the sample molecules do not move out from the well into the buffer solution.

BUFFER SYSTEMS

The buffer system has a profound effect on the electrophoresis. It affects the power conditions, separation and resolution. Two kinds of buffer system are used:

CONTINUOUS BUFFER SYSTEM

1. In this case, the same buffer is used in gel and electrode reservoirs. The sample is loaded on the gel in which separation occurs. The molecules migrate through the pores of gel and they are fractionated according to mobility.
2. A gel with homogenous concentration is used in this system.
3. The main limitation of this system is the low resolution. The best resolution is obtained only when a very high concentration of samples is used. Normally, it is used when nucleic acid and proteins have a concentration of 1mg/ml or more.

DISCONTINUOUS BUFFER SYSTEM

1. In this case, different buffer solutions are used in gel and in electrode chamber.
2. It is high resolution technique.
3. Gels of two different concentrations are used, i.e. stacking gel (low concentration and large pores) and resolving gel (high concentration and small pores).
4. An example of the discontinuous system includes Ornstein and Davis model.

ORNSTEIN AND DAVIS MODEL OF DISCONTINUOUS BUFFER SYSTEM

In 1964, Ornstein and Davis developed high resolution discontinuous PAGE for separation of proteins. It uses two different buffers solutions containing different anions and common cations to separate proteins **(Figure 8.6)**. It consists of 4 parts:

1. **Stacking gel:** It has large pores (4% T) and gel is made in 0.125 M Tris-Cl at pH 6.8

2. **Resolving gel:** It contains small pores (5-30% T) and gel is made in 0.375 M Tris-Cl at pH 8.8.

3. **Electrode buffer:** Tris-glycine is used as the electrode buffer.

4. **Sample:** Sample is loaded in the system i.e. placed in wells of gel. The ionic strength of sample should be low compared to the buffers.

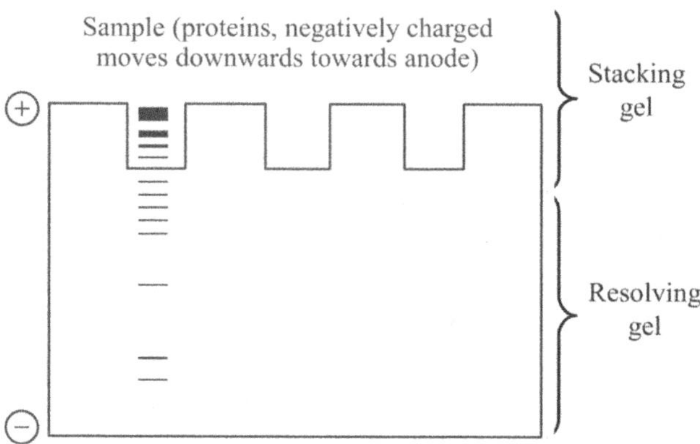

FIGURE 8.6 Representation of Ornstein and Davis model

Principle and Working

The samples are applied in the wells of large pore stacking gel. The stacking gel has minimal sieving properties and it mainly acts as anti-convection medium. The ionic molecules in the sample move in forward direction. Buffer ions in the gel form the front that moves ahead of sample ion. The electrode buffer ions form a front that trails behind the sample. So, the sample ions are stacked between two buffer fronts (of gel and of electrode) **(Figure 8.7)**. The sample molecules form extremely narrow zones arranged in the order of decreasing mobility. In other words, sample molecules rapidly "stack" into a very narrow zone. Thereafter, stacked samples move from large pore stacking gel into small pore resolving gel (separating gel). Once in the resolving gel, sieving becomes predominant and on the basis of size and charge, the stacked sample molecules are separated.

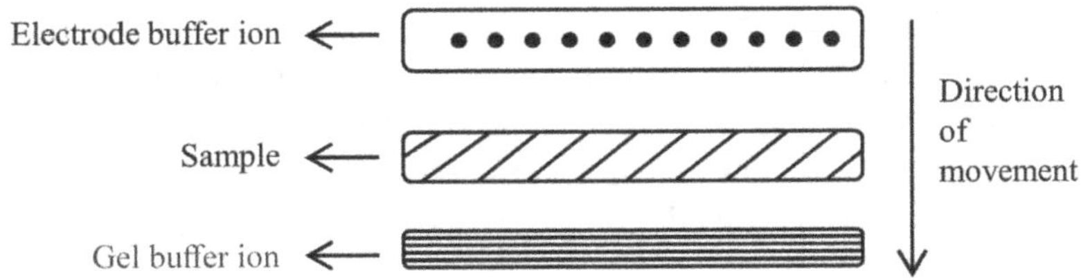

FIGURE 8.7 Stacking of sample between gel buffer ion and electrode buffer ion in discontinuous gel electrophoresis

SDS–PAGE (DISCONTINUOUS BUFFER SYSTEM)

SDS–PAGE is another type of discontinuous buffer system. It has similar arrangements as discussed in Ornstein Davis model including stacking gel, resolving gel, electrode buffer etc. However, the unique point of SDS-PAGE is that excess of SDS is added to the protein sample to denature them. SDS-protein sample is heated so that proteins are separated into smaller peptides. Thereafter, these peptides are uniformly coated with negatively charged SDS molecules. All peptides take up charge depending on their size and assume similar charge density (charge to mass ratio). Furthermore, these peptides also assume similar shape. Therefore, these peptides are of similar shape and charge, but only differ in size. These peptides are separated from one another on the basis of their size (shape and charge being similar) in gel electrophoresis. The larger the size of the peptide, the lesser the distance travelled by it in the gel. Therefore, distance traveled is inversely proportional to size (or molecular mass). Accordingly, this method is particularly used to determine the molecular weight of proteins.

The distance travelled by a particular peptide is measured to calculate its molecular weight. The distance travelled by the test sample is compared to that of the standard to estimate the molecular weight with the help of a standard plot. Relative migration distance (R_f) is used as a measure of distance travelled by the sample **(Equation 8.8)**.

$$R_f = \frac{\text{Distance travelled by sample}}{\text{Distance travelled by tracking dye}} \qquad .....(8.8)$$

DETECTION METHODS

There are different detection methods depending on proteins or nucleic acid:

1. Detection of Nucleic acids (DNA or RNA)

   (i) ***Ethidium Bromide:*** It is the most commonly used dye for detecting nucleic acids. It is a fluorescent dye, which intercalates between stacked

bases of DNA and RNA. A dye-nucleic acid complex could be detected for fluorescence with UV illumination. The fluorescence observed on exposing the gel to UV light from beneath is pink/orange in color. However, it is carcinogenic, so, it needs to be handled with caution, which is the only disadvantage of using it as the detecting agent **(Figure 8.8)**.

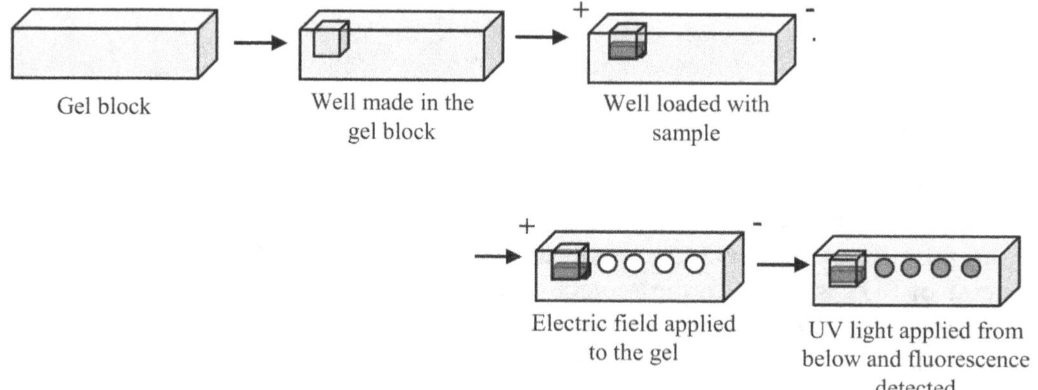

FIGURE 8.8 Method for ethidium bromide staining

(ii) ***Methylene blue:*** The use of methylene blue as the staining agent for the DNA and RNA fragments is relatively easy and safe method. This dye is positively charged, and binds to the DNA and RNA fragments which are negatively charged. This stains the fragments blue and can be easily detected in the gel. Methylene blue may be used either as a dilute solution at the concentration of 0.025% or as a concentrated solution (0.1%).

The gel is submerged in the dilute methylene blue solution for up to 16 hours so as to allow diffusion of stain into the gel and binding to the DNA fragments. In case of using concentrated solution of methylene blue, only the surface of the gel is covered with the solution. The gel is allowed to stay in contact with the solution for 5 minutes. The excess stain is then rinsed off, and gel is allowed to stand for 16 hours so as to ensure diffusion of the stain into the gel. To enhance the contract between the background and the stained fragments, the gel is rinsed with water repeatedly.

2. Detection of proteins

(i) ***Coomassie Brilliant Blue:*** It is the standard dye used for detecting proteins. It is a sensitive method as it can detect proteins as low as in micrograms. This dye can stain proteins in the concentration range of 0.1-1µg protein/band.

(ii) ***Silver staining***: It can detect proteins at a concentration of nanograms, thus, making it the most sensitive method. The test protein is oxidized in potassium dichromate, dissolved in dilute nitric acid. After washing, silver nitrate is added. Silver binds to oxidized proteins. The silver attached to the oxidized proteins is reduced to metallic silver by treating with alkaline formaldehyde. Thus formed metallic silver is visualized in the form of silver color.

(iii) ***Copper staining***: It is a rapid and single step staining. It shows an intermediate sensitivity. In this staining, copper chloride ($CuCl_2$) is added to gel and incubated for 5 minutes. After incubation, it is washed with water, thus, obtaining blue green precipitates of copper hydroxide in the gel except where there is high concentration of SDS bound to proteins. Clear protein bands can be seen against blue green background. Hence, it is a negative staining. Major advantage of this staining is that it is a reversible type of staining, wherein clear gel could be retrieved by chelation of copper with the help of ethylenediaminetetraacetic acid (EDTA). Therefore, it prevents wastage of gel and it could be used more than once. Moreover, it is useful for preparative type of gel electrophoresis because sample proteins are not stained and remain intact.

ISOLATION OF NUCLEIC ACIDS OR PROTEINS FROM ELECTROPHORESIS GEL

In preparative type of gel electrophoresis, nucleic acid or proteins are separated on gel and thereafter, these separated molecules are isolated from gel and are used. The different methods to isolate sample molecules from gel include:

1. **Passive diffusion:** Passive diffusion is a process in which the substance moves from higher concentration to lower concentration without consumption of energy. After carrying out electrophoresis, the gel is cut in slices containing the fragments of DNA/proteins. Each slice is added to a separate buffer solution. If the gel is agarose, agarase enzyme is added to break the gel and free the compound by melting the gel at 65°C. For obtaining the sample from polyacrylamide gel, either cross linker is added to the gel or it is crushed with pestle and mortar. This breaks the bonds of polyacrylamide gel, freeing the DNA and RNA fragments **(Figure 8.9)**.

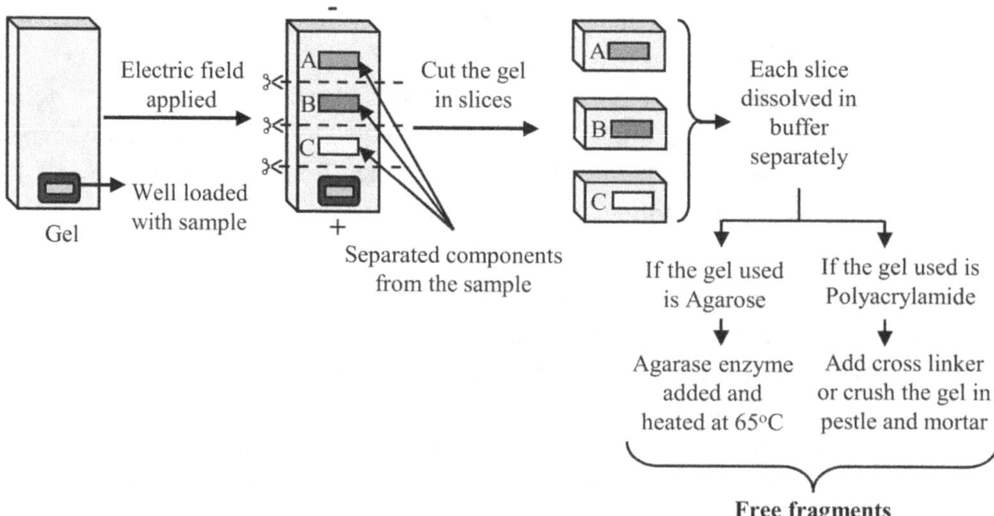

FIGURE 8.9 Passive diffusion for isolation of nucleic acids or proteins

2. **Electroelution:** This method of extracting the macromolecules employs application of electric field to the smallest area of the gel in the buffer. As described in passive diffusion, after separation of molecules, the gel is cut in slices containing the fragments of DNA/proteins. The small pieces of gel are placed in a buffer solution and electric field is applied. The application of electric field transfers the molecule from gel to the solution. Thereafter, the solution is precipitated to obtain the extracted DNA **(Figure 8.10)**.

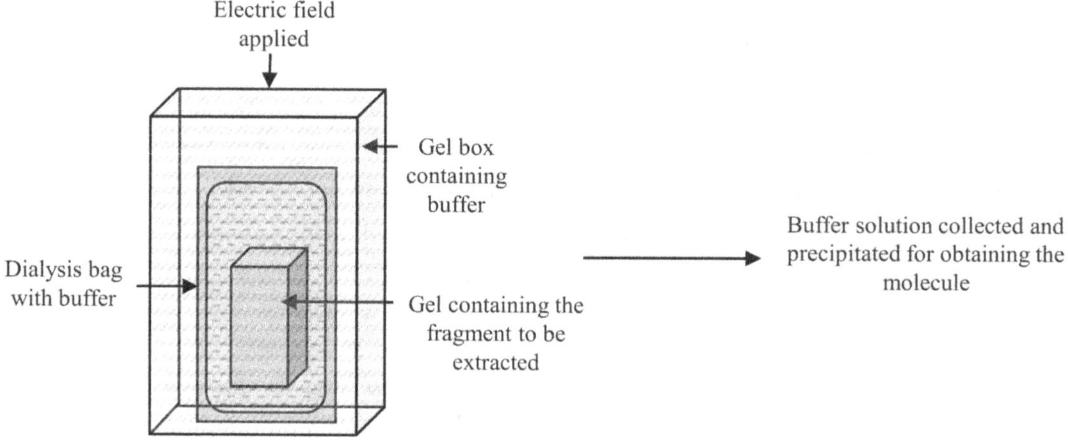

FIGURE 8.10 Extraction of nucleic acids or proteins by electroelution

3. **Continuous Elution:** Instead of cutting gel and isolating samples from gel pieces, gel electrophoresis is allowed to run continuously till all fragments move out from the gel and this process is called as 'continuous elution'. Continuous application of electric field to the gel allows the molecules to transfer from the gel to the buffer solution after the separation of the molecules. These molecules may be collected in different beakers separately for further analysis (**Figure 8.11**).

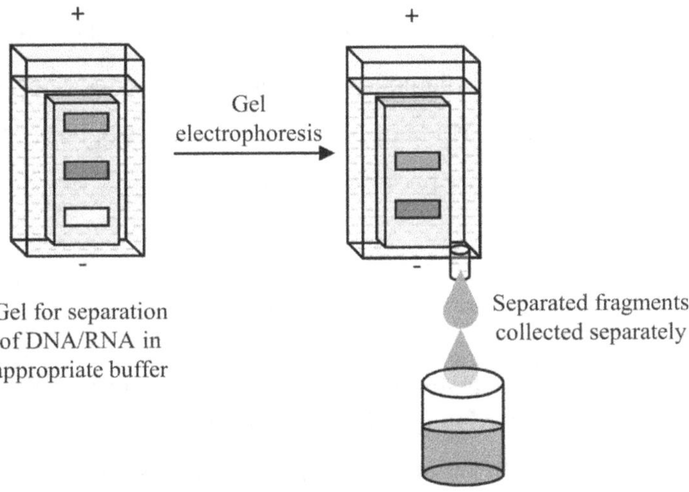

FIGURE 8.11 Continuous elution to separate different fragments of nucleic acids/ proteins

REVIEW QUESTIONS

TWO MARKS QUESTIONS

1. What is the difference between agarose and polyacrylamide gel in terms of pore size?

2. How are proteins detected using silver staining?

3. How may DNA be detected using ethidium bromide?

4. How is agarose gel formed?

5. How is polyacrylamide gel formed?

6. Define gel electrophoresis?

7. What is the difference between discontinuous and continuous buffer system in gel electrophoresis?

8. What do you mean by a tracking dye in gel electrophoresis? What is its use?

9. What is percentage T and percentage C in PAGE?

10. What is the role of free radicals in formation of polyacrylamide gel?

FIVE MARKS QUESTIONS

1. What is discontinuous buffer system method in gel electrophoresis?

2. What are different methods of protein detection in gel electrophoresis?

3. How may nucleic acids be detected in gel electrophoresis?

4. How may sample proteins or nucleic acids be isolated in gel electrophoresis?

TEN MARKS QUESTIONS

1. What is gel electrophoresis? What is its basic principle? What are different gels used in gel electrophoresis?

2. What are the different techniques to detect sample molecules in gel electrophoresis?

MULTIPLE CHOICE QUESTIONS

1. Which of following is the most sensitive method of protein detection?
   - (a) Silver staining
   - (b) Copper hydroxide
   - (c) Coomassie brilliant blue
   - (d) Methylene blue

2. Which of following method is used for staining in preparative gel electrophoresis?
   - (a) Silver staining
   - (b) Copper hydroxide
   - (c) Coomassie brilliant blue
   - (d) Methylene blue

3. Which of following is used as tracking dye?
   - (a) Bromophenol blue
   - (b) Ethidium bromide
   - (c) Coomassie brilliant blue
   - (d) Methylene blue

4. Which of following has large sized pores?
   - (a) Resolving gel
   - (b) Stacking gel
   - (c) Both a and b
   - (d) None of above

5. SDS-PAGE may be used for determining the molecular weight of following?
   - (a) Proteins
   - (b) DNA
   - (c) RNA
   - (d) None of above

6. The separation of molecules in gel electrophoresis depends on
   - (a) Charge
   - (b) Size
   - (c) Shape
   - (d) All the above

7. The purpose of gel in gel electrophoresis is?
   - (a) Anti-convective media
   - (b) Sieving actions
   - (c) A and B
   - (d) None of above

8. Which of followings are used in sample preparations?
   - (a) SDS
   - (b) Mercaptoethanol
   - (c) Glycerol
   - (d) All the above

9. Which of following is not true for discontinuous buffer system?
   - (a) It uses two types of gels
   - (b) It uses different buffers
   - (c) It is low resolution
   - (d) It may be used for molecular mass determination

10. Which of following is carcinogenic dye?
    - (a) Bromophenol blue
    - (b) Ethidium bromide
    - (c) Coomassie brilliant blue
    - (d) Methylene blue

CHAPTER 9

Gene Therapy

CHAPTER OUTLINE

Introduction and General Features

Types of Gene Therapy
In vivo Gene Therapy
Ex vivo Gene Therapy
Somatic Cells Gene Therapy
Germ line Gene Therapy

Methods of Gene Delivery
Viral Vectors
Non-viral Vectors

Problems Faced in Gene Therapy

Applications of Gene Therapy

INTRODUCTION AND GENERAL FEATURES

Gene therapy (human gene transfer) refers to a therapeutic technique, which targets human gene. The alteration of genes in the body is the basis for treating a disease in gene therapy. It may be defined as introduction of fully expressible gene in the body or deletion of an over-expressing gene to cure the disease. The first approved successful gene transfer in humans was performed in May 1989 and the first therapeutic use of gene transfer in humans was performed in a trial in 1990. Till now, gene therapy based therapeutics is in clinical trials and more than 2,300 clinical trials have been conducted. Most of these are in phase I and none has been approved for treatment in patients.

TYPES OF GENE THERAPY

Gene therapy has been classified into different types. Depending on the method of delivery, gene therapy may be of two types **(Table 9.1)**. The genes for providing the gene therapy are delivered to the patient in the following ways:

1. ***In vivo* Gene Therapy:** This method involves addition of gene along with a 'vector' inside the body. In other words, genes are delivered in the body. After entering in the body, gene travels in the blood and is delivered to

TABLE 9.1 Types of Gene Therapy depending on delivery methods

S. No	*Ex vivo* Gene Therapy	*In vivo* Gene Therapy
1.	Genes are introduced inside the isolated cells	Genes are introduced directly in the body
2.	The modified cells are implanted in the body and gene is delivered to tissue/organ	Gene travels in the blood and is delivered to target cell
3.	It is mainly used to deliver genes to dividing cells such as bone marrow	It is mainly used to deliver genes to non-dividing cells such as brain

target tissue. The vector replicates inside the patient's body to help cure the disease. This type of therapy is adapted when the genes are to be introduced in non-dividing cells or those cells, which are difficult to remove such as brain cells.

2. ***Ex vivo* Gene Therapy:** In this method, cells are removed from the body of the patient and the removed cells are treated using biotechnological techniques to perform addition or deletion of genes from the cells. Later, the treated cells are carefully transplanted (to the same location where from where they were initially obtained from) in the patient's body. For example, stem cells are isolated from the bone marrow and therapeutic genes are added in the cells. The modified cells are reintroduced inside the body of the patient. This type of therapy is followed when the gene is to be introduced inside the dividing cells.

Gene therapy may also be divided into two types depending on the types of cells used or to be altered in the process **(Table 9.2)**.

1. **Somatic cells gene therapy:** This therapy involves introduction of genetic alterations in somatic cells of the patient. Somatic cells refer to non-gonadal cells only. Since no changes are introduced in the somatic cell, therefore, the gene alteration does not pass on to the next generation. This is the type of gene therapy, which is permitted ethically.

2. **Germ line therapy:** The germ cells are targeted in this therapy to bring about changes in the genome. Germ cells include sperms or ova. Because the alterations are made in the genome of the cells, which are responsible for carrying the characteristics from one generation to another, the future generations are also affected due to germ line therapy. Therefore, this method is banned due to non-ethical outcomes. No experimentation based on this principle is allowed due to ethics reasons.

TABLE 9.2 Types of gene therapy depending on the types of targeted cells

S. No	Somatic Cell Gene Therapy	Germ Line Gene Therapy
1.	Genes are introduced in somatic cells (non-gonadal cells)	Genes are introduced in germ cells (sperms or ova). Because the alterations are made in the genome of the cells, which are responsible for carrying the characteristics from one generation to another, the future generations are also affected due to germ line therapy. Therefore, this method is banned due to non-ethical outcomes. No experimentation based on this principle is allowed due to ethics reasons.
2.	Gene alteration does not pass on to the next generation	Genes pass to next generation and future generations may be affected
3.	Only this form of gene therapy is permitted ethically	This form of gene therapy is banned due to non-ethical outcomes

METHODS OF GENE DELIVERY

The delivery system used for delivering the genes to the patient is considered ideal if,

(a) The delivery system is able to accommodate a wide range of size of insert (target) DNA

(b) It could be produced in a concentrated form

(c) Is specific to certain types of cells i.e., able to deliver the genes to specific cells

(d) Provide gene expression for an extended period of time

(e) Is non-toxic and does not initiate an immunogenic response on administering to the subject

However, a delivery system with all the above mentioned desired qualities has yet not been developed and hence, no vector (carrier of gene) is ideal. Nevertheless, there is ongoing research to develop a delivery system, which is near ideal for this purpose. At present, a number of viral and non-viral vectors are being employed for transferring the gene into the patient's genome. Some of the vectors from both the categories are discussed below:

VIRAL VECTORS

Viruses have received a great deal of attention of the scientists as vectors for gene therapy due to their natural life cycle. Naturally, the genetic material inside the virus is transferred (delivered) to the host cell during an infection. Inside the host cell the genes encoded on the viral genome expresses itself and causes infection to the subject. This characteristic of viruses i.e., delivering the genes to host cells has been exploited in the gene therapy. For viruses to be used as effective vectors, several functions of viruses need to be toned down (reduced) or altered such as replicating functions of viruses has to be removed. Thus, replication incompetent viruses are created, which can deliver genes to cells; however, these are unable to replicate and cause infection. The removal of genes responsible for replication also creates space for incorporation of target DNA.

Different aspects need to be kept in mind while selecting the most appropriate vector for the purpose. The life cycle of the virus, certain biological characteristics, the viruses' ability to infect the target cell (known as tropism), etc are a few of the aspects to be considered closely. Tropism to some extent also depends on expression of specific cell surface receptors present on the host cell. These receptors work as a site for the attachment of infecting virus to the host cell. Some of the viral vectors used for gene therapy are discussed below **(Table 9.3)**:

I. Retroviruses

These small viruses have RNA as their genetic material. They are capable of incorporating their own genetic material into the DNA of the host cell. Moreover,

TABLE 9.3 Comparative details of viral vectors employed for gene therapy

Viral vectors	Target cells	Advantages	Disadvantages
Retrovirus	Dividing cells	(a) Efficient delivery to dividing cells (b) Long term expression	(a) Ineffective for non-dividing cells (b) Safety issues
Adenovirus	Dividing and non-dividing cells	(a) Safer (b) Broad host range	(a) Short term expression (b) immunogenic
Adeno-associated virus	A wide variety of dividing and non-dividing cells	(a) Broad host range (b) Long term expression (c) Does not initiate immune response (d) Safer	(a) Small size of gene can be incorporated (b) Less efficient
Lentivirus	Both dividing and non-dividing cells	(a) Can infect both dividing and non-dividing cells (b) Stable gene expression (c) Can incorporate Approx. 8 kb size of gene	(a) Safety issues
Herpes simplex virus	Non-dividing cells	(a) Can carry large sized genes	(a) Relatively more toxicity

they have the ability of infecting and replicating within living cells exclusively. Given to this, retroviruses can be used as successful vectors only in certain types of target cells.

Characteristics of retroviruses as vectors

1. For the retroviruses to be used as vectors without inducing an immune response in the host, the virulence producing genes are removed prior to incorporation. Moloney murine leukemia virus (MMLV) is the major source of retroviral vectors.

2. Retroviruses are generally used as the vector for transferring the gene *ex vivo* or for treatment of cancer in an investigational manner. In other words, retroviruses can be used to deliver genes to dividing cells only.

3. The genes delivered by retroviruses are integrated within DNA of host cells. Due to integration of target genes in host chromosome, there is long term expression with this vector.

4. Retrovirus is capable of incorporating a gene of the size of up to 8 kb (kilobase).

Key features of retroviral genome and life cycle events in host cells

1. The RNA genome of retroviruses is composed of three viral genes. These three genes (gag, pol, and env) are responsible for replication and packaging of the new viruses.

2. For the genes in the genome of the retroviruses to express themselves successfully, they first need to be reverse-transcribed into double stranded DNA (dsDNA). This dsDNA then gets incorporated into the DNA of the host cell and the genes begin their expression. This takes place under the effect of enzymes reverse transcriptase and integrase, respectively. These two enzymes are also present in the retrovirus itself.

3. Once the DNA of the retrovirus is incorporated into the host DNA, it is called 'provirus'. Thereafter, provirus uses the host cells components for transcription of mRNA, its processing, and hence translation into viral proteins.

4. The encapsulation of the RNA with proteins is meditated by encapsidation signal *psi* (ø). This is also present within the viral genome. The viral genome is packaged by viral proteins and new viruses are formed **(Figure 9.1)**.

5. The genome of retrovirus has region known as long terminal repeat (LTR). 5'LTR regions perform promoter and enhancer functions and help in initiating replication or transcription. On the other hand, 3'LTR regions serve to stop transcription.

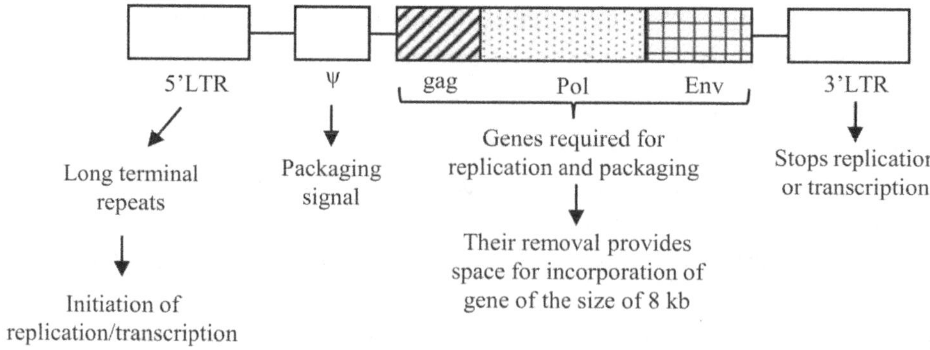

FIGURE 9.1 Representation of genome of Retrovirus

Modification of retroviral genome for gene therapy

The genome of retroviruses is modified in such a manner that it can carry gene of interest (therapeutic gene), but virus is unable to replicate (replication incompetent) (**Figure 9.2**).

1. For the production of vector from the retrovirus, gag, pol and env genes are removed. This makes space for incorporating the therapeutically active gene. The therapeutic gene is added in empty space created after removal of replicating genes. Removal of these creates about 8kb of space, therefore, therapeutic gene up to the size of 8 kb can be inserted in retrovirus vector.

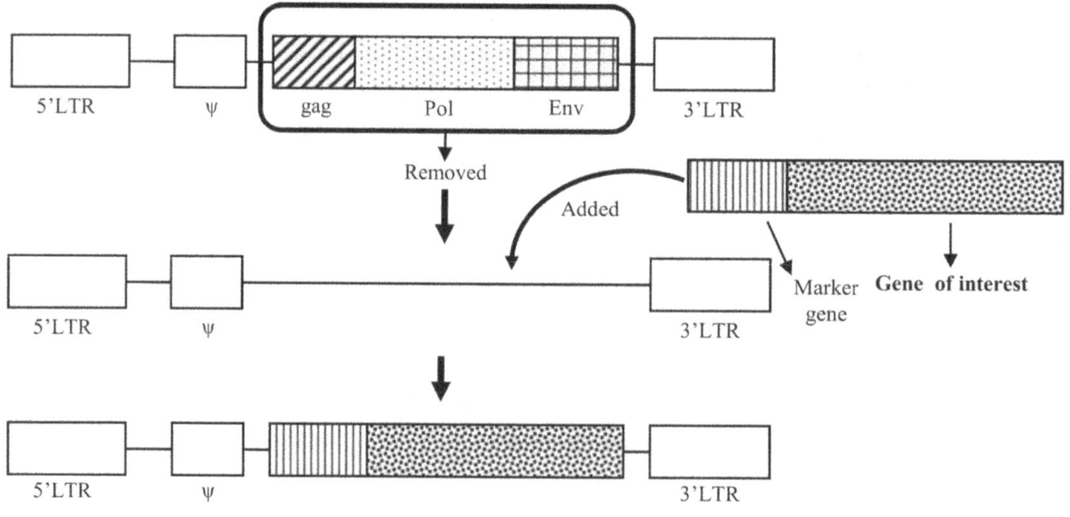

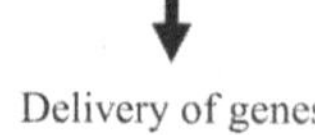

FIGURE 9.2 Incorporation of gene of interest after removal of gag, pol and env

2. Removal of genes responsible for replication also puts a halt to the viral replicating function and virulence producing ability. Thus, viruses become replication incompetent. Hence, the immune response is not initiated on its administration into the patient's body.

3. The LTR regions are retained, which help in efficient expression of the vector in the host cell.

4. The encapsulation signal *psi* (ø) is also retained, which helps in packaging the modified genome to form vector.

Limitations and Adverse Effects

There are certain limitations for these retroviruses. Moreover, using retrovirus for therapy is not completely free of risks and disadvantages. Some of the limitations and adverse effects related to the use of retrovirus as vector for gene transfer are:

1. It can transfer the gene of interest to dividing cells only. It is not effective for gene transfer in non-dividing cells.

2. There is also a safety issue related to its use. Although these viruses are made replication incompetent, yet these may obtain (gain) the replication genes after interacting with wild type of viruses. Due to acquisition of these genes, retroviruses can replicate and produce disease in the patient.

3. The genes delivered by retroviruses are inserted in host chromosomes. Due to insertion of genes, these retroviral vectors may produce 'insertional mutagenesis' in the host DNA, which may give rise to tumors.

Advantages of Retroviruses

Despite the disadvantages discussed above, retroviruses also prove to be advantageous on some bases, which are:

1. It efficiently delivers genes to dividing cells.

2. Insertion of genes into the host chromosome enables its long term expression.

Therefore, long lasting effects of gene therapy may be provided to the patient using retrovirus as the vector.

II. Adenovirus

These viruses have DNA as their genetic material. It is capable of incorporating gene of size equal to or less than 7.5 kb. Mostly this virus is known to produce respiratory infections in animals, such as cold.

Modification of genome for gene therapy

Similar to retroviruses, the genome of adenoviruses is modified by removing the gene responsible for replication and inserting the gene of interest (therapeutic gene) in empty space. This also serves to make the viruses as replication-incompetent.

Disadvantages:

1. The gene carried by the adenovirus vector does not integrate into the host DNA. Hence, there is short term expression of gene. Thus, short period of relief to the patient.

2. This virus is immunogenic and immune response is activated in the body. The immune response is responsible for producing side effects.

3. The activation of immune response against viral vectors tends to eliminate the vector from the body. This further decreases the expression time of vector in the body.

Advantages:

1. Since genes delivered by adenovirus remain episomal (does not integrate and remains separate from host chromosome), therefore, there is no risk of insertional mutagenesis unlike retrovirus. Thus, it is safer in comparison to retrovirus.

2. It has a broad host range, that is, it efficiently delivers therapeutically engineered genes to the dividing as well as non-dividing cells.

III. Adeno-associated virus (AAV)

Although it has a limited carrying capacity of 5.2 kb, it is the most commonly employed virus for gene therapy because it exhibits the desirable features of both retrovirus and adenovirus. Due to a number of desirable features, it is one of the most commonly employed viral vectors for gene therapy.

Disadvantages:

1. The size of gene that it can accommodate is very less, that is 5.2 kb.

2. It is not as efficient in production as retrovirus and adenovirus.

Advantages:

1. The broad host range provides a great advantage so that it efficiently transfers gene to dividing as well as non-dividing cells.

2. It incorporates (integrates) the genes into the DNA of the host cell, therefore providing long term expression, like retroviruses. However, the incidences of insertional mutagenesis are very rare as compared to retroviruses. Therefore, it is a safer alternative to retroviruses.

3. It does not initiate an immune response, unlike adenoviruses. Hence, it is better tolerated and provides even more long term expression.

IV. Lentivirus

These viruses belong to the class of HIV group. Their capability allows them to lodge gene of the size of 8 kb. Due to safety issues, these are not generally employed in gene therapy.

Disadvantages:

1. Since it belongs to the group of HIV, there is always a safety issue associated with it and there is a risk of causing HIV in the patient.

Advantages:

1. It can easily infect both dividing as well as non-dividing cells.

2. The expression of the gene is stable and there is long term expression.

3. The approximate size of gene that it can accommodate is 8 kb.

V. Herpes simplex virus

It has a very large carrying capacity (20-30 kb), so it can be effectively used for transfer of large sized genes. Another important feature of this virus vector is that it has a very high affinity for nerves. Therefore, it is mostly used for delivering genes to the nervous system, where it delivers genes with high specificity. However, the major disadvantage of using *Herpes simplex* as a vector is the cytotoxicity.

NON VIRAL VECTORS

To overcome the immunogenic response, mutagenesis and other adverse effects of viral vectors, non viral vectors have been evolved. These vectors have advantage that these are much safer than viral vectors. However, these vectors mainly suffer from the problem of poor delivery. These are not able to efficiently transfer genes to host cells. The different non-viral methods include:

I. Un-complexed DNA

This type of DNA without any complex is also known as 'naked DNA'. A purified DNA (therapeutic gene) is injected straight into the tissues. This results in expression of the gene in that tissue. This method is mostly used to deliver genes in muscle tissue or superficial skin. The major applications of this type of delivery include:

(i) An example of this type of delivery include DNA vaccination, in which instead of delivering 'antigen', gene responsible for producing antigen is injected. This technique may be of a great help in preventing various infectious diseases.

(ii) This type of delivery may also be used for ectopic synthesis of proteins. For example, gene for synthesis of erythropoietin (EPO) is injected into the muscles of the patient suffering from anemia due to chronic renal failure. Indeed, EPO is released from kidneys and its level decrease during renal failure leading to development of anemia. In this condition, muscles may be used as source of EPO synthesis (ectopic site) by injecting EPO gene in muscles to bring the levels of EPO back to normal.

***Disadvantages*:**

1. It provides short term expression only, since the gene remains separate from host chromosome and it is not integrated with host DNA.
2. The delivery of genes is possible only to the superficial tissues, for example, skin or muscles.

***Advantages*:**

1. It is the simplest method.
2. Its implementation does not require any special methods or equipments.

II. DNA-Coated Gold Particles

The DNA of interest (therapeutic gene) may be fixated onto the surface of the gold particles of diameter approximately 1 micron by co-precipitating DNA with gold particles. These gold particles coated with DNA are then loaded into the gene gun. An electric spark or a blast of pressurized gas (motive force) helps in accelerating and shooting these accelerated DNA-coated gold particles into the superficial tissues, such as skin or melanomas (tumors of skin) **(Figure 9.3)**.

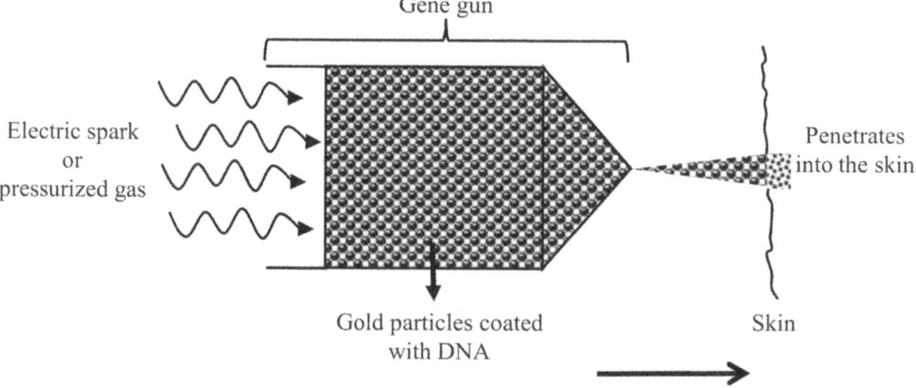

FIGURE 9.3 Administration of DNA-coated gold particles by gene gun

***Disadvantages*:**

1. The genes delivered by this method are expressed only for a short period of time. This is not due to a shortcoming of the method, rather it is due to the physiological behavior of the targeted cells. In skin cells, the sloughing of the cells results in loss of the gene expression relatively quicker.
2. Non-integration of genes with the host chromosome is also responsible for short term expression.
3. Delivery of the genes is possible to superficial tissues such as to the skin cells.

Advantages:

It is ideal method for the delivery of immunization-based genes (DNA vaccines), when the body needs to be exposed to the antigen only for a short time period.

III. Liposomes

Plasma membrane is made up of lipids, thus rendering it non-polar. On the other hand, DNA is polar in nature because of the charged molecules. Hence, delivering a hydrophilic or polar molecule inside the cells through a hydrophobic system is difficult. Therefore, DNA (hydrophilic) is coated with lipid layers in the form of liposomes for its passage through lipophilic membrane. The membrane of liposomes integrates (fuses) with the cell membrane due to similar structural properties, thus simplifying the entry of the DNA from liposomes to target cell **(Figure 9.4)**.

Liposomes are spherical molecules synthesized from different types of lipids. They may be unilamellar (with just one layer) or multilamellar (with multiple layers). The liposomes have been classified into anionic or cationic liposomes on the basis of net charge on them.

1. ***Anionic liposomes***: Firstly, anionic liposomes were used to deliver the gene responsible for the production of insulin. It was found in the animals that

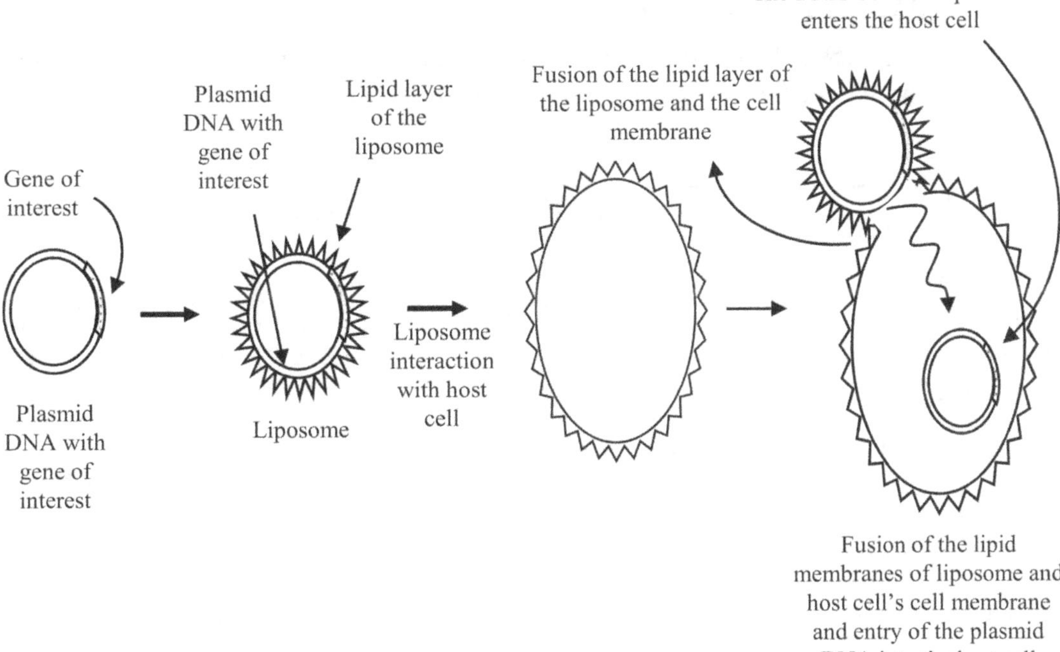

FIGURE 9.4 Formation of liposomes and transfer of plasmid DNA into the target host cell

after being administered with these insulin gene containing anionic liposomes, the level of insulin increased and the levels of glucose in the blood declined. However, it had some disadvantages related with it. On being administered intravenously, the primary target of these liposomes is the reticuloendothelial cells of the liver. These anionic liposomes are up-taken by macrophages and hence, very less numbers of liposomes are able to bind to other cells.

2. ***Cationic liposomes***: The liposomes with net positive charge on their membrane are known as cationic liposomes. They are different from anionic liposomes in a number of properties. On administration of cationic liposomes into the afferent blood vessels (taking blood to the organ) or by intravenous route, the organs are able to take up the genes from liposomes. The cationic liposomes are advantageous in that they can be administered through aerosol or intra-airway injection to target the lung epithelium.

Disadvantages:

1. The process of manufacturing is complex because for therapeutic gene DNA needs to be encapsulated inside the liposomes.

2. The efficiency of encapsulation is low. This is because the size of the gene to be incorporated into the host cell is large in comparison to that of the liposomes.

IV.   DNA-Protein Complex

The DNA of interest is combined with a protein moiety specific to the receptors present on the desired cells to be targeted. This combination of the two forms

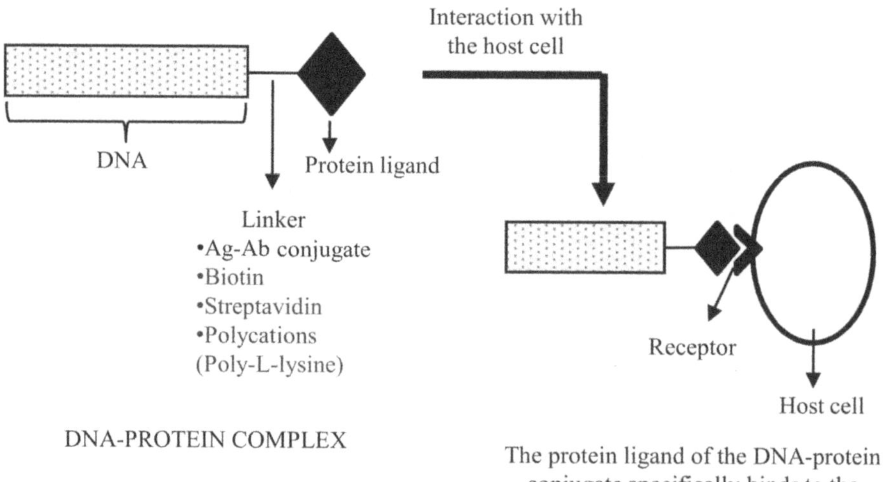

FIGURE 9.5 DNA-Protein Complex and its interaction with surface receptors on the host cell

a DNA-protein adduct, which is modified to specifically deliver the gene of interest to the target cells (site specific delivery). The linkers used for linking the DNA to the protein are polycations (Poly-L-lysine), antigen-antibody conjugates, biotins, streptavidin, etc **(Figure 9.5)**.

Obstacles in Gene Therapy as Therapeutic Approach

Gene therapy is the latest technology used for treating certain diseases, which are generally related to dysfunction of genes. Since it is relatively new therapy, therefore, there are certain problems related to gene therapy. Some of the obstacles are:

1. **Pharmacokinetics and the delivery of DNA:** The gene transfer has to be designed while keeping an eye on the pharmacokinetics of the DNA. The fate of the DNA inside the body affects the duration of expression of the gene inside the body. The gene has to go through all the phases that a usual chemical drug undergoes. Therefore, there are number of obstacles such as route of delivery of gene, bioavailability, stability of gene in the blood, nonspecific uptake by non target cells, delivery of gene inside the cell of target cells, integration of gene with host DNA.

2. **Duration of gene expression:** It is very important to understand the duration of time during which the gene remains inside the body and expresses itself. Moreover, the factors which affect its duration are also important to consider. In some diseases, long term expression is required such as in inherited disease (e.g. SCID). In this condition, it is required that gene expression is stable and for long duration. Long term expression is achieved using vectors which integrate themselves within the genome of the host cell e.g. retrovirus and adeno-associated viral vectors. On the other hand, long term expression may be hazardous in treating curable diseases such as malignancies and in these cases, short term expression is sufficient. In these cases, adenoviruses may be useful because genes delivered by this method are not integrated with host DNA.

   The activation of immune system of the body also plays a vital role in determining the duration of gene expression. If a vector initiates an immune response, it has a greater chance of being swooped away by the macrophages, resulting in short term expression.

3. **Adverse Effects related with gene expression:** It is very much expected to have some adverse consequences arising due to gene therapy. However, it cannot be predicted in advance that what events would occur. However, some of the effects are sure to be anticipated irrespective of the gene expressed.

   (i) One of the predicted side effects is activation of an immune response. Not that it is only due to the vector introduced in the body (which is very common), but it may also be due to the protein produced as a result of the expression of the gene. The more important point is the extent of the immune response. A very rigorous immune response could even inactivate a released product (protein) or begin an autoimmune reaction in the corresponding tissues.

(ii) Retroviruses are particularly responsible for inducing insertional mutagenesis, which may lead to development of cancers.

(iii) The gain of replicating genes from wild type viruses may add replication functions in replication-incompetent viruses. Once viral vectors start replicating, these may lead to development of diseases.

4. **Ethical issues:** It has been a matter of long debate regarding ethical issues associated with gene therapy. To overcome these issues, stringent laws and rules have been formulated and such therapy is conducted under proper supervision. It is ensured that gene therapy is meant for treatment of disease, not for other purposes.

APPLICATIONS OF GENE THERAPY

Initially, gene therapy was used extensively for treating inherited disorders, but over time it has been used to treat acquired disease (cancer, infectious diseases, etc) as well. Some of the applications of gene therapy are discussed below. However, most of them are still in clinical trials and are not being used clinically in patients routinely.

1. **Ectopic Protein Synthesis:** Many diseases are a result of deficiencies of various proteins either in the form of growth factors, hormones, enzymes, etc. Therefore, to treat such diseases it is required to replenish the deficient proteins. For this, the gene responsible for the production of this protein is injected in the ectopic tissue (which normally does not produce this protein). These tissues take up the genes and start producing proteins. Most commonly employed tissue for this purpose is skeletal muscle because of its large size and easy accessibility. Some diseases related with protein deficiency are described as under:

(i) *Erythropoietin (EPO) production:* Chronic renal failure is generally associated with deficiency of EPO. This glycoprotein is responsible physiologically for the production of RBCs. In the case of its deficiency, the number of RBCs decline dramatically and the patient becomes anemic. Therefore, to maintain optimum levels of RBC in patients the level of EPO needs to be kept adequate by frequent administration of EPO. The gene for EPO is either directly injected into the muscles or skin, or using gold coated DNA through gene gun. Inside the body, the

EPO gene integrates itself into the host DNA and starts producing EPO from the muscle or skin cells.

(ii) ***In hemophilia:*** Hemophilia is a congenital disorder and is a consequence of deficiency of factors VIII and IX. These factors are a part of the blood coagulation cascade. In case of their deficiency, blood loses its ability to coagulate. Hemophilia A arises due to the deficiency of factor VIII and hemophilia B due to deficiency of factor IX. Preclinical studies have used administration of genes to the skeletal muscles which show sustained expression of these factors.

(iii) ***Others:*** Studies have been successfully performed in animals for providing long term expression of hormones (growth hormone) and growth factors (insulin like growth factors) using gene therapy.

2. Treatment of Immunodeficiency disorders: Treatment of many congenital immune deficiency disorders has employed *ex vivo* gene therapy including SCID, severe combined immunodeficiency disorder. SCID is characterized by deficiency of both B and T cells. It may occur due to two reasons:

(i) ***Mutation of gene encoding for γ-chain (γc) of cytokine receptor:*** In this type, γc gene present on the X-chromosome is mutated. Mutation of this gene leads to dysfunction of cytokine receptors and lymphocytes fail to mature. This leads to the development of fatal immunodeficiency syndrome, which is characterized by defective differentiation of lymphocytes (both B and T) **(Figure 9.6)**. Therefore, as per recent studies, to treat SCID the normally functioning γc gene is incorporated into the stem cells, which were then administered to infants suffering from SCID-X1. Since the gene of interest is incorporated into the stem cells outside the body, it is called *ex vivo* technique of administration of genes.

(ii) ***Deficiency of Adenosine Deaminase (ADA):*** The second reason for SCID may be deficiency of ADA, which also leads to decline in the number of B and T lymphocytes in the blood. Although ATP, ADP, AMP and adenosine are vital for various functions in our body, but their unduly high concentration is toxic for lymphocytes. Normally, ATP is metabolized to adenosine, which further in the presence of ADA undergoes deamination and gets completely metabolized. But due to deficiency of ADA, the metabolism of adenosine is affected, resulting in rise in the level of ATP, ADP, AMP and adenosine. This leads to killing of lymphocytes. The patients with this condition have a very weak immune system, which makes them fall prey to several infectious diseases time and again **(Figure 9.6)**.

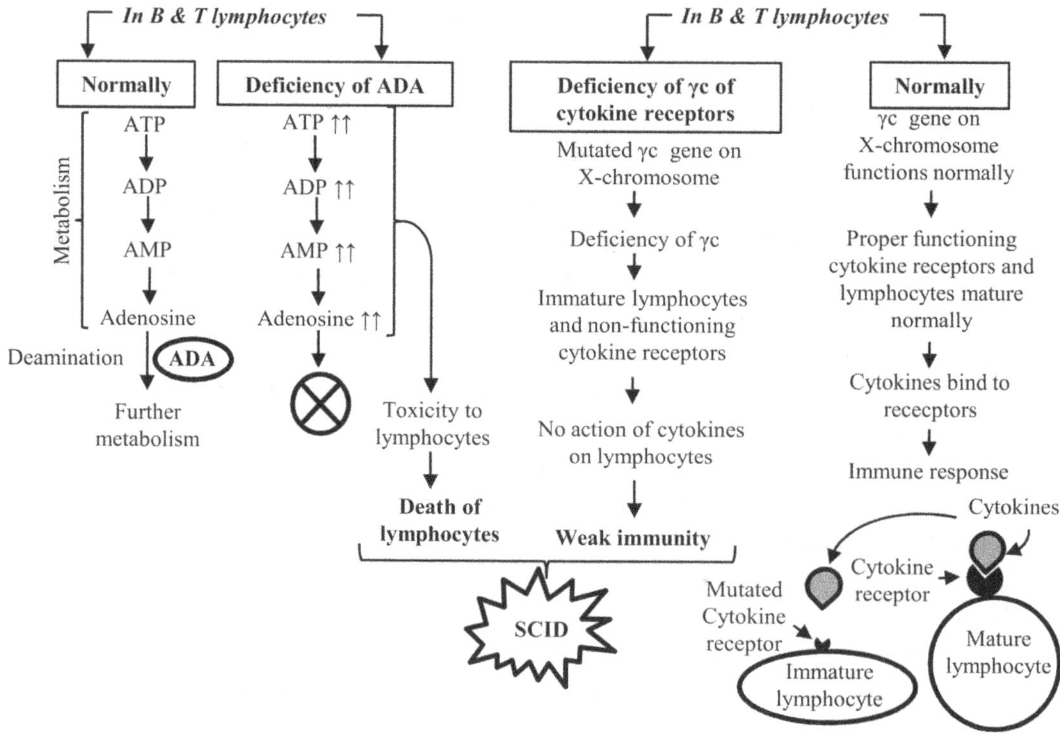

FIGURE 9.6 Development of SCID either due to deficiency of α-chain (αc) of cytokine receptor or adenosine deaminase deficiency

To treat this disease, bone marrow stem cells are isolated and ADA gene is added in these stem cells (*Ex vivo* gene therapy). The modified cells are re-implanted in bone marrow and these stems differentiate to form lymphocytes with normal ADA enzyme. The clinical trials have been successful in alleviating the symptoms of the disease.

3. **Respiratory disorders:** Gene therapy for treating respiratory diseases is beneficial as the genes may be delivered specifically to the respiratory tissues through aerosols and inhalational methods. However, despite the route being easy and specific, there are commonly experienced hindrances with this route. The respiratory system is very sensitive to any foreign material and has several protective mechanisms to prevent the entry of an antigen. Therefore, adeno-associated virus due to its natural bias affinity for respiratory epithelial tissue has been considered the most suitable for being chosen as a vector in case of gene therapy for respiratory diseases.

(i) *Emphysema*: In this disease, the respiratory tissues become vulnerable to proteases released from the neutrophils during inflammation. This is due to α_1-antitrypsin deficiency. The enzyme α_1-antitrypsin is important for regulating the action of trypsin, a proteolytic enzyme. In the absence of α_1-antitrypsin, trypsin is released in increased amounts from the neutrophils in response to an inflammatory stimulus. The proteolytic enzyme, trypsin begins digesting the cells walls of the alveoli, thus decreasing the surface area for effective breathing. This poses difficulty in respiration **(Figure 9.7)**. The standard treatment for emphysema in humans is use of recombinant α_1-antitrypsin. However, it is very expensive and is not free of risks.

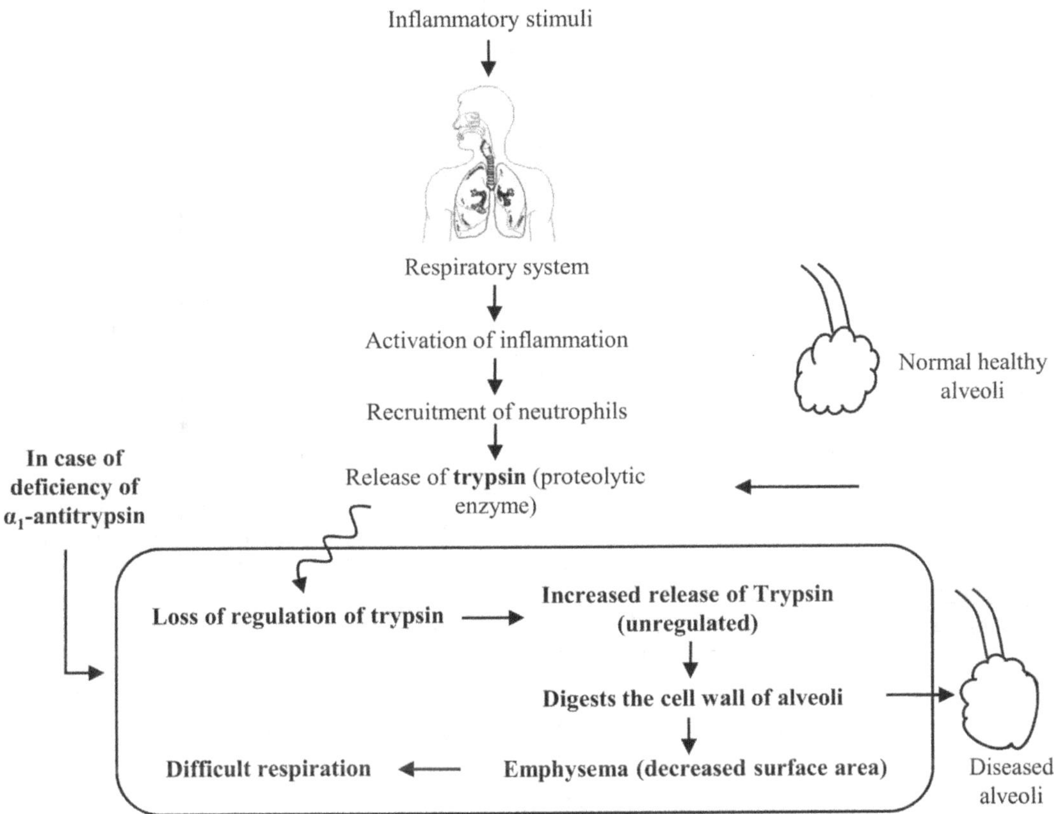

FIGURE 9.7 Cause and changes in alveoli during emphysema

As per some pre-clinical studies, α_1-antitrypsin gene can also be delivered to the respiratory tissues as cationic lipid-DNA conjugate via bloodstream or through inhalational methods. But it has been observed that the gene expression in the mucus membranes of the nose cause local inflammation, which is absent in intravenous administration of the gene.

(ii) ***Cystic fibrosis***: It is a genetic disease characterized by deficiency of 'CFTR gene'. The inability of the CFTR gene expression results in failure of chloride channels in the respiratory epithelium. This leads to thickening of the mucus. The person feels difficulty in breathing because of blockage of the airway passages due to lodging of thick mucus. Also, formation of mucus plugs pose risk for recurrent respiratory infections **(Figure 9.8)**. For delivery of CFTR gene into the patient generally AAV is preferred given to its bias affinity for respiratory epithelium. Use of liposomal gene transfer systems are also being studied and clinical trials are being carried out.

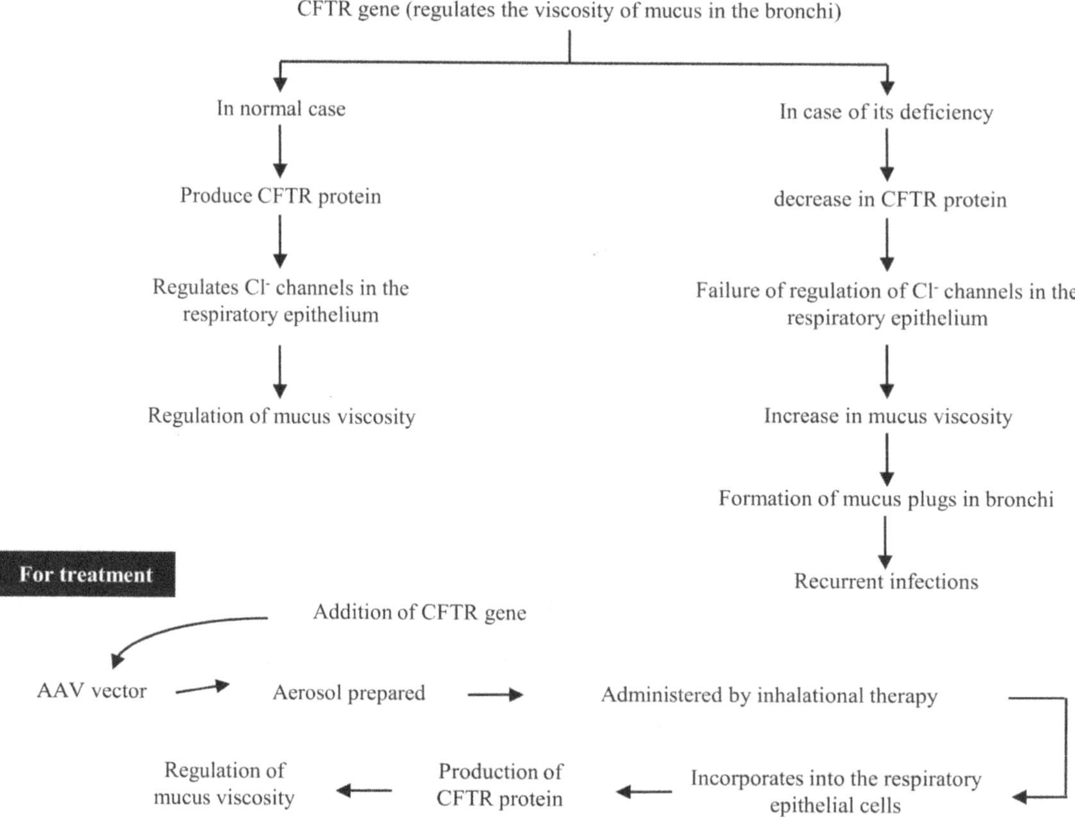

FIGURE 9.8 Pathogenesis of CFTR and its treatment

4. **Cancer** : Treatment of cancer is based on three approaches, namely, inactivation of oncogenes, over-expression of tumor suppressor genes and making the cells more resistant to chemotherapy.

   (i) ***Inactivation of oncogenes:*** Proto-oncogene is a normal growth promoting gene. However, under the effect of carcinogenic stimuli proto-oncogenes are converted to oncogenes. These oncogenes express and produce oncoproteins, which are responsible for formation of tumors, causing cancer. Gene therapy suppresses the oncogenes, thus preventing the production of oncoproteins and consequently cancer. For example, suppression of erb-2 genes is used to treat breast cancer.

(ii) ***Tumor suppressor genes:*** Activation of these genes naturally suppresses the growth of tumor. Over-expression of these tumor suppressor genes (for example, p53 gene) decreases the growth of cancer in the cells.

(iii) ***Making the cells resistant to side effects of chemotherapy:*** Multi-drug resistance gene (MDR) present in the genome encodes for P glycoprotein efflux pump on the cells. These pumps protect the non-cancerous cells from the toxic effects of chemotherapeutic agents by pumping out the drug from the cell. The over-expressing this MDR gene in the bone marrow allows fast efflux (removal) of chemotherapeutic drugs from the cells of the bone marrow. This prevents toxicity of anti-cancer drugs to the bone marrow.

5. **Duchene muscle dystrophy (DMD):** It is a congenital genetic X-linked recessive disorder. Due to deficiency of dystrophin gene, there is decrease in dystrophin in the muscles. It leads to degeneration of skeletal muscles, resulting in weakening of muscles. The person generally dies by the age of twenty due to loss of various muscular functions including respiratory muscles. To treat DMD, the missing gene can be replenished by incorporating 14 kb long dystrophin gene in *Herpes simplex* vector. Administration of this gene carrying vector leads to integration of gene into the host's cells.

REVIEW QUESTIONS

TWO MARKS QUESTIONS

1. What do you mean by ex vivo gene therapy?
2. What is the difference between somatic and germ line gene therapy?
3. How may gene therapy be useful in muscle disorders?
4. What are the limitations of retroviruses as vectors of gene in gene therapy?
5. What are the limitations of adenoviruses as vectors?
6. What are the advantages and limitations of non-viral vectors?
7. How gene therapy may be useful in chronic renal failure-induced anemia?
8. What is gene gun? What is its use in gene therapy?
9. What are liposomes? What is their role in gene therapy?
10. What are the advantages of adeno-associated viruses for gene therapy?

FIVE MARKS QUESTIONS

1. How may gene therapy be useful in different cancers?
2. How may blood disorders be managed using gene therapy?
3. What are different non-viral methods of delivering genes in patients?
4. How may retrovirus be used as vector for gene therapy?
5. What are different viral vectors employed in gene therapy?

TEN MARKS QUESTIONS

1. What is gene therapy? What are its different types? What is the current status of this therapy? What are the hurdles in the success of such therapy?

2. Write a note on different viral and non-viral vectors employed in gene therapy?

3. What are the potential uses of gene therapy in management of diseases?

MULTIPLE CHOICE QUESTIONS

---

1. Which of following vector has the potential of inducing insertional mutagenesis?
    (a) Retrovirus   (b)   Adenovirus
    (c) Adeno-associated virus   (d)   Electroportion
2. Which of following is non integrating viral vector?
    (a) Retrovirus   (b)   Adenovirus
    (c) Adeno-associated virus   (d)   Electroportion
3. Which of following disease may be managed by using Multidrug resistant gene?
    (a) Cancer   (b)   Muscular dystrophy
    (c) SCID   (d)   Cystic fibrosis
4. The addition of adenosine deaminase gene is used to treat
    (a) Cancer   (b)   Muscular dystrophy
    (c) SCID   (d)   Cystic fibrosis
5. EPO gene is inserted to manage
    (a) Cancer   (b)   Muscular dystrophy
    (c) SCID   (d)   Anemia

6. Which of following gene therapy is banned?
    (a) Somatic cell   (b) Germ line
    (c) *In vivo*   (d) *Ex vivo*

7. The cells are isolated from body to insert a gene in cells. This is done in following
    (a) Somatic cell   (b) Germ line
    (c) *In vivo*   (d) *Ex vivo*

8. p53 gene is
    (a) Tumor suppressor gene   (b) Oncogene
    (c) Protooncogene   (d) Apoptosis controlling gene

9. Addition of antitrypsin gene is done to treat
    (a) Emphysema   (b) Cystic fibrosis
    (c) SCID   (d) Anemia

10. Herpes simplex is used to deliver genes to
    (a) Respiratory system   (b) Bone marrow
    (c) Nerves   (d) Skin

CHAPTER 10

Polymerase Chain Reaction

CHAPTER OUTLINE

Definition and General Features

Requirements for Polymerase Chain Reaction

Steps Involved in Polymerase Chain Reaction
Denaturation
Annealing
Extension

Efficiency of PCR

Different Types of Polymerase Chain Reaction

Reverse Transcriptase-Polymerase Chain Reaction (rt-PCR)
Real Time-Polymerase Chain Reaction (RT-PCR)
Allele Specific PCR
Inverse PCR
Anchored PCR
Asymmetric PCR

Applications of Polymerase Chain Reaction

DEFINITION AND GENERAL FEATURES

Polymerase chain reaction (PCR) is a fast *in vitro* enzymatic process for amplification of DNA. It was invented by Kary Mullis in 1984. PCR has become one of the most commonly employed techniques in molecular biology. It is characterized by three 'S' i.e., specificity, sensitivity and speed. It is a highly specific process, where in same copies of original DNA are produced. This is also a sensitive technique for amplifying DNA, as initial requirement of DNA is very small. Only a small amount of DNA (as starting material) is required for its amplification. Even very few bases of DNA are sufficient for successful implementation of PCR. It is a very fast technique as within few hours a large amount of DNA may be obtained from a very small amount of DNA **(Table 10.1)**. Another distinguishing feature of PCR is that even broken DNA may be amplified. A variant of PCR termed as 'Jumping PCR' is employed to amplify broken DNA. In this method, the initial DNA strand is in broken state; however, intact DNA is formed after amplification with PCR.

TABLE 10.1 Three Key Characteristic Features of PCR

S. No	Characteristic Feature	Comments
1.	Sensitivity	Requirement of initial DNA is very less
2.	Specificity	Only desired DNA is amplified
3.	Speed	Very fast amplification;takes less than an hour to few hours to complete PCR

REQUIREMENTS FOR POLYMERASE CHAIN REACTION

The process of polymerase chain reaction requires equipment, raw materials and enzymes etc and they are explained below:

1. **Instrument:** The specific instrument required for carrying out this process of DNA amplification is known as '**thermocycler**' or '**thermal cycler**' or '**PCR machine**'. It is an instrument in which temperature changes over a regular period of time. Indeed, the temperature in this instrument is regulated automatically at regular time intervals. The change in temperature is set in accordance with the requirement at each step of PCR. The process is fully automated. The addition of materials is not required during the process as all the materials are added in excess in the beginning of the process itself.

2. **Sample DNA:** It refers to DNA that has to be amplified. It may also be termed as target DNA or initial DNA. Even a small amount of starting

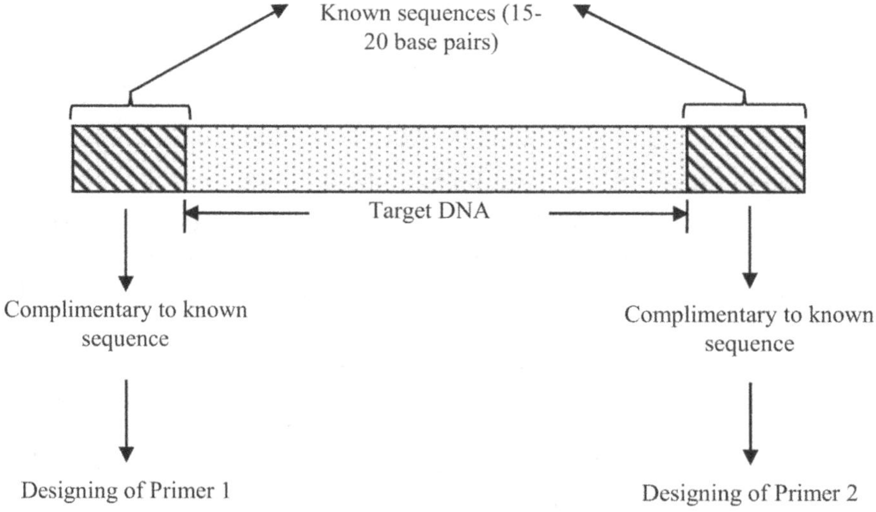

FIGURE 10.1 Requirement of two known sequences flanking the target DNA

DNA is sufficient for the amplification process because of high sensitivity of this method. There is a special requirement about the sample DNA that the small sequence of nucleotides at each end of DNA has to be known. In other words, small portion of DNA sequences flanking (surrounding) the target DNA must be known. These known sequences may be 15-20 base pair (bp) long **(Figure 10.1)**. It helps in synthesizing two primers, complementary to these known sequences.

3. **Two Primers:** Primers are approximately 15-20 base pair long oligonucleotides that serve as a starting point for DNA synthesis. Primers are essential for DNA synthesis (replication) because DNA polymerases (enzyme required for DNA amplification) can only add new nucleotides to an existing strand of DNA. In other words, enzyme can only carry out extension of already existing DNA strand. Therefore, primer is used as existing DNA strand and it is extended to form full length DNA molecule **(Figure 10.2)**.

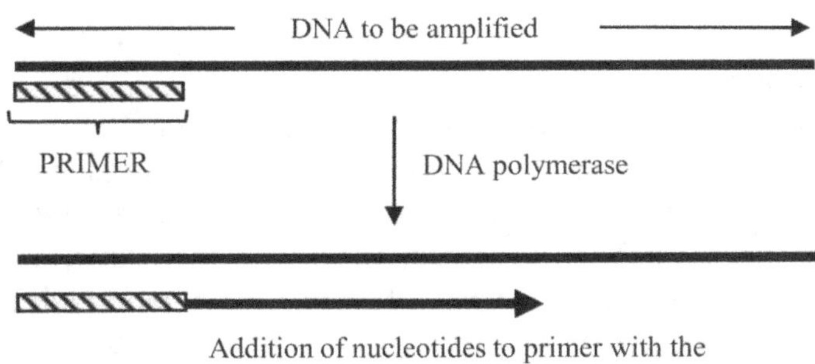

Addition of nucleotides to primer with the
help of enzyme

FIGURE 10.2 Extension of primer by enzyme to form full length DNA

For carrying PCR, two primers are required and these are complementary to the known sequences on each end of the sample/target DNA **(Figure 10.1)**. These two primers anneal at the specific sites (complementary sequence) on the target DNA. The specificity of PCR depends on specific binding of primers to desired site i.e., known sequence around the target DNA. In case of non-specific binding of primer, the wrong form of DNA (non specific DNA) will be amplified. Primers are put in excess in the thermocycler in the beginning of the process. These primers act as initiators and addition of new incoming deoxyribonucleotides (dNTPs) extend the primer to form new DNA strand.

4. **DNA Polymerase:** These are enzymes which are required for the synthesis of DNA from deoxyribonucleotides. Deoxyribonucleotides are the building blocks of DNA. With the help of this enzyme, one nucleotide is added at a time to the 3'-end of the strand in PCR and addition of a number of deoxyribonucleotides leads to formation of full DNA strand. Several

polymerases have been isolated from different sources and some of these employed in PCR include **(Table 10.2)**:

(i)   Klenow fragment: It is obtained from *E. Coli* and it shows optimum activity at 37 °C. Klenow fragment is seldom used as DNA polymerase because of number of limitations.

(a)   It is used for non-automated PCR as the process cannot be automated using this enzyme.

(b)   It lacks proof reading ability. Proof reading is the ability of a DNA polymerase to check whether a correct deoxyribonucleotide is added or not.

(c)   There are chances of formation of non-specific DNA due to higher chances of misincorporation (addition of wrong form of deoxyribonucleotides). The chances of misincorporations are directly linked with temperature of DNA amplification. At low temperature, the chances of misincorporation are increased (such as at 37° with klenow fragment). On the other hand, amplification at high temperature leads to decrease in misincorporation (such as at 72° with Taq polymerase).

(ii)   Taq Polymerase: Taq polymerase is the most commonly employed DNA polymerase for PCR. It is obtained from a heat resistant bacterium, *Thermus aquaticus*. Physiologically, the bacteria use this enzyme for synthesis of its DNA. The optimal activity of this enzyme is obtained at 72°C. However, it can even withstand temperatures as high as 95°C. Therefore, there is no requirement of enzyme addition at the beginning of each new cycle. Due to these properties, PCR process can be automated, the chances of misincorporation are less and specific form of DNA is formed. Another major advantage of using this enzyme is its ability to withstand repeated cycles of heating and cooling. Only shortcoming of this enzyme is its inability to proof read the newly formed DNA.

(iii)   DNA polymerase from Sulfolobus acidocaldarius: The enzyme obtained from these bacteria optimally acts at 100°C; therefore, chances of misincorporation are comparatively less.

(iv)   DNA polymerase from Thermus thermophillus (Tth polymerase): The polymerase obtained from these bacteria show an additional reverse transcriptase activity in presence of $MnCl_2$. However, in the absence of $MnCl_2$ it shows only DNA polymerase activity. This polymerase may be used when the sample is RNA. The RNA is treated with manganese chloride ($MnCl_2$) and *Thermus thermophillus*. The reverse transcriptase activity of this enzyme converts the RNA sample into DNA. After the conversion, $MnCl_2$ is removed using a chelating agent. This allows the enzyme to act as a DNA polymerase at this stage.

(v) DNA polymerase from Thermus litorates (Tli polymerase): The enzymes from this bacterium optimally act at 98°C and these have the ability of proof reading.

TABLE 10.2 Comparison of different DNA polymerases on the basis of their major characteristics

S. No	DNA polymerase & its source	Characteristics	
		Optimum Temperature	Proof reading ability
1.	Klenow fragment from *E. Coli*	37°C	Absent
2.	Taq polymerase from *Thermus aquaticus*	75-80°C	Absent
3.	*Sulfolobus acidocaldarius*	70-75°C	Absent
4.	Tth polymerase from *Thermus thermophillus*	75°C	Absent
5.	Tli polymerase from *Thermococcus litoralis*	98°C	Present

5. Others: There is requirement of four different deoxyribonucleotide triphosphates (dNTPs), dATP, dGTP, dCTP and dTTP as these are the building blocks for DNA replication. DNA polymerase adds these nucleotides to the new growing DNA strand according to the sequence of original DNA strand. Moreover, buffer system of optimum pH is required in which all reactions take place. It is essential to add magnesium chloride in buffer system as Mg^{2+} acts as a co-factor for Taq polymerase and influences its enzyme activity **(Table 10.3).**

TABLE 10.3 Different Requirements for executing PCR

S. No	Items	Functions/Characteristics
1.	Thermocycler	An instrument with repeated changes in temperature
2.	Target DNA	DNA to be amplified with known sequences from its two ends
3.	Primers	Two primers which are complementary to known sequences from two ends of target DNA
4.	DNA Polymerases (Mostly, Taq Polymerase)	Amplify the target DNA by incorporating dNTPs
5.	dATP, dGTP, dCTP and dTTP along with buffer system containing Magnesium chloride	dNTPs are building blocks for new DNA strand; Mg^{2+} is a co-factor for Taq polymerase

STEPS INVOLVED IN POLYMERASE CHAIN REACTION

The process of PCR is carried out in three main steps i.e, denaturation, annealing and extension. These steps are repeated in a cyclical manner again and again to amplify and form a larger amount of DNA **(Table 10.4)**. In an automated PCR, DNA sample, primers (in excess), deoxynucleotides, and DNA polymerase enzyme are added into the thermocycler. Thereafter, there are repeated changes in temperature after a constant interval of time and DNA is amplified. The different steps involved in DNA amplification are **(Figure 10.3)**:

1. **Denaturation:** Denaturation of DNA refers to separation of two strands of DNA. In other words, DNA duplex is unwound to single stranded DNA (ssDNA). Unlike proteins, denaturation of DNA is reversible and two single strands can again form DNA duplex. Generally, DNA denaturation is done by heating the DNA.

   In PCR, DNA denaturation is the first step and it involves heating the DNA sample at 90-95°C for 1 minute to denature the DNA (in layman language, to melt the DNA). At this step, the double stranded DNA (dsDNA) gets separated into two individual strands. These separated strands are used as a template for synthesis of new DNA stands. Since the separated strands may be joined back to form dsDNA by cooling or decreasing the temperature to 40°C, close monitoring of temperature is required to avoid reversing of denaturation (renaturation).

2. **Annealing:** It is the process for the attachment of two primers to the single stranded DNA templates. The temperature used for annealing is generally kept at 55-60°C and annealing is carried for 1 minute. As discussed above, two primers are complementary to known sequences surrounding the target DNA. Therefore, these primers are attached to these known sequences. The separated DNA strands also have the ability to self-anneal, but it is prevented by addition of primers in large quantities. Primers serve as initiators for extension process.

3. **Extension:** This step involves addition of deoxynucleotides to the primers to form full length DNA strand. The addition of nucleotides is guided by the nucleotide sequence of template DNA. The extension is carried at an optimal temperature at which the particular DNA polymerase acts most effectively i.e., 72°C (for Taq polymerase). DNA polymerase helps in adding dNTPs to the primer to form corresponding complimentary strand. One cycle of extension is generally complete within 1.5 minutes.

TABLE 10.4 Three steps involved in PCR

S. No	Steps	Characteristics		
		Temperature	Features	Time
1.	Denaturation	90-95°C	Denaturation of DNA (dsDNA → ssDNA)	1 minute
2.	Annealing	55-60°C	Attachment of primers to the template	1 minute
3.	Extension	72°C	Addition of dNTPs to extend the complimentary strand	1.5 minute

4. **Cyclical Repetition of Three Steps:** The extension step is again followed by denaturation of DNA, annealing of primer and extension of primer. These steps continue in cyclical manner in thermocycler, in which temperature changes periodically from 95°C (denaturation) to 55°C (annealing) to 72°C (extension). After completion of one cycle of PCR, there is formation of two DNA molecules from a one DNA molecule. In second cycle of PCR, four molecules of DNA are formed from two DNA molecules. Thus,

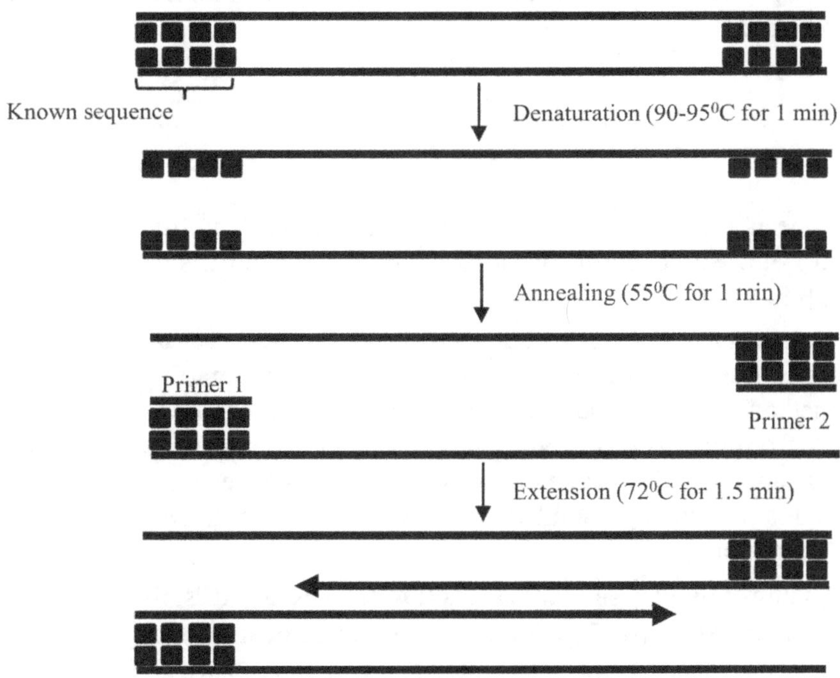

FIGURE 10.3 Three steps of PCR

multiplication of the DNA molecules in PCR occurs in exponential manner. These three steps (denaturation, annealing and extension) keep repeating as long as the substrate molecules (primers and dNTPs) exist in the reaction mixture. Therefore, the substrate's amount has to be adjusted in beginning to obtain the desired amount of DNA.

EFFICIENCY OF PCR

The efficiency of a Polymerase Chain Reaction depends on following factors:

1. Initial amount of DNA

2. Number of cycles

3. Final amount of DNA

The formula used is for calculation of its efficiency is (Equation 10.1):

$$N = n(1 + \varepsilon)^c \qquad \qquad .....(10.1)$$

N = Final amount of DNA; n = initial amount of DNA; ε =Efficiency (0.60-0.93); c = number of cycles

For example, for amplification of approximately 10^9-fold of the sample DNA, at least 30 cycles followed by an extended 10 minute round for DNA synthesis will be required.

DIFFERENT TYPES OF POLYMERASE CHAIN REACTION

PCR has been evolved in various ways depending on its utility, specificity, substrate, etc. Some of the various types have been discussed below (**Table 10.5**):

1. **Reverse Transcriptase-Polymerase Chain Reaction (rt-PCR):** This process differs from the conventional PCR in that the starting material in this method is mRNA. The enzyme reverse transcriptase is used to synthesize cDNA from the given mRNA sample. This cDNA molecule is used for amplification using the same method discussed in the previous section. This method is particularly useful for qualitative and quantitative detection of RNA expression.

2. **Real Time-Polymerase Chain Reaction (RT-PCR):** It is also known as 'Quantitative PCR' (qPCR) as it is used for quantification of the amount of DNA in the given sample. It is called as real time PCR because in this process the amplification of a targeted DNA molecule is monitored during

the PCR process i.e. in real-time, and not at its end, as in conventional PCR. The final amount of DNA formed is directly proportional to initial DNA fed into the thermocycler (**equation 10.2**).

$$\frac{Final_S}{Final_{UK}} \alpha \frac{Initial_S}{Initial_{UK}} \qquad .....(10.2)$$

Initial $_S$ = Initial concentration of Standard DNA (known initial amount); Initial $_{UK}$ = Initial concentration of sample (unknown amount); Final $_S$ = Final concentration DNA of Standard (calculated during PCR); Final $_{UK}$ = Final concentration DNA obtained of sample (calculated during PCR).

The estimation of DNA in real time PCR is done using two common methods:

(i) Employment of fluorescent dyes that intercalate with double-stranded DNA and gives fluorescence. The intensity of fluorescence is directly proportional to amount of DNA formed

(ii) Employment of sequence-specific fluorescently labeled DNA probes. These probes bind with amplified DNA and give fluorescence. The intensity of fluorescence may be used to calculate the amount of DNA.

3. Allele specific PCR: It is a highly specific form of PCR and as its name suggests, this method is preferably used to specifically amplify only one of the two alleles of a given gene. Alleles refer to alternative forms of a gene. These are very similar (approximately 99.99%) to one another and there may be a difference of one or two base pairs. Therefore, the primer is such that it selectively binds only to the alleles and hence, that allele is selectively amplified. For example, in case of blood group AB, the A and B are two alleles. Using allele specific PCR, one of two alleles may be selectively amplified.

4. Inverse PCR (IPCR): Inverse PCR is employed to amplify DNA when the sequence at the ends of the target region is unknown. In this case, sequences from the ends of DNA are not known; rather seqeunce within DNA are known. It is in comparison to the classic PCR, where the sequence on either sides of the target is known. To execute inverse PCR, the DNA fragment (to be amplified) is circularized using ligases. The circularized DNA is cut using specific restriction endonuclease in the known region such that the linear DNA fragment is formed and it has two known ends with unknown region in between the known sequences. Now, two primers may be designed on the basis of known sequences present at the ends of DNA and PCR may be carried in usual manner (**Figure 10.4**).

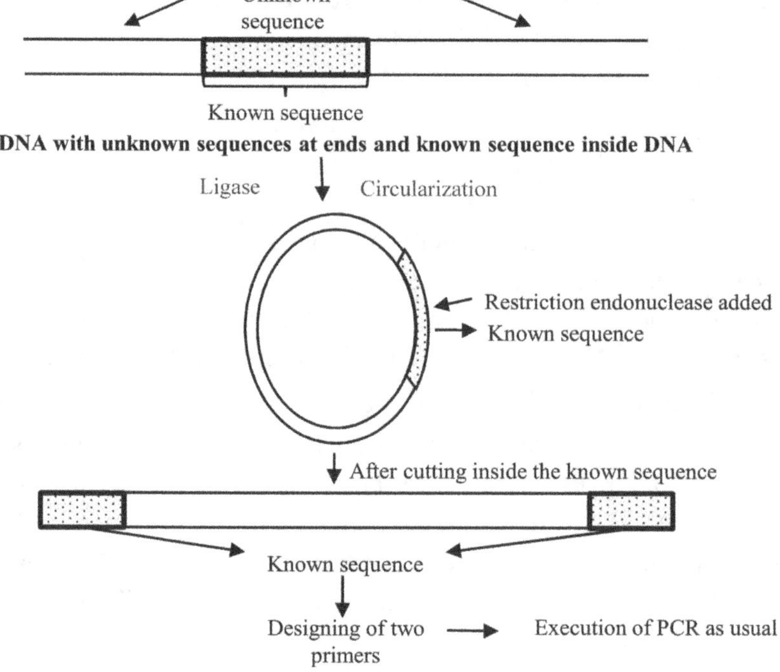

FIGURE 10.4 Procedure of Inverse PCR

5. Anchored PCR: When the sequence only on either one side of the target region is known, this is the method of choice. To provide another known site

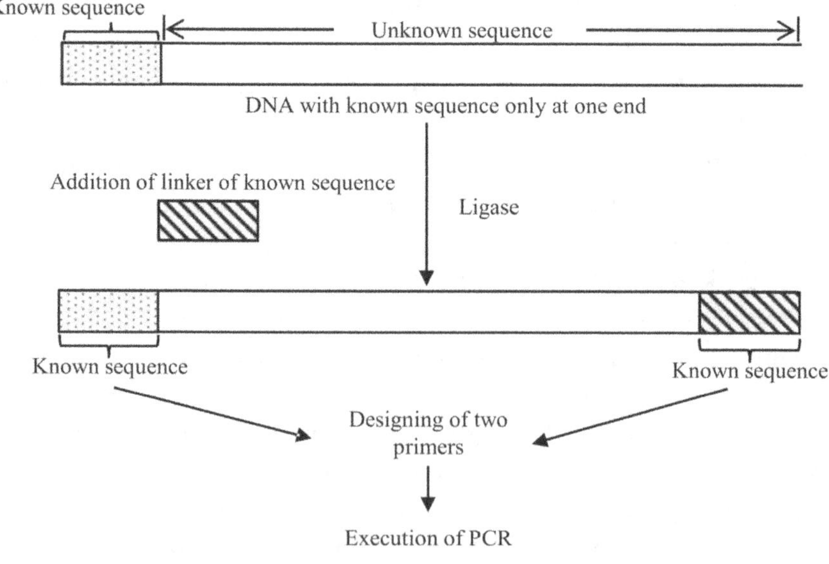

FIGURE 10.5 Anchored PCR

for the addition of primer, a linker (also known as anchor) composed of known sequence is added. This provides two known priming sites as in the classic PCR **(Figure 10.5).**

6. **Asymmetric PCR:** This method is also known by the term 'sequencing'. This involves selective amplification of only one of the two DNA strands. This is done by adding one of the primers in excess in comparison to other primer. The primer added in excess is labeled with biotin and this processing is termed as 'tagging'. The preferred single strand (selectively amplified) product is selectively removed by adding streptavidin, which is specific for biotin.

TABLE 10.5 Summarized discussion of different types of PCR

S. No	Types of PCR	Characteristics
1.	rt-PCR(Reverse transcriptase PCR)	• It is used when the sample is mRNA. • Used for qualitative and quantification of RNA expression
2.	RT-PCR(Real Time PCR)	• When the amount of DNA needs to be determined • Quantification of DNA in sample in real time (during PCR, not at the end of PCR)
3.	Allele specific PCR	• Used when only one of the allele is to be amplified
4.	Inverse PCR (IPCR)	• Sequence around target region are unknown from both ends • Circularization and then cutting to have known sequences at ends
5.	Anchored PCR	• When sequence only on one of the two sides is known • Linker with known sequence is attached to unknown end
6.	Asymmetric PCR	• Selective amplification of one strand using one of the primers in excess quantity • Used during DNA sequencing

APPLICATIONS OF POLYMERASE CHAIN REACTION

The technique, PCR has evolved vastly over the years since its invention. The requirement of very small samples, consumption of less time, and automated process are some of the advantages of PCR, which makes it a widely applied technique in various fields of science. Some of its applications are discussed below:

1. **Disease Diagnosis:** PCR has been widely used in diagnosis of various diseases:

(i) **Genetic diseases**: PCR is used in the diagnosis of inherited genetic diseases (Duchenne muscular dystrophy, sickle cell anemia) as well as diseases due to spontaneous genetic mutations. It has also been used to diagnose diseases even before birth using tissue samples from the chorionic villi or fetal tissue from the amniotic fluid.

(ii) **Other Diseases:** PCR has also been found to be very useful in diagnosing cancers. PCR is very sensitive technique and it can amplify specific DNA sequences, occurring in some cancers. On the similar lines, PCR is a useful tool for diagnosis of other diseases, and pathogen detection, including AIDS, viral and other infectious diseases.

2. **Genetic Fingerprints:** Genetic fingerprints refer to specific pattern of DNA, which is unique for every individual and vary from person to person. PCR has been used in creating genetic fingerprint (DNA profiling) by taking tissue samples from the body such as blood, semen, or hair. These fingerprints have been useful in paternity testing, and in tissue typing for organ transplantation.

3. **Quantification of Gene Expression:** PCR has been a very useful tool to quantify gene expression and extent of gene expression has been linked with disease development. For example, inflammatory diseases have been directly related to increased expression of cytokines and thus, increased expression of cytokines (measured by PCR) indicates presence of inflammation in body. Similarly, development of fever has been linked with increased expression of interleukin 1, which increase prostaglandins in the body to produce fever.

4. **Forensics:** PCR is very useful for amplifying the little amount of even an old sample of DNA obtained from a crime scene, which could be the only evidence helpful in identifying the criminal. The amplified DNA may be used for DNA fingerprinting. DNA is about 99.9% same in all humans, but it differs only because of some highly specific regions known as polymorphic regions, namely, D-loop of mitochondrial DNA, tandemly repeated minisatellites, and HLA (Human Leukocyte Antigen). These polymorphic regions are amplified, studied and identified so as to isolate the person to whom the DNA sample belongs to.

5. **Archeology:** PCR has been used to amplify DNA from fossils, which in turn has helped to know about extinct species such as dinosaurs.

6. **Identification of new members of a receptor family:** The technique of PCR is also useful in identifying new members of a pre-existing receptor family using 'degenerate primers'. In this case, PCR is carried in such a way that a number of related DNA sequences, present in a tissue, are amplified with the help of related, but different primers (degenerate primers).

REVIEW QUESTIONS

TWO MARKS QUESTIONS

1. What is PCR? What is the most commonly employed DNA polymerase for PCR?
2. What is the role of primers in PCR?
3. What are the particular features of Taq polymerase that make it the most commonly employed enzyme in PCR?
4. What are different steps involved in PCR?
5. What is real time PCR?
6. What do you understand by reverse transcriptase-PCR?
7. What do you understand by annealing process of PCR?
8. What is denaturation of DNA? How is it achieved?
9. What is inverse PCR?
10. What is the significance of PCR in quantification of gene expression?

FIVE MARKS QUESTIONS

1. What is PCR? What are its characteristic features? What are different steps involved in PCR?
2. What are different requirements for conducting PCR?
3. What are the applications of PCR?
4. What are the different variants (types) of PCR?

TEN MARKS QUESTIONS

1. Write a note on PCR with special emphasis on its requirement, methodology and applications?

MULTIPLE CHOICE QUESTIONS

1. Which of the following enzymes optimally acts at 37° C
   (a) Taq polymerase   (b) Klenow fragment
   (c) Tth polymerase   (d) Tli polymerase

2. Which of the following is most commonly employed enzyme in PCR?
   (a) Taq polymerase   (b) Klenow fragment
   (c) Tth polymerase   (d) Tli polymerase

3. Which of the following enzymes has additional reverse transcriptase activity?
   (a) Taq polymerase   (b) Klenow fragment
   (c) Tth polymerase   (d) Tli polymerase

4. Extension process is generally carried out at
   (a) 37 °C   (b) 72 °C
   (c) 55 °C   (d) 95 °C

5. Denaturation of DNA is carried at
   (a) 37 °C   (b) 72 °C
   (c) 55 °C   (d) 95 °C

6. Annealing of primers with DNA template is done at
   (a) 37 °C   (b) 72 °C
   (c) 55 °C   (d) 95 °C

7. The chances of misincorporation is minimized by carrying extension at
   (a) 37 °C   (b) 72 °C
   (c) 55 °C   (d) 95 °C

8. Which of the following is not true about PCR?
   (a) Specificity   (b) Slow
   (c) Sensitivity   (d) Selectivity

9. Which of the following is not a requirement for PCR?
   (a) Thermocycler   (b) Buffers
   (c) DNA polymerase   (d) DNA ligase

10. Which of the following is not required for extension process using Taq polymerase?
    (a) Primers   (b) Mg^{2+}
    (c) dNTPS   (d) Restriction endonuclease

CHAPTER 11

ELISA and Micro Array Technique

CHAPTER OUTLINE

ELISA
Definition and General Features
Types of ELISA

Direct ELISA

Indirect ELISA

Sandwich ELISA

Competitive ELISA
Applications of ELISA

Microarray Technology
Definition and General Features
Principle of Microarray Analysis
Procedure of Microarray Analysis
Applications of Microarray Technology

ELISA

DEFINITION AND GENERAL FEATURES

ELISA stands for 'Enzyme-Linked Immunosorbent Assay' and it is also known as 'Enzyme Immunoassay' (EIA). ELISA is defined as a biochemical technique used for detection or quantification of antibody or antigen in a sample. This technique has been extensively used nowadays to detect or quantify proteins in a given sample using enzyme linked antibodies and observing color changes. The color change is produced due to action of enzymes on substrates. ELISA was developed as an alternative to another immunoassay named 'Radioimmunoassay' (RIA). RIA has health hazards due to use of radioactive substances. The radioactive signals of RIA are replaced with non-radioactive signals in ELISA, such as, color or fluorescence changes. Therefore, ELISA is a safer method of analysis.

The operational feasibility of ELISA has been based on evolution of two concepts.

1. One of the concepts includes linking (conjugation) of enzymes to a suitable antibody **(Figure 11.1)**. The linking of an enzyme with antibody was described by Stratis Avrameas and G.B Pierce.

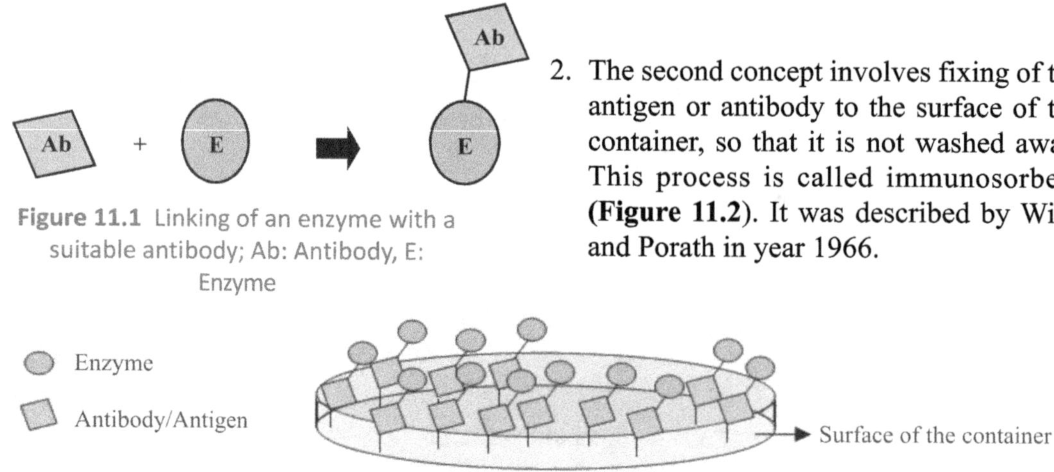

Figure 11.1 Linking of an enzyme with a suitable antibody; Ab: Antibody, E: Enzyme

2. The second concept involves fixing of the antigen or antibody to the surface of the container, so that it is not washed away. This process is called immunosorbent **(Figure 11.2)**. It was described by Wide and Porath in year 1966.

FIGURE 11.2 The process of immunosorbent

These two concepts linking of antibody to the enzyme and immunosorbent, led to the advent of ELISA in 1971 **(Figure 11.3)**. ELISA was described by Peter Perlmann, Eva Engvall (Sweden) and Anton Schuurs.

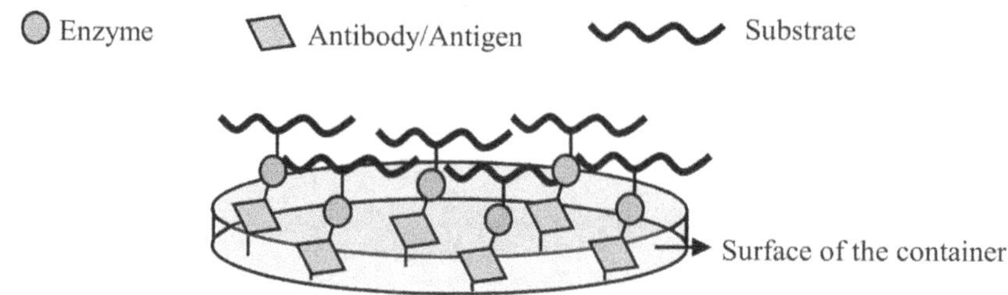

FIGURE 11.3 The principle of ELISA: Linking of antibody/antigen to the enzyme and immunosorbent

TYPES OF ELISA

There are four types of ELISA: Direct ELISA, Indirect ELISA, Sandwich ELISA and Competitive ELISA

I. Direct ELISA

It is a simpler form of ELISA and it requires few reagents and steps. However, it is not a commonly employed ELISA due to its less sensitivity, high background noise and reduced flexibility. In this type of ELISA a single antibody is used, which is conjugated to some enzyme. The steps involved in this process are as follows **(Figure 11.4)**:

1. An antigen is immobilized on the ELISA plate.

2. A concentrated solution of non-interacting protein (Bovine serum albumin or casein) is added to the plates. This process is known as blocking. Non-interacting protein binds and blocks all potential protein binding sites on the plate. This step is critical as it reduces the background noise.

3. Primary antibody, which is specific for antigen to be detected, is added. Primary antibody is labeled with an enzyme such as Horse radish peroxidase (HRP).

4. It is followed by washing so that unbound primary antibody is washed. After washing, antigen bound antibody will remain on plate.

5. Thereafter, HRP specific substrate is added to obtain color (chromogenic) or light (chemilumniscent). HRP catalyzes the conversion of chromogenic substrates such as TMB (3,3',5,5'-Tetramethylbenzidine), DAB (3,3'-Diaminobenzidine), ABTS (2,2'-azino-bis(3-ethylbenzothiazoline-6-sulphonic acid) into colored products. On the other hand, HRP produces light when it acts on luminol (chemiluminescent substrate) **(Table 11.1)**.

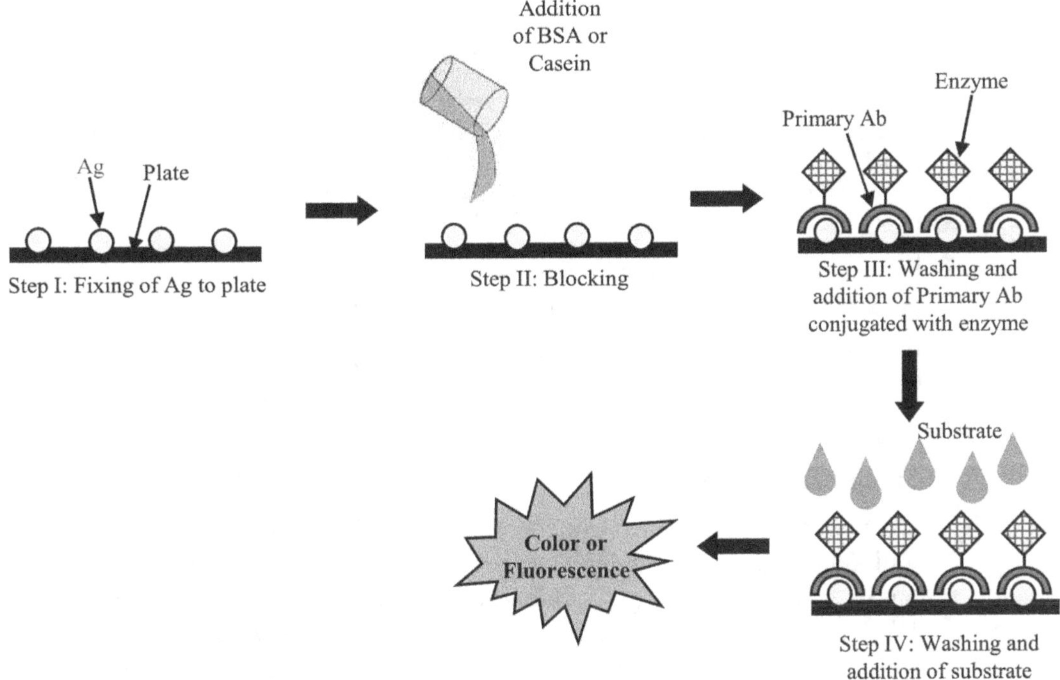

FIGURE 11.4 Steps involved in direct ELISA

Advantages of Direct ELISA

Direct ELISA detection is much faster than other ELISA techniques as it requires fewer steps.

Disadvantages of Direct ELISA

1. Higher background noise is observed in comparison to indirect ELISA. The high noise is because all proteins in the sample, including the target protein, bind to the plate.

2. Direct ELISA is less flexible since a specific conjugated primary antibody is needed for each target protein.

3. This procedure does not use secondary antibody, therefore, there is no signal (detection) amplification. This is responsible for its reduced sensitivity.

TABLE 11.1 Commonly employed enzymes as non-radioactive labels along with substrate and detection signals

S. No	Enzyme	Substrate	Signal
1.	Horse Radish Peroxidase	• TMB (3,3',5,5'-Tetramethyl benzidine)· • DAB (3,3'-Diamino-benzidine) • ABTS (2,2'-azino-bis (3-ethylbenzothiazoline-6-sulphonic acid)	Chromogenic signal, color
		• Luminol	Chemiluminescent, light
2.	Alkaline Phosphatase	• 5-Bromo- 4-Chloro-3-Indolyl Phosphate (BCIP) and Nitroblue Tetrazolium (NBT) • PNPP (p-nitrophenyl phosphate)	Chromogenic signal, Blue color
		• MUP(4-Methylumbe-lliferylphosphate)	

II. Indirect ELISA

In this type, antigens are bound to an ELISA plate (microtiter plate) and two antibodies are employed. Primary antibody (detection antibody) is unlabelled and is specific for antigen, which is bound to plate. Secondary antibody is labeled with some enzyme (e.g. HRP or alkaline phosphatase) and it is specific against primary antibody. The steps involved in this process are as follows **(Figure 11.5)**:

1. A sample of known concentration of antigen (Ag) is applied to the well of microtiter plate. The antigen is made immobile by fixing to the surface of the microtiter plate by simple adsorption.

2. Thereafter, a concentrated solution of non-interacting protein (Bovine serum albumin or casein) is added to the plates. This process is known as blocking.

Non-interacting protein binds and blocks all potential protein binding sites on the plate. This step is critical as it reduces the background noise.

3. Thereafter, the plate is washed.

4. It is followed by addition of primary (detection) antibody specific to antigen attached to the plate. The detection antibody specifically binds to the specific antigen. This antibody is unable to bind non-specifically to the ELISA plate because all potential protein binding sites were blocked by bovine serum proteins (non-interacting proteins, or blocking proteins).

5. The plates are washed to remove any unbound detection antibody. Therefore, only antigen-antibody complex remains attached to the well.

6. In the next step, labeled secondary antibodies specific against primary antibodies are added.

7. The plates are washed to remove the excess unbound enzyme-antibody conjugate.

8. Thereafter, depending on the label on the secondary antibody, specific substrate is added. This produces color, fluorescence or light which may be detected. In case of HRP enzyme, various chromogenic substances such as TMB, DAB, ABTS may be added to give colored products. On the other

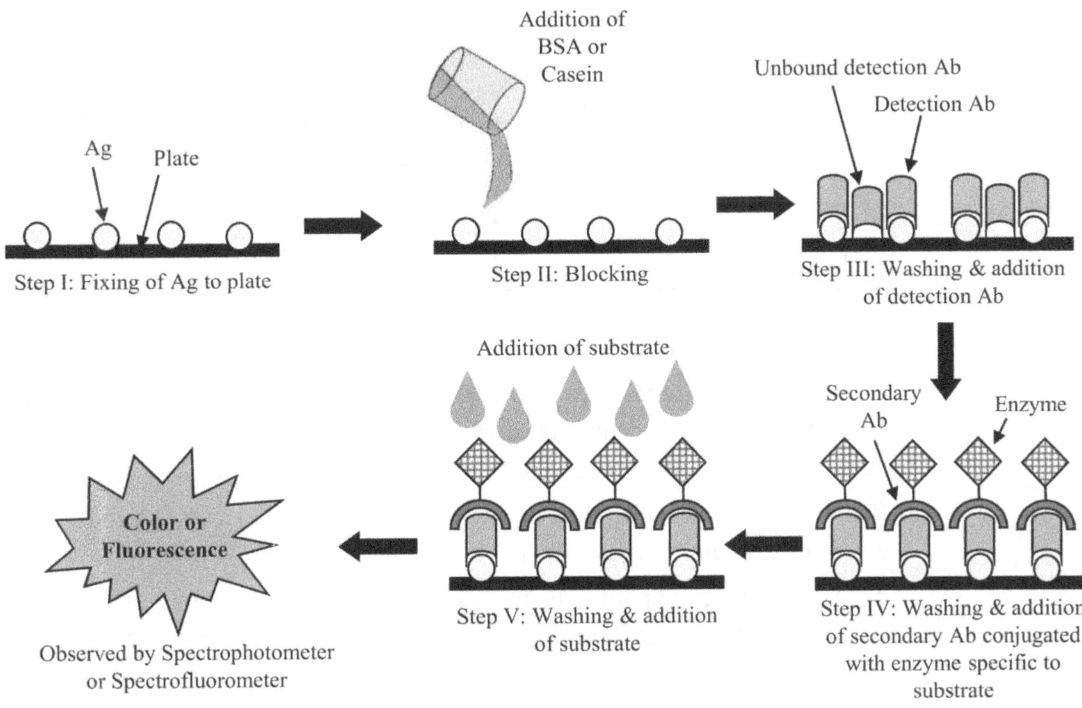

FIGURE 11.5 Steps involved in Indirect ELISA

hand, chemiluminescent substrate such as luminol may be added to obtain light as the detection signal.

Alkaline phosphatase is another commonly employed enzyme in ELISA. In this case, 5-Bromo-4-Chloro-3-Indolyl Phosphate (BCIP) and Nitroblue Tetrazolium (NBT) are used as chromogenic substrates. Alkaline phosphatase acts on these chromogenic substrates to give blue color, which is used as detection signal **(Table 11.1)**.

Employment of Indirect Assay for Quantitative Estimation of antibodies:

Apart from qualitative assays, the indirect assay may be used to quantify the amount of antibodies in a given sample. For example, indirect ELISA is routinely used for the determination of HIV antibodies in the serum sample in the form of diagnostic test for HIV. The salient points of quantitative indirect assay include:

1. A standard graph is plotted by keeping the antigen in fixed amount (and in excess) and varying the amount of antibodies **(Table 11.2)**. In making a standard plot, the known amount of antibodies is added in each well. The antigens are attached to the wells of the plate and antibodies bind to antigens attached on the plate.

TABLE 11.2 Standard plot for indirect assay, in which fixed amount of antigen is added in each well and concentration of antibody is varied

S. No	Concentration of Antigen (Ag) (x)	Concentration of Antibody (Ab) (y)	Signal
Well 1	X	y1	
Well 2	X	y2	Increasing Signal Intensity
Well 3	X	y3	
Well 4	X	y4	

1. With increase in the concentration of Ab (y), more Ags are bound. This results in more number of secondary Abs binding to the primary Ab. Therefore, addition of substrate gives intense color, the absorbance for which is determined using spectrophotometer **(Figure 11.6)**.

2. The concentration of the Ab in the unknown sample can be obtained from the standard plot **(Figure 11.7)**.

3. However, the results obtained through indirect assay are also confirmed by Western blotting, which also determines the concentration of antibodies.

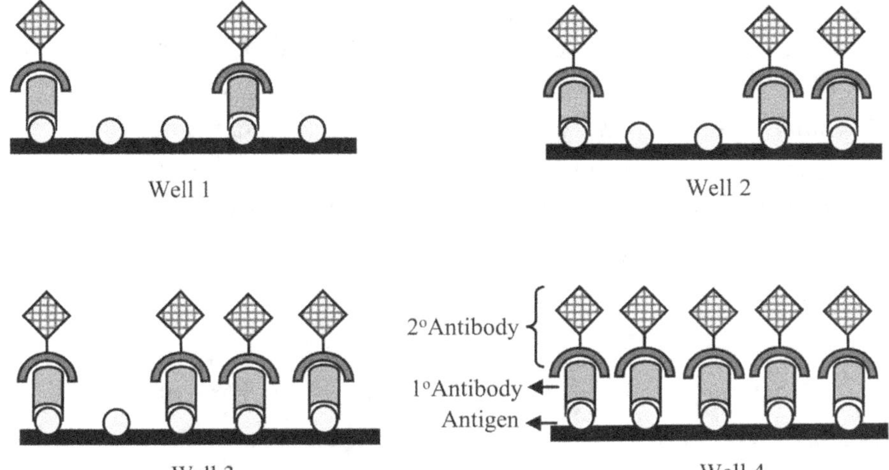

FIGURE 11.6 Increase in concentration of antibodies from well 1 to well 4. Higher the concentration of antibody, stronger is the signal

III. Sandwich ELISA

This is a more commonly employed technique of ELISA. It is called sandwich ELISA because antigens are sandwiched between two layers of antibodies. The steps involved in this type of ELISA are as follows **(Figure 11.8)**:

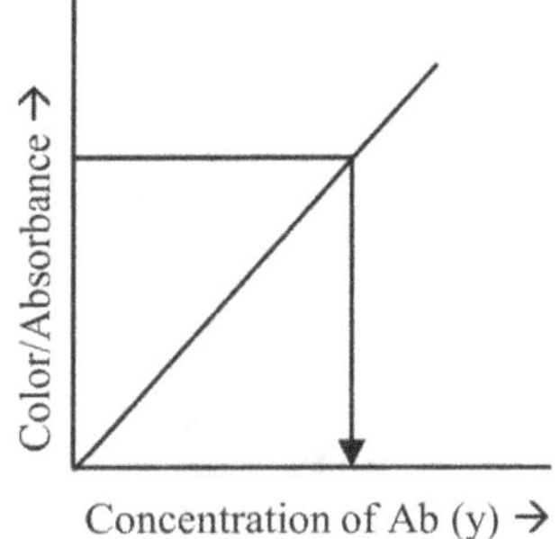

FIGURE 11.7 Standard plot for indirect assay between absorbance and concentration of Ab (y)

1. The titer plate (microplate or ELISA plate) is coated with a known quantity of Ab. This type of antibody attached to plate is termed as 'capture antibody'.

2. Non-specific binding sites on the ELISA plate are blocked by adding BSA or casein in a process termed as 'blocking' as described in indirect ELISA (step 2).

3. Thereafter, serum sample containing antigen (to be determined) is added. The antigens bind to the capture Ab.

4. The plate is washed to remove any unbound Ag.

5. In this step, primary antibodies are added, which bind specifically to the Ag.

6. Washing is done to get rid of free (unbound) primary Abs.

7. Antigens are sandwiched between two layers of antibodies, capture antibodies and primary antibodies. Therefore, this process is termed as 'sandwich ELISA'.

8. Secondary antibodies conjugated with enzyme (labeled secondary antibodies) specific for primary antibody are added. Thus, secondary antibodies are attached indirectly to antigens through primary antibodies.

9. Washing is done to remove excess or unbound secondary antibody.

10. Depending on enzyme attached to secondary antibody, substrate is added. Reaction of substrate with the enzyme on the secondary Ab produces color, fluorescence or chemilumniscent **(Table 11.1)**.

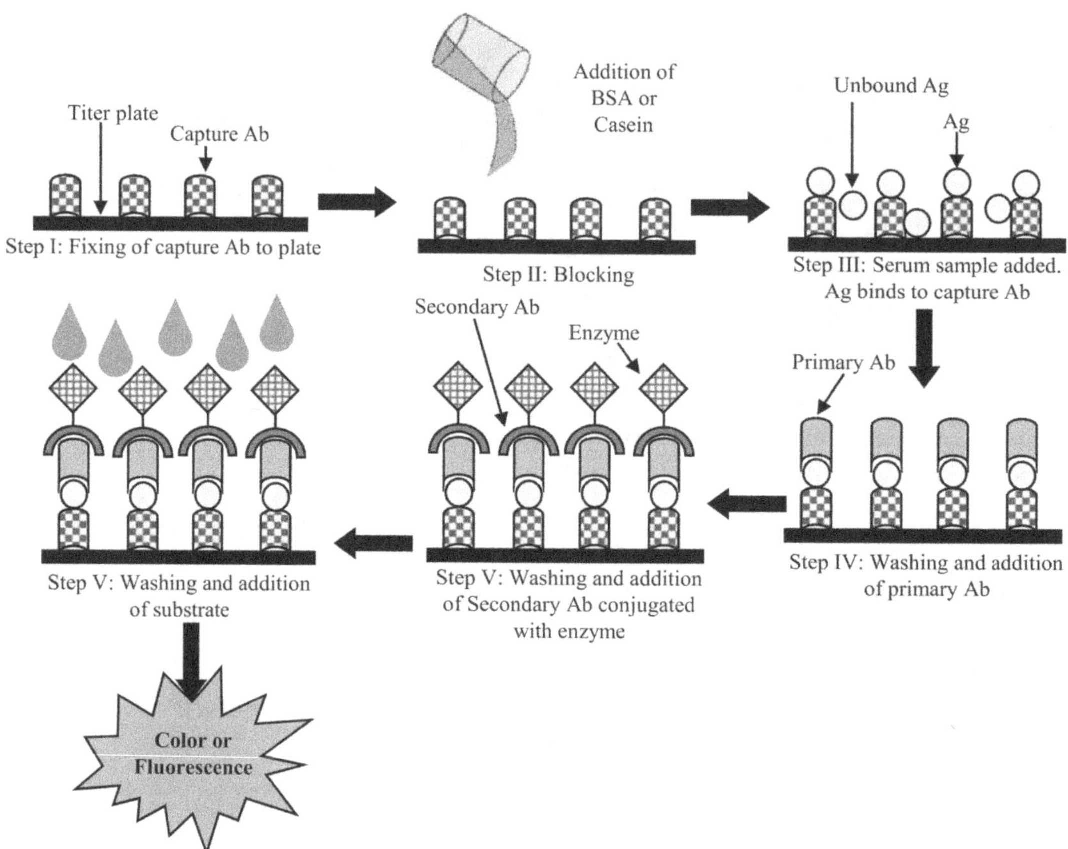

FIGURE 11.8 Steps involved in Sandwich ELISA

Quantitative assay of antigens using Sandwich assay

This assay may be used to quantify the amount of Ag in the sample. It may be used for detecting HIV by measuring the concentration of HIV antigen (HIVgp120, HIV-1p24) in serum sample. The important features of this method are discussed **(Figure 11.9)** below:

1. For plotting a standard curve, the amount of antigen (x) is varied while that of antibody (y) is kept constant **(Table 11.3)**. Here, antibodies are in excess and are attached to the wells in the plate.

TABLE 11.3 Standard plot for sandwich assay

S. No	Concentration of (Ag) (x)	Concentration of (Ab) (y)	Signal
Well 1	X_1	Y	
Well 2	X_2	Y	Increasing Signal Intensity
Well 3	X_3	Y	
Well 4	X_4	Y	

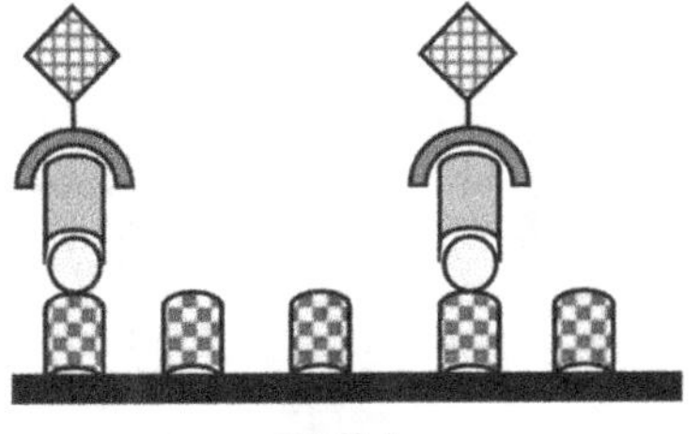

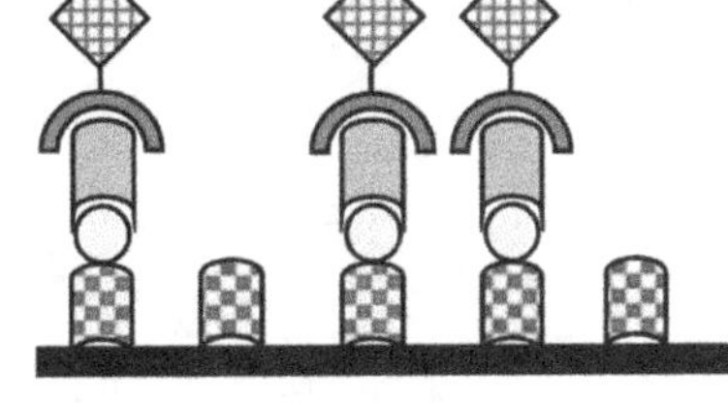

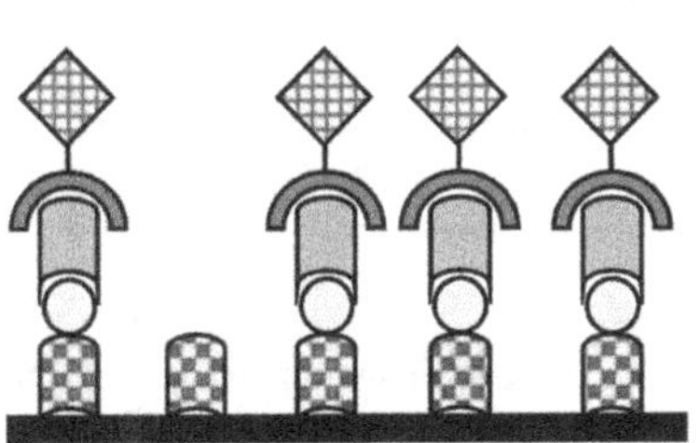

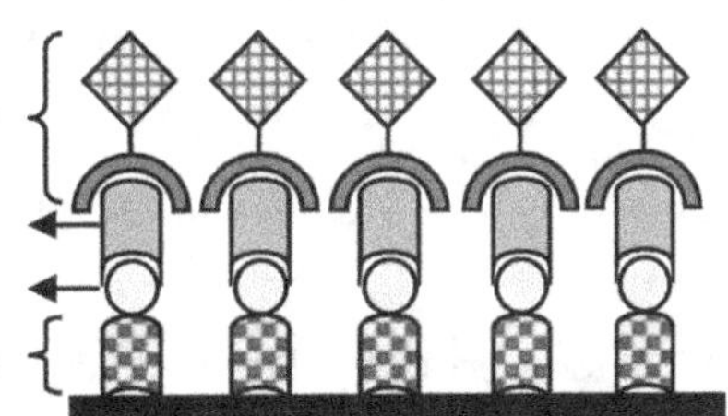

FIGURE 11.9 Increase in concentration of Ag from well 1 to well 4. More the concentration of Ag, stronger is the signal.

2. With increase in the concentration of Ag, the binding of primary Ab and consequently, secondary Ab increases. Secondary Ab linked with enzyme reacts with the substrate added producing color. Higher the concentration of Ag, stronger is the signal

3. This concentration of the Ag in the unknown sample may be determined from the standard plot obtained between the absorbance and concentration of Ag **(Figure 11.10)**.

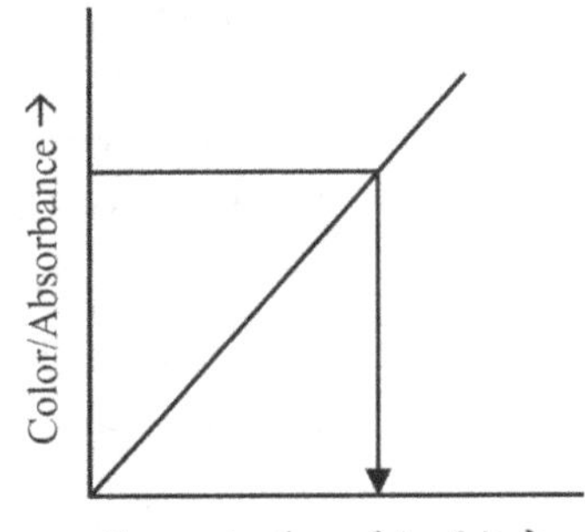

FIGURE 11.10 Standard plot for Sandwich assay between absorbance and concentration of Ag (x)

IV. Competitive ELISA

In this type of ELISA, there is a competition between antibodies to bind with antigens in the sample or antigens attached to plate wells. The steps involved in competitive ELISA are as following **(Figure 11.11)**:

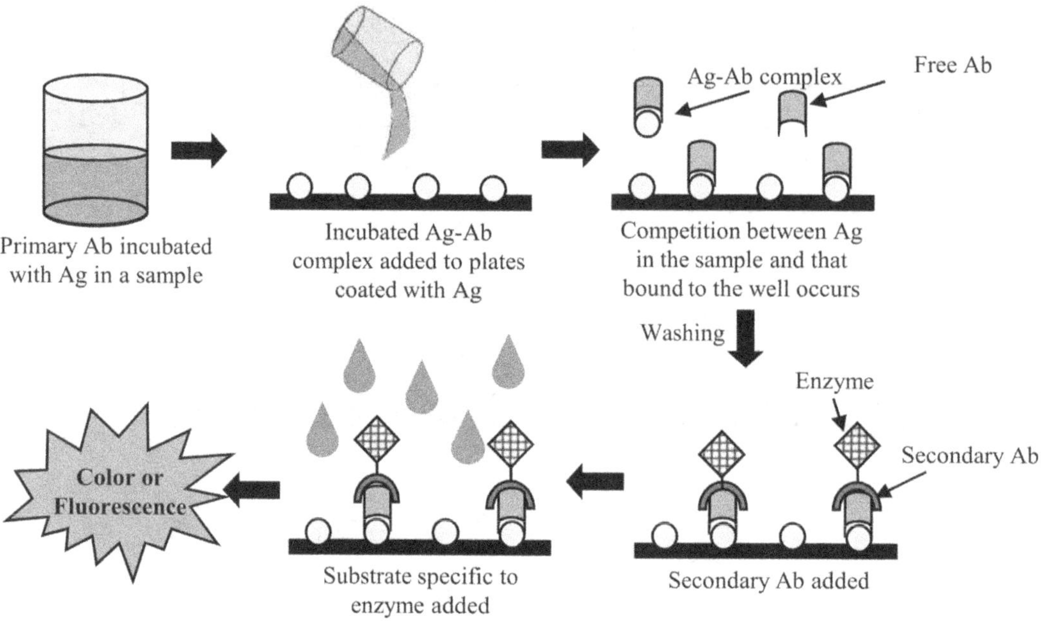

FIGURE 11.11 Steps involved in Competitive ELISA

1. The microtitre plate is coated with antigen as described in indirect ELISA.

2. Unlabeled antibodies (primary antibodies) are incubated with antigens and Ag-AB complex is allowed to form in a sample.

3. The Ag-Ab complex is added to the wells coated with Ag. Upon addition of Ag-Ab complex, competition arises for primary antibodies to bind with Ag in a sample or with Ag attached to well. The degree of binding of antibody with Ag on the well is dependent on amount of Ag in the sample. More the amount of Ag in the sample, lesser will be the Ab binding to the Ag in the well. Conversely, lower the amount of Ag in sample, higher is binding of Ab to Ag on wells.

4. The plates are washed to remove unbound Ab.

5. Secondary Ab specific to primary Ab is added.

6. The enzyme specific substrate is added, which gives color on reacting with the enzyme attached with secondary antibody. The color obtained is used to calculate the concentration of Ag in the sample using spectrophotometer and the standard curve.

7. Higher the concentration of Ag in the sample, the weaker would be the signal obtained. This is so because Ag in the sample binds to the Ab in the Ag-Ab complex. Therefore, lesser Ab is available for binding to Ag coating the well.

Quantitative Assay for Determining Antigens/Antibodies using Competitive Assay

Like indirect and sandwich assay, competitive assay may also be used for quantifying the antigens or antibodies in sample. The steps in competitive ELISA include:

1. Antigens are added to well and these are allowed to attach to well.

2. A standard graph is plotted by varying the amount of antigen (x) and keeping the concentration of antibody (y) as constant and excess **(Table 11.4)**.

TABLE 11.4 Standard plot obtained for competitive ELISA

S. No	Concentration of (Ag) (x)	Concentration of (Ab) (y)	Signal
Well 1	X_1	Y	Increasing Signal Intensity
Well 2	X_2	Y	
Well 3	X_3	Y	
Well 4	X_4	Y	

3. With increase in number of Ag present in the sample, the amount of free Ab decreases because more amount of Ab binds to the Ag present in the sample. Lesser free Abs are available for binding with antigens on the well. Accordingly, the signal is strongest when the less amount of Ag is present in the sample **(Figure 11.12)**.

4. Secondary Ab linked with enzyme reacts with the substrate and produce color.

5. A standard plot helps in determining the concentration of the Ag present in the sample from the standard plot obtained between the absorbance and concentration of Ag **(Figure 11.13).**

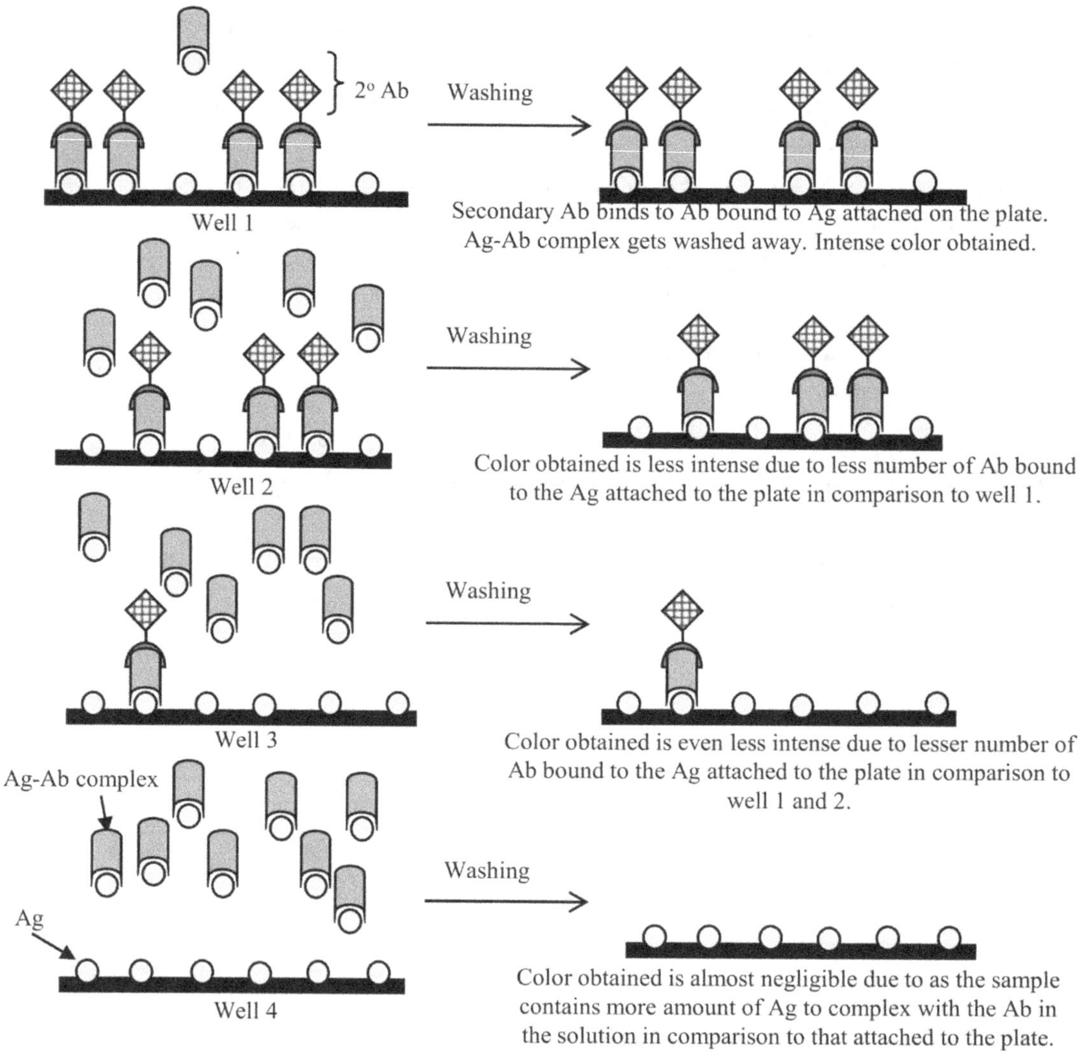

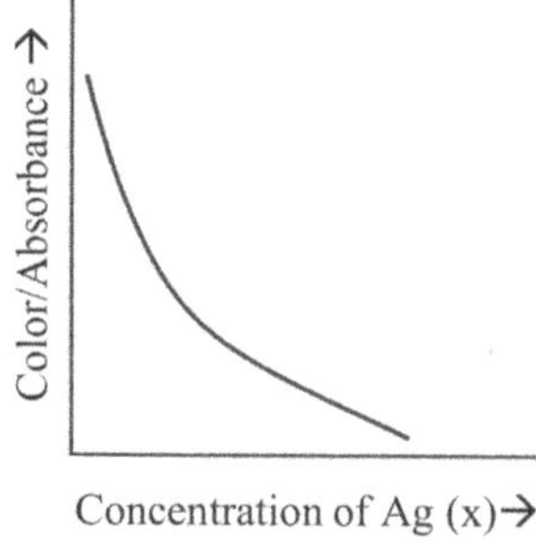

FIGURE 11.12 Increase in concentration of Ag from well 1 to well 4. More the concentration of Ag, weaker the signal

FIGURE 11.13 Standard plot for Competitive assay between absorbance and concentration of Ag (x)

Applications of ELISA

There are various known applications of ELISA in various fields such as in research, clinics and forensics, etc **(Figure 11.14)**:

1. **Blood bank screening:** Viral contamination in the blood stored in the blood banks is detected using ELISA. For example, detection of HIV-1, HIV-2 (by presence of anti-HIV antibodies), Hepatitis-C (by presence of antibodies), Hepatitis-B (by presence of both antigen and antibody) is routinely done using ELISA. This helps in prevention of transmittance of these diseases to the patient to whom blood will be transfused.

2. **Endocrinology:** ELISA is widely used for detecting:

    (i)   Human Chorionic Gonadotropin (hCG), which serves as a successful test for pregnancy

    (ii) Detection of Luteinizing hormone (LH), which serves to explore time of ovulation

    (iii) Thyroid Stimulating Hormone (TSH), triiodothyronine (T_3) and tetraiodothyronine (T_4), as indicators of thyroid function

    (iv) Detection of anabolic steroids, as dope test in athletics.

3. **Detecting Infections:** Several infections such as HIV, syphilis, Hepatitis B and C, *Toxoplasma gondii* (causative agent for toxoplasmosis), etc. are detected in the various body fluids using different types of ELISA. For instance, sandwich ELISA is used to detect the presence of antigen in the blood, urine or other body fluids of the patient, and indirect ELISA employs detection of antibodies for particular antigens in the blood sample e.g. in detection of anti-HIV antibodies. Determination of H1N1 (Swine flu virus) by measuring the concentration of antigen in serum sample of the patient is another application of ELISA.

4. **Measurement of allergen in food or house dust:** Allergens are one of the main causes of threat to many sensitive patients. ELISA proves to be very useful in measuring the level of allergens in food or house dust.

5. **Measurement of Rheumatoid factor:** Rheumatoid factor (RF) is an important biomarker for diagnosis of Rheumatoid in patients and ELISA is a useful technique for its detection and estimation.

6. **Measurement of auto-antibodies in systemic lupus erythematosus (SLE):** The measurement of auto-antibodies formed in response to the immune system is a useful diagnostic test for SLE, which is an inflammatory autoimmune disorder manifested by rashes typically on the face and extremities along with several other symptoms.

7. **Detection of Narcotics:** ELISA is also used in measuring the level of narcotics, such as opium, cocaine, morphine, etc in the body fluids. It is very helpful for forensic purposes.

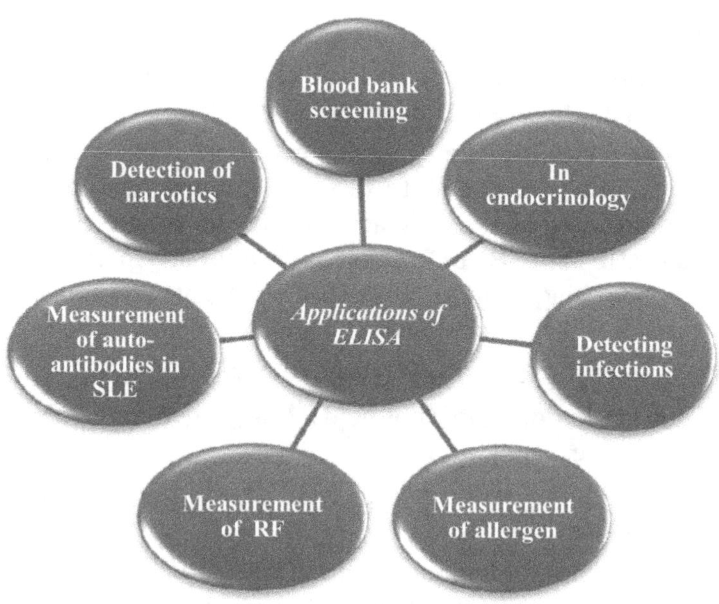

FIGURE 11.14 Applications of ELISA

MICROARRAY TECHNOLOGY

DEFINITION AND GENERAL FEATURES

DNA microarray technology (DNA chips or biochips) is one of the latest breakthroughs in experimental molecular biology. Patrick Brown and his colleagues at Stanford University first described the application of DNA microarray technology in 1995. DNA microarray technology may be defined as a high-throughput and versatile technology used for parallel gene expression analysis for thousands of genes. Indeed, it is one of the types of gene expression methods. Conventional gene expression methods involve southern or northern blotting; reverse transcriptase-PCR (RT-PCR) etc. However, these are best suited for analyzing a limited number of genes and samples at a time. Like Southern blots, microarrays use hybridization (target DNA and probe, i.e. detecting DNA) to detect a specific DNA in a sample. However in southern blot, a single probe is used to search target DNA; whereas, DNA microarray uses a large number of different probes to identify the specific DNA in sample (**Table 11.5**).

TABLE 11.5 Differences between southern Blotting and microarrays

S. No	Southern Blotting	Microarrays
1.	A single probe is used to search target DNA	A large number of different probes to identify the specific DNA
2.	The target DNA is immobilized on a membrane	The probes are fixed to the slide or chip
3	Only a limited number of genes and samples may be analyzed at a time	It is high throughput screening method and it may analyze a large number of genes at a time
4.	Hybridization is performed on membranes	Hybridization is performed on slides or chips

In microarray technology, the terms probe and target is used interchangeably. However, in this chapter, the term 'probe' means DNA which is used for detection and it is attached to slide. The term 'target' DNA means sample DNA, which is to be identified.

PRINCIPLE OF MICROARRAY ANALYSIS

These are actually miniaturized hybridization assays for studying thousands of nucleic acid fragments simultaneously. The hybridization between labeled target (sample DNA) and probe (attached to slide) is carried out. All microarray systems have the following key components:

1. **Microarray:** It contains immobilized nucleic acid sequences (probes). Indeed, microarray is a pattern of single stranded DNA (ssDNA) probes which are immobilized (bound) on a surface called a chip or a slide. The probes are designed and placed on an array in a regular pattern of spots. The size of these spots is less than 200 µm in diameter. A glass slide acts as the solid support onto which up to tens of thousands of spots can be arrayed in a total area of a few square centimeters.

2. **Labeled Sample:** Sample DNA i.e. DNA which needs to be investigated is isolated and is labeled. The sample labeled DNA is allowed to hybridize with probes on microarray. This requires that sample DNA and probes are single-stranded and accessible to each other.

3. **Detection System:** Depending on the label, appropriate detection system is used to quantify the hybridization signal. Fluorescent dyes, especially Cy3 and Cy5 dyes are used as the predominant label in microarray analysis. Fluorescence has the advantage that more than one signal may be detected by using labels of different fluorescence colors. This allows investigators to perform comparative analysis of two or more samples in one microarray.

PROCEDURE OF MICROARRAY ANALYSIS

There are four major steps in performing a typical microarray experiment, sample preparation and labeling; hybridization; washing and image acquisition **(Figure 11.15)**.

1. **Sample Preparation and Labeling:** There are a number of different ways in which a DNA microarray sample is prepared and labeled. The sample is prepared by isolating messenger RNA, which represents a quantitative copy of genes expressed at the time of sample collection. The overall success of microarray experiment depends on the quality of the RNA. The purity, homogeneity and uniformity of the mRNA are the critical factors in the hybridization performance. The sample mRNA extracted from the biological sample is converted into complementary DNA (cDNA) using a reverse-transcriptase enzyme. Thereafter, cDNA is labeled with fluorescent dyes Cy3 and Cy5.

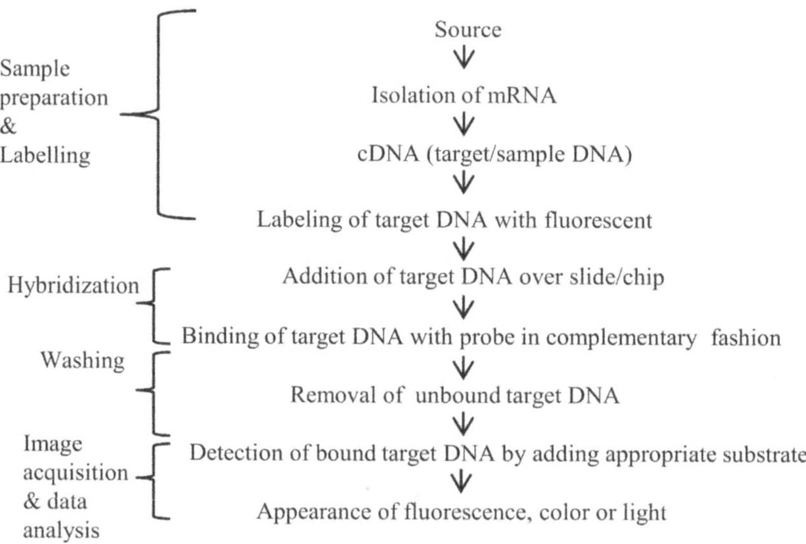

FIGURE 11.15 Different steps involved in microarray experiments

2. **Array Hybridization:** Hybridization is the process of joining two complementary strands of DNA to form a double-stranded molecule. In this step, the labeled cDNA (sample) is added over a slide on which probes have been attached. It leads to hybridization of sample DNA and probe on slide **(Figure 11.16)**. Hybridization is carried under stringent conditions so as hybridization takes place only between complimentary base pairs and there is no cross hybridization. The stringency is increased by increasing the temperature or lowering the ionic strength of the buffers.

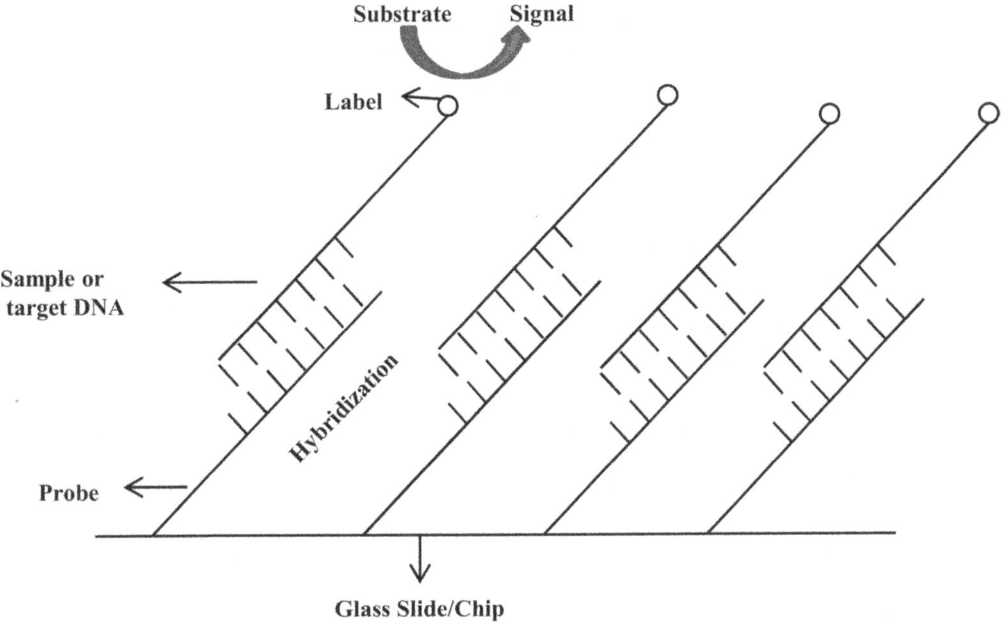

FIGURE 11.16 Hybridization between probe and target DNA in microarray technology

3. **Washing:** It is necessary to remove unbound sample DNA from the slide. In other words, sample DNA which fails to bind with probe, are removed during washing.

4. **Image Acquisition and Data Analysis:** It is the final step of microarray experiments and in this step, an image of the surface of the hybridized array is obtained. Depending on the label, appropriate technique is used to determine how much labeled cDNA is bound to probe. The fluorescence, color or light may be used as signals depending on the labels employed during the process **(Table 11.1).**

APPLICATIONS OF MICROARRAY TECHNOLOGY

Due to versatility of microarray analysis, it has rapidly emerged as a general molecular biology analytical technique.

1. **Gene Expression Analysis**

   (i)   It allows the analysis of the composition of cellular messenger RNA populations. The identity of genes may be revealed using microarrays.

   (ii) Microarray gene expression analysis may be used to compare the relative gene expression in two different samples.

(iii)   The effects of different chemicals or other environmental stimuli on gene expression may be done using microarrays. For example, the effect of regulatory factors on gene expression (over expression or under expression) may be analyzed. In cancer research, microarrays have been used to find changes in gene expression in transformed cells (cancer cells).

2. Genomic Analysis

(i)   Microarrays are very useful tools for genomic analysis. These are routinely used to identify new genes by examining nucleic acid sequences.

(ii)   It may be used to understand gene regulation by elucidating transcription factor gene interactions.

3. Drug Discovery: These have been found to provide useful information at different stages of the drug discovery process.

(i)   These may be used to identify potential drug targets by understanding the relationship between metabolic pathway and gene expression. The protein targets of drug treatments can be identified by finding a protein that causes the same changes as a drug when removed from cells.

(ii)   These can also be used to the toxic properties of drugs by examining changes in expression profiles due to drug treatment.

(iii)   Different functions of drugs may be identified on the basis of changes in gene expression.

REVIEW QUESTIONS

TWO MARKS QUESTIONS

1. Define ELISA.
2. What does immunosorbent signify in ELISA? What are different antibodies employed in ELISA?
3. What are the different types of ELISA?
4. What do you mean by blocking? What is its significance in ELISA?
5. Why is sandwich ELISA?
6. What are the most commonly employed enzymes and substrates for detection purposes in ELISA?
7. What is the difference between microarray and southern blotting?

8. Enlist different steps involved in DNA microarray.

9. What do you understand by microarray technology?

10. What are traditional methods of detecting gene expression? What are the advantages of microarray over traditional methods?

11. Define microarray.

12. What is the role of microarray in drug discovery?

FIVE MARKS QUESTIONS

1. Write a brief note on Sandwich ELISA.

2. Differentiate between Indirect and Competitive ELISA.

3. Explain the principle of microarray technology?

4. What are the applications of microarray?

5. Explain the main steps involved in microarray technology.

TEN MARKS QUESTIONS

1. Explain sandwich and competitive methods of ELISA.

2. What is indirect ELISA? Write applications of ELISA?

3. What is microarray? Explain its principle, procedure and applications.

MULTIPLE CHOICE QUESTIONS

1. In microarray technology, glass slides are attached with
   - (a) Sample DNA
   - (b) Probe DNA
   - (c) It remains free
   - (d) None of above

2. Microarray is based on
   - (a) Hybridization
   - (b) Denaturation
   - (c) DNA amplification
   - (d) None of above

3. Microarray is carried in
   - (a) High stringent conditions
   - (b) Low stringent conditions
   - (c) Does not matter
   - (d) None of above

4. A large number of genes may be analyzed using
   - (a) Microarray
   - (b) Southern blotting
   - (c) Both a and b
   - (d) None of above

5. Which of following is not application of microarray?
   (a) DNA replication   (b)   Drug discovery
   (c) Gene analysis   (d)   Cancer research
6. Which of following is attached to ELISA plate in indirect ELISA?
   (a) Antigen   (b)   Antibody
   (c) Antigen-antibody complex   (d)   None of above
7. Which of following is attached to ELISA plate in sandwich ELISA?
   (a) Antigen   (b)   Antibody
   (c) Antigen-antibody complex   (d)   None of above
8. What is the influence of increasing antigen concentration in a sample on detection signal in competitive ELISA?
   (a) Increase in signal   (b)   Decrease in signal
   (c) No influence   (d)   Can increase or decrease
9. In which of following methods, a single antibody is used?
   (a) Direct ELISA   (b)   Indirect ELISA
   (c) Competitive ELISA   (d)   Sandwich ELISA
10. In ELISA, which of following antibodies are labeled with enzymes?
   (a) Primary Antibodies   (b)   Secondary antibodies
   (c) Capture antibodies   (d)   None of above

CHAPTER 12

Western Blotting

CHAPTER OUTLINE

Definitions and General Features

Transfer Methods
Diffusion Blotting
Capillary Blotting
Vacuum Blotting
Electrophoretic Blotting
Semidry Blotting
Bidirectional Blotting

"The Blotting Procedure"

Membranes used for Blotting

Detection Systems

Applications of Western Blotting

DEFINITIONS AND GENERAL FEATURES

Blotting is a technique to characterize the biomolecules (DNA, RNA and Proteins) after their separation by gel electrophoresis. In other words, the bands (spots) of biomolecules obtained after performing gel electrophoresis are characterized by blotting. Indeed, these separated biomolecules are transferred from the gel onto some membranes (e.g. nylon membrane) and this process of transfer of biomolecules on the membrane is known as 'blotting'. After the transfer of these biomolecules on a membrane, these biomolecules are characterized using probes (for DNA or RNA) or antibodies (for proteins). Depending on the biomolecules, blotting may be of four types:

 (i) **Southern Blotting:** for DNA

 (ii) **Northern Blotting:** for RNA

 (iii) **Western Blotting:** for Proteins

 (iv) **Eastern Blotting:** For post-translational modifications such as glycosylation, phosphorylation

The names of these blotting techniques are not based on directions, rather, southern blotting was named after the name of scientist 'Southern'. Thereafter, the names of other types of blotting were given by convention only (not on scientists).

TRANSFER METHODS

Blotting has been classified into various types, based on the method of transfer of biomolecules on to the immobilizing membrane. The following are some types:

1. **Diffusion blotting:** The principle of this type of blotting is simple diffusion. The gel surface is covered with the blotting membrane to which the protein components are transferred. The components move from higher concentration i.e. from gel surface to the lower concentration i.e. blotting membrane. This method is successful especially, when gels with large pores are used e.g. agarose gel in isoelectric focusing. While in case of gels with small pore size, such as polyacrylamide gel, a weight is generally kept on top of the blotting membrane to allow diffusion of biomolecules from the tight pored gel to the blotting membrane **(Figure 12.1)**.

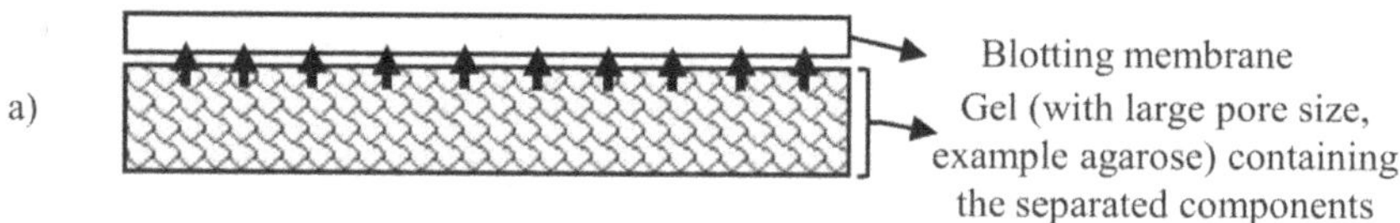

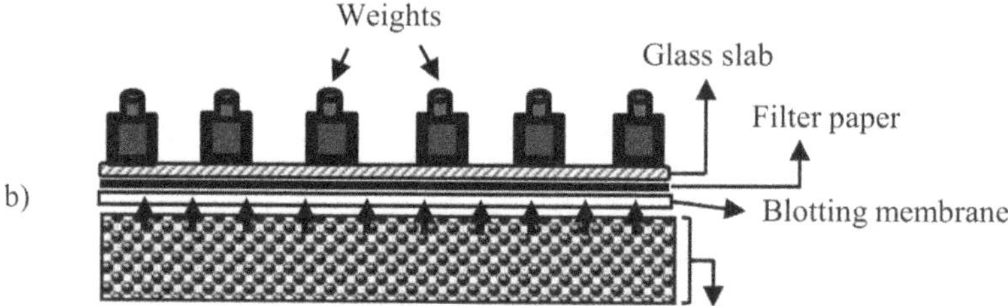

FIGURE 12.1 Arrangement in diffusion blotting in case of (a) gel with large pore size (b) gel with small pore size. A piece of filter paper followed by a glass slab is placed over the gel. A weight is placed over the glass plate to allow diffusion of molecules from gel to membrane.

2. **Capillary blotting:** It is a simple technique for efficient transfer of proteins from the gel to the membrane. The setup exploits the capillary action produced by continuous flow of buffer. The constant flow of buffer maintains a low concentration zone, which facilitates effective and fast transfer of proteins from the gel onto the membrane. In this setup, gel is sandwiched

between two glass plates. The gel is in direct contact with the blotting membrane and a long strip of filter paper runs below it. One end of this filter paper is soaked in a container containing buffer, while the other end hangs free **(Figure 12.2)**. This filter paper allows continuous flow of buffer from the system, assisting the transfer process.

This system may also be used for some temperature sensitive proteins, for which the whole arrangement is kept inside the refrigerator throughout the process. This method takes approximately 2 hours for complete transfer of proteins.

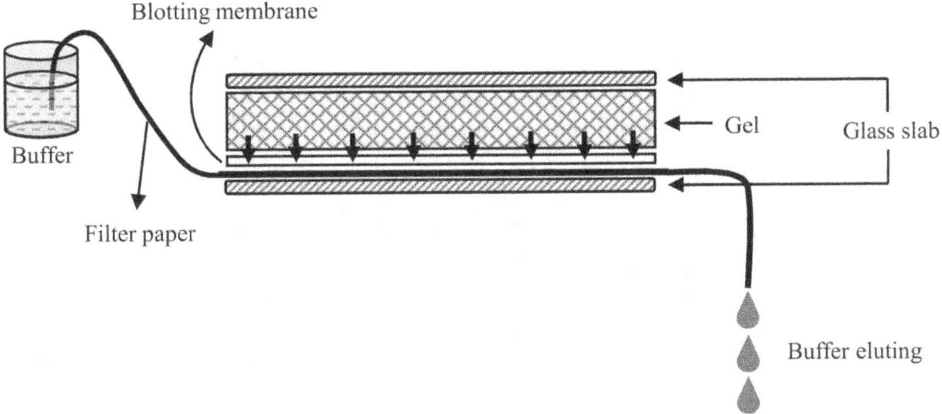

FIGURE 12.2 The setup and process of capillary blotting

3. **Vacuum blotting:** This method employs use of vacuum for hastening the transfer process. However, this method is not preferable when polyacrylamide gel is used for protein separation. This is because polyacrylamide gel sticks to the blotting membrane inseparably. **(Figure 12.3)**

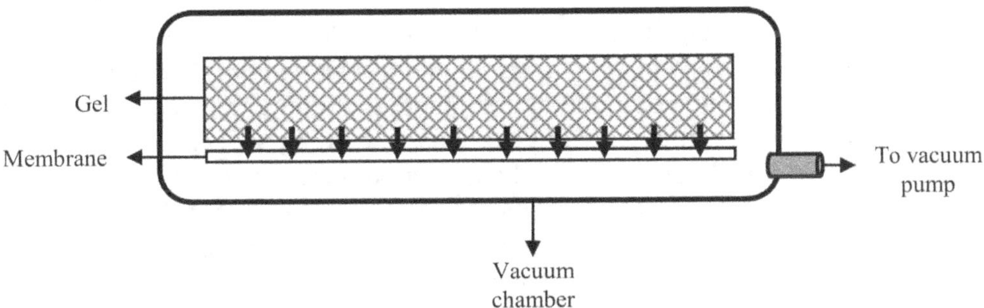

FIGURE 12.3 Vacuum blotting

4. **Electrophoretic blotting:** It is also known as electroblotting. This technique uses the electrophoresis for drawing protein components from the gel onto

the membrane. This method is exceptionally beneficial, when polyacrylamide gel is used due to small pore size. The application of electric current allows easy extraction of proteins from the gel. This method enables rapid transfer. **(Figure 12.4)**

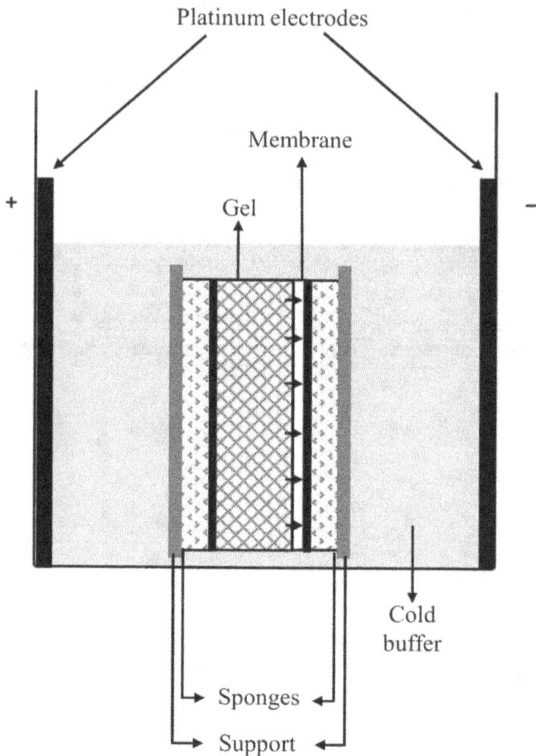

FIGURE 12.4 Electrophoretic blotting

5. **Semidry blotting:** This system is much simplified, less costly, and requires less time to complete. Moreover, use of dry gel is beneficial because dry gel entraps the transferred proteins much more efficiently. The setup for semidry blotting is similar to that of electrophoretic blotting with only difference in terms of electrodes. In this method, electrodes are made up of graphite and the system does not need to be immersed in the buffer **(Figure 12.5)**. Moreover, there is no need to cool the buffer system during blotting process. However, it is recommended that the current does not exceed 0.8 amperes per centimeter squared (cm^2). Above this amount of current, the gel might get heated up leading to denaturation of proteins. The transfer by this method is generally complete within 1 hour.

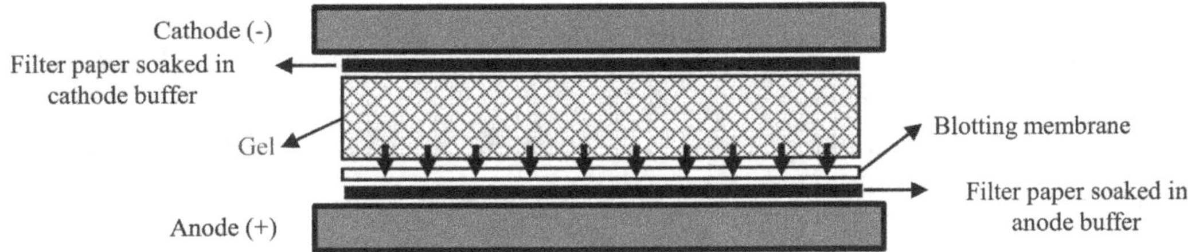

FIGURE 12.5 Semidry blotting

6. **Bidirectional blotting:** In this method, a replica of blotting can be obtained using bidirectional blotting. It includes a sandwich composed of blotting membrane, filter paper, paper towel and glass slab on either side of the gel. The transfer from the gel to the blotting membranes is facilitated by putting a weight on the glass slab on top. Thus obtained two identical blots from one gel may be used for effective characterization of proteins.

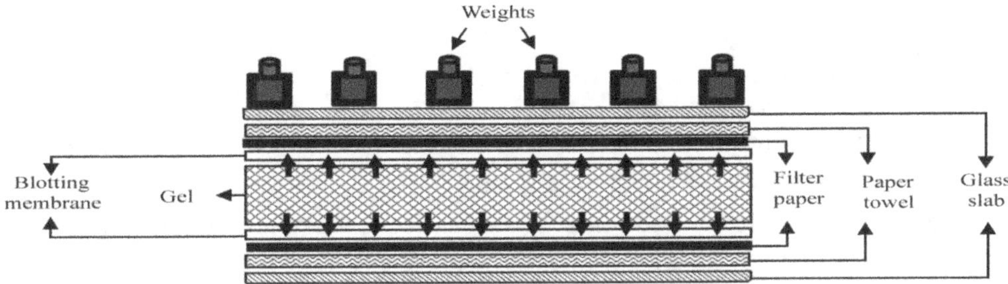

FIGURE 12.6 Bidirectional blotting

THE BLOTTING PROCEDURE

Western blotting is carried out in order to characterize the separated proteins using the following procedure **(Figure 12.7):**

(a) The protein molecules are separated by subjecting the sample to gel electrophoresis.

(b) The separated components are transferred on to a suitable blotting membrane (discussed later under the **membranes used for blotting** section).

(c) It is followed by 'blocking' step. This step is done to prevent non-specific binding of the detecting antibody to the blotting membrane.
If these sites are not blocked, the antibody binds to the membrane and yields faulty results. Blocking is performed using bovine serum albumin (BSA) or non fat milk (having protein), which binds to the membrane. Thus, antibodies can bind only with proteins attached to the membrane.

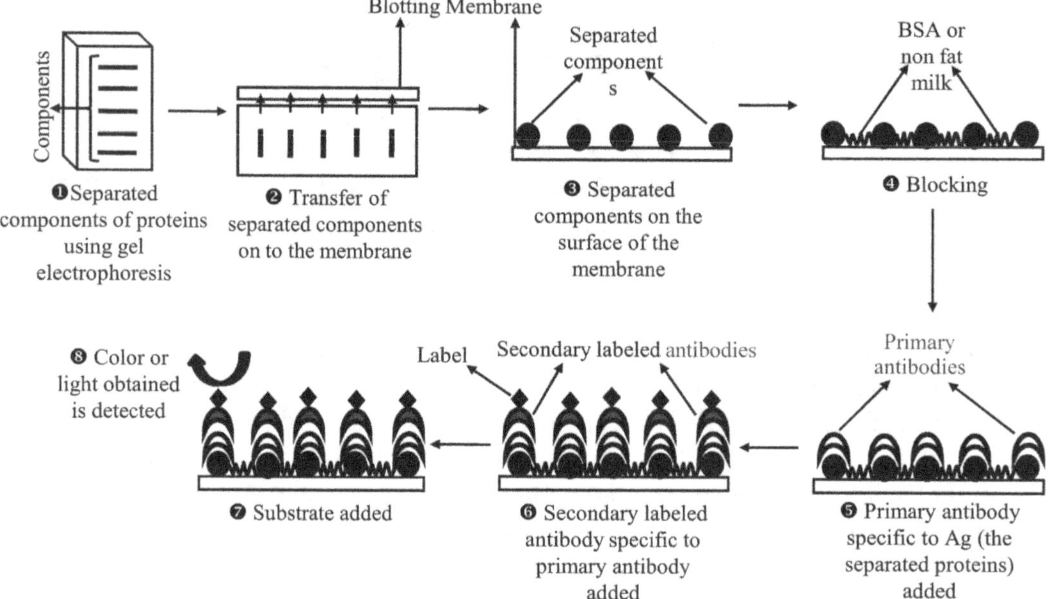

FIGURE 12.7 Steps involved in Western Blotting

(d)   Primary antibodies are added to membrane. These antibodies are specific to the proteins attached on the membrane.

(e)   It is followed by addition of labeled secondary antibodies, which are specific to the primary antibody. Labeling is done for detection purpose.

(f)   Thereafter, a substrate corresponding to the label is added, which after reaction with label give color, fluorescence or light.

MEMBRANES USED FOR BLOTTING

There are various membranes available commercially for blotting. The membrane chosen for blotting depends upon the material to be transferred, the method used for the transfer and the strength of binding required. Despite advancement in the manufacture of blotting membranes, no membrane is ideal to allow complete 100% transfer of protein components from the gel to the membrane. The small sized fragments easily seep through the gel to the membrane, while large sized fragments are hard to transfer. Some of the several membranes are discussed below:

1. **Nitrocellulose:** It is the most commonly used membrane. The pore size of this membrane varies from 0.05–0.45 microns. The pore size affects the binding capacity of the membrane. Higher binding capacity is obtained with

membranes with smaller pore size. However, its low mechanical stability and broad range of binding capacity (non specific) makes its use limited. For drying this membrane, it is baked at 80°C in vacuum for 2 hours.

2. **Nylon (Polyamide):** It is another membrane which is widely used for blotting. These have some advantages over nitrocellulose membranes:

 (i) These have higher mechanical stability and are less fragile. Therefore, they are less likely to crack while handling. Unlike nitrocellulose membranes, they do not disintegrate on using them again and again.

 (ii) Nylon membrane is positively charged, which allow protein sample to covalently bind to the membrane. This prevents leaching out of the sample from the membrane during blotting and also decreases the transfer time considerably. On the other hand, nitrocellulose membrane initially binds the sample semi-permanently followed by permanent immobilization on baking at 80°C.

3. **Polyvinylidenedifluoride (PVDF):** These membranes with Teflon as base are similar to nylon membranes. These have very high binding capacity and better mechanical stability.

4. **Ion exchange membranes:** The membranes in this class include diethylaminoethyl (DEAE) or carboxymethyl (CM).

DETECTION SYSTEMS

Detection of the proteins using labeled antibody uses following systems. The secondary antibodies are labeled with various types of labels and these include:

1. **Radiolabeling:** The secondary antibodies are labeled with radioactive substance. This enables easy detection as the radioactive signal detected on X-ray films. The films obtained are known as 'autoradiographs' and the process is called 'autoradiography'. However, special care has to be taken while handling radioactive substances due to safety issues. Special instruments and containers are required for its safe handling. Therefore, this method is not commonly used in laboratories.

2. **Non-Radioactive Labeling:** It is a safer alternative to radioactive labeling. This method of labeling employs various enzyme and substrate combinations. These systems are useful for both colorimetric and chemiluminescent type of substrates. On reaction with corresponding enzyme, the chromogenic substrate gives off a colored product. On the other hand, chemiluminescent substrates give light on reacting with the enzyme. These color and light signals are used for determining the   presence or absence of proteins. The commonly used non radioactive labeling systems are:

(i) ***Horseradish peroxidase system (HRP):*** Horseradish is a metalloenzyme obtained from the roots of the plant horseradish. The secondary antibody is attached to HRP using polyethyleneimine and 1% glutaraldehyde (cross linker). This labels the secondary antibody.

In presence of chloronapthol (chromogenic substrate) the HRP gives purple color. And when luminal (chemiluminescent substrate) is used as the substrate light is given out **(Figure 12.8)**. The degree of color or light recorded tells about the amount of proteins present in the sample. If the amount of protein is less, the site available for primary antibodies is less. Hence, the secondary labeled antibodies (enzyme substrate complex, example HRP) show lesser binding giving rise to weaker signal.

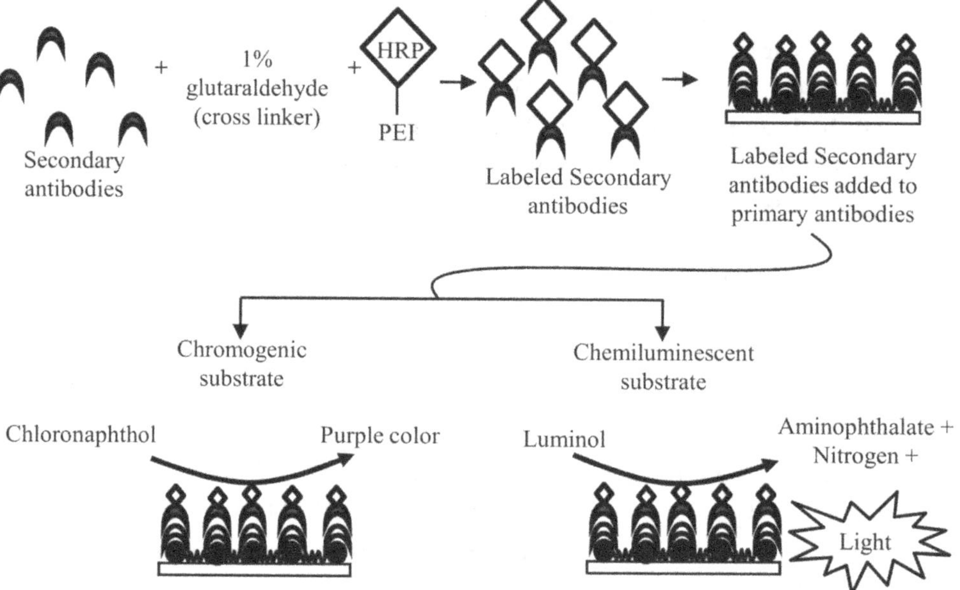

FIGURE 12.8 Labeling of secondary antibodies with HRP and its reaction with chromogenic and chemiluminescent substrate

(ii) ***Digoxigenin-antidigoxigenin System and Biotin streptavidin System:*** These two systems utilize the property of alkaline phosphatase. The enzyme alkaline phosphatase removes the phosphate group on the substrate and converts it into an intense colored dye (chromogenic) or a product which gives out light (chemilumniscent). These reactions are depicted in **Figure 12.9.** Chemiluminescence method of detection is more favored in comparison to chromogenic method because it is more sensitive than chromogenic dyes.

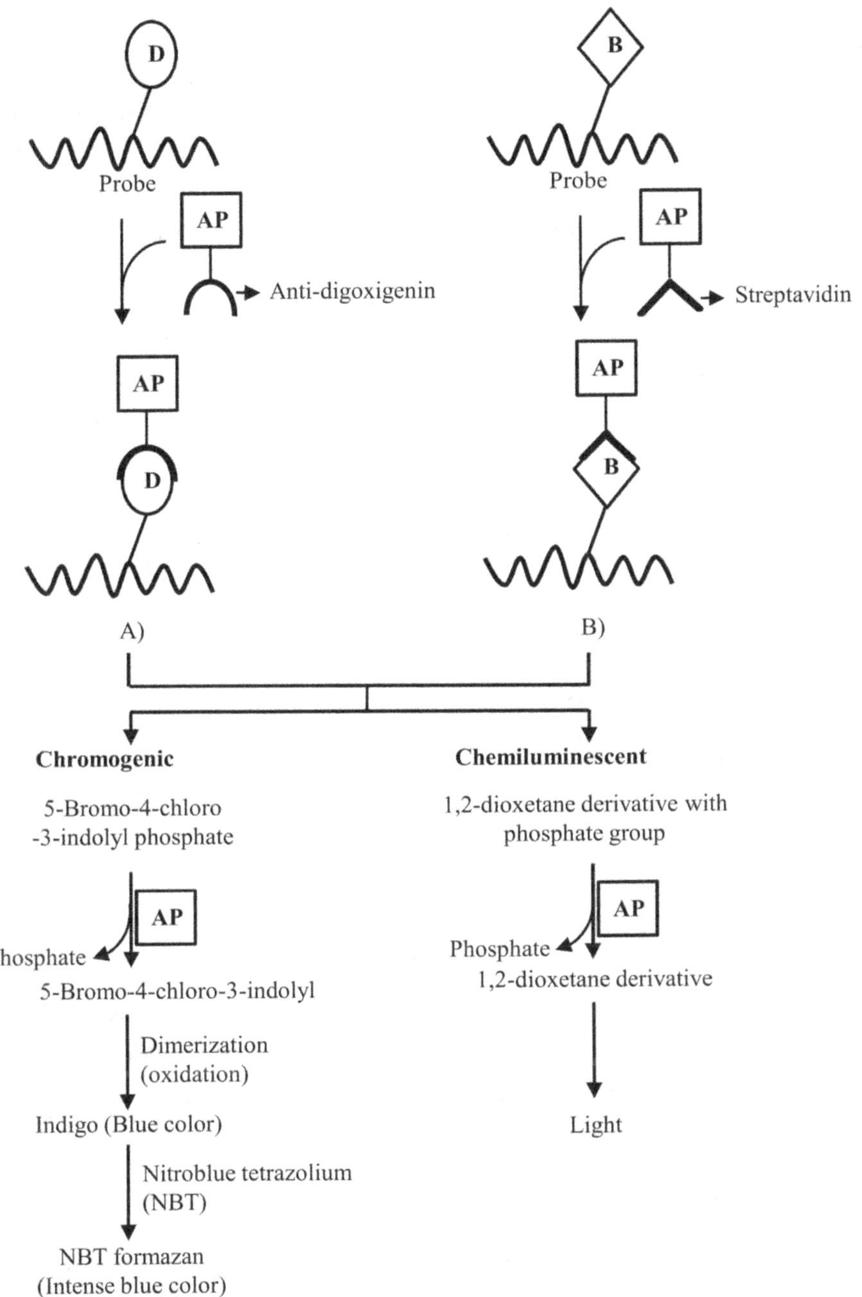

FIGURE 12.9 Depiction of chromogenic and chemiluminescent detection methods using (a) Digoxigenin-antidigoxigenin system and (b) Biotin-streptavidin system. D: Digoxigenin; AP: Alkaline phosphatase; B: Biotin.

APPLICATIONS OF WESTERN BLOTTING

Western blotting is very commonly employed technique to determine the presence of specific protein in blood or tissue or any sample. Thus, the main use of western blotting is qualitative detection of proteins.

1. It is routine test to confirm the HIV infection. Indeed, ELISA is carried to detect the presence of HIV infection. Later, confirmatory test is done using western blotting. In this test, the presence or absence of anti-HIV antibodies is checked in blood of a patient. The presence of anti-HIV antibodies is a confirmatory test for HIV infection.

2. Western blotting is also used as a confirmatory test to diagnose other viral or bacterial diseases such as viral hepatitis B, herpes simplex, Creutzfeldt-Jakob Disease and Lyme disease.

3. It is also routinely used to characterize the proteins produced by recombinant DNA technology

4. It is also used to identify 'blood doping' in which athletes consume substances to increase RBC or hemoglobin for better performance.

REVIEW QUESTIONS

TWO MARKS QUESTIONS

1. Define blotting.
2. What are different types of blotting techniques?
3. What are the most commonly employed membranes in blotting?
4. What is the advantage of nylon membrane over nitrocellulose membrane?
5. What is the importance of blocking process in blotting?

FIVE MARKS QUESTIONS

1. What are the different detection systems employed in western blotting?
2. What are the different steps involved in western blotting?
3. What are the different methods of transferring the proteins from gel to blotting membrane?

TEN MARKS QUESTIONS

1. What is blotting? What are the methods of transfer in blotting? What are the applications of blotting?

MULTIPLE CHOICE QUESTIONS

---

1. Proteins are characterized using
   (a) Southern blotting (b) Northern blotting
   (c) Western blotting   (d) Eastern blotting
2. DNA is characterized using
   (a) Southern blotting (b) Northern blotting
   (c) Western blotting   (d) Eastern blotting
3. Which of following is used as membrane for blotting?
   (a) Nylon   (b) Nitrocellulose
   (c) Polyvinylidenedifluoride (d) All the above
4. The employment of radioactive label yields:
   (a) Autoradiograph   (b) Chemilumniscence
   (c) Color change   (d) None of above
5. Blocking is done in blotting by:
   (a) Non fat milk   (b) Fat milk
   (c) Primary antibody   (d) Secondary antibody

UNIT - 3

Pharmacogenomics

13. Gene Mapping and Genetic Variations 213

14. Polymorphisms Affecting Drug Metabolism
and Drug Transporters 227

15. Proteomics Sciences 237

Gene Mapping and Genetic Variations

CHAPTER OUTLINE

Gene Mapping and Cloning of Genes
Definitions and General Features
Biochemical Approach (Functional Cloning)
Positional Cloning

Genetic Variations and Role in Pharmacology
Definitions and General Features
Genetic Polymorphism
Single Nucleotide Polymorphism (SNP)
Pharmacogenetics and Pharmacogenomics
Potential Applications of Pharmacogenetics/ Pharmacogenomics

Genetic Variations in G-Protein Coupled Receptors
Introduction and General Features
Genetic Variations in N-terminal Domain
Changes in Receptor Binding Affinity
Variations in Down-Regulation of Receptors
Variations in Transmembrane Domains
Variations in Intracellular Loop Domains
Variations in C-Terminal Domain
Variations in Non-coding Regions

GENES MAPPING AND CLONING OF GENES

DEFINITIONS AND GENERAL FEATURES

There are a number of diseases whose pathogenesis is not clear or there are gene-linked diseases, whose genes have not been identified. Therefore, it is important to identify and clone the genes responsible for diseases. Thus, cloning of genes helps in clear understanding of pathophysiology of a disease, which in turn is essential for its better management. Gene mapping has been explained in unit I **(Chapter 2)**. Cloning of diseased genes can be done by two methods:

1. **Biochemical Approach:** There are certain diseases which produce clear and well known biochemical alterations. For these diseases, cloning of genes is done using biochemical approach. This technique is also termed as functional cloning.

2. **Positional Cloning:** However, in certain disease no biochemical alterations are observed. Therefore, in these cases, genes are cloned by noting their position on chromosomes.

BIOCHEMICAL APPROACH (FUNCTIONAL CLONING)

This method is adapted if a disease is associated with alteration with functionality of protein. For example, phenylketonuria is characterized by decrease in phenylalanine hydroxylase activity and TaySachs disease is characterized by decrease in hexosaminidase A activity. The different steps in this approach include **(Figure 13.1):**

1. In the first step, the protein (whose function is altered) is isolated and purified.

2. Thereafter, the sequences of amino acids are determined in a protein.

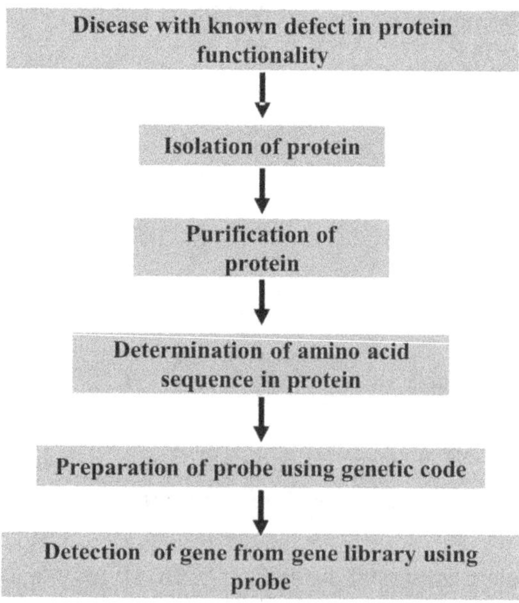

FIGURE 13.1 Different steps involved in cloning of gene using biochemical approach (Functional cloning)

3. Based on the amino acid sequence in protein, a sequence of nucleotides is prepared using the genetic code.

4. This nucleotide sequence is used to design a DNA probe. This probe is single stranded oligonucleotides (15-20 base pair long), which is used to search a DNA library.

5. Thus, probe may identify and detect the presence of specific desired gene from a DNA library.

POSITIONAL CLONING

This approach is used to clone diseased gene, whose function is not unknown. The positional cloning is also termed as 'reverse genetics'. In positional cloning, the identification of gene is done on the basis of differences in DNA sequence between affected (diseased person) and unaffected (normal) individuals. It is very useful technique when nothing is known about genes. However, it is very tedious and difficult technique to perform. The different steps involved in this process are as follows **(Figure 13.2)**:

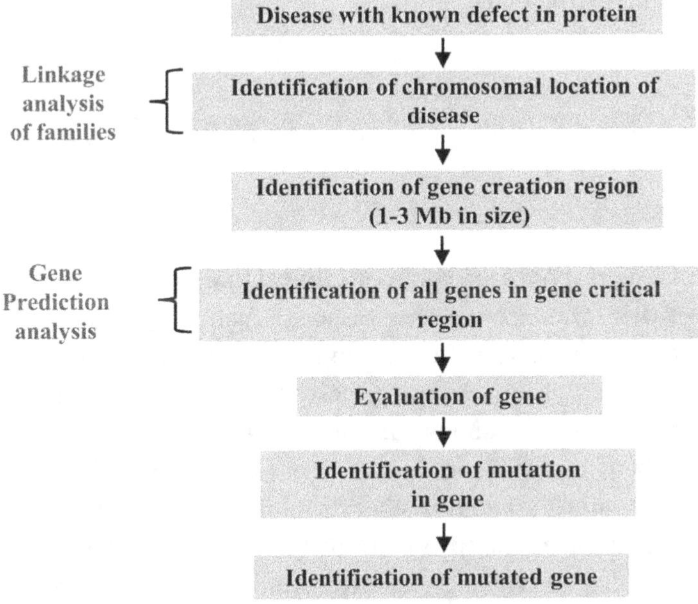

FIGURE 13.2 Steps involved in positional cloning of gene

1. **Identification of the Chromosomal Location of a Disease**: A 'linkage analysis' is performed to narrow the location of the disease to a specific chromosome. In this linkage analysis, many families are studied to follow a pattern between disease and genes.

2. **Identification of Gene Critical Region:** Once a disease is linked to some specific chromosome, the next step is to identify the area on chromosome, where diseased genes may reside. The small region where there is a strong possibility of identifying the desired gene is termed as 'gene critical region'. The gene critical region is around 1-3 Mb in size and this region must have defined borders.

3. **Identification of genes in gene critical region:** In this step, all genes located in gene critical region are identified. There may be around 25 genes in about 1000 kb of DNA. These genes are identified usually using gene prediction computer programs.

4. **Evaluation of Genes and identification of mutations in candidate genes:** After identification of all genes in the gene critical region, it is required that all genes are evaluated to identify the most promising candidate gene. The expression pattern of these genes in the body may be identified using northern blotting. Thereafter, mutations are identified in genes using techniques involving PCR.

GENETIC VARIATIONS AND ROLE IN PHARMACOLOGY

DEFINITIONS AND GENERAL FEATURES

Variations in drug response are common clinical findings in patients. There are many factors that influence the drug response such as age, gender, ethnicity, nature and severity of disease, co morbidities (other diseases), diet, patient compliance and life style etc. Amongst these factors, there is another important factor that influences the response of drugs in patients i.e. genetic variations. About 15–30 % of variations in drug response are attributed to these genetic variations. A separate branch of pharmacology has emerged to study the influence of genetic makeup on the drug response and it is termed as 'Pharmacogenetics'. Pharmacogenetics studies the influence of genetic variations on both pharmacokinetics and pharmacodynamics. The variations in drug metabolism and drug transportation may introduce variability in plasma levels of drug i.e. alters pharmacokinetics. On the other hand, variations in drug targets (receptors, ion channels etc) may alter the drug response and side effects i.e. pharmacodynamics. Amongst these, the variations in drug metabolism affecting the drug response have been widely studied.

GENETIC POLYMORPHISM

Genetic polymorphism refers to existence of many forms of a given gene. No two individuals are same and there are always some genetic variations between individuals. The genetic variability is due to variations in the DNA sequence of the genome. Therefore, there may be a change in any given gene due a variation in DNA sequence. These variable forms of a gene are called as 'alleles. An allele is also defined as a variant of a given gene or alternative form of a gene. For example, the ABO type of blood grouping is based on presence of specific antigens (A, B, AB, or none) on RBC. At the genetic level, these antigens are expressed by three different alleles, I^A, I^B, and i. Genetic polymorphism refers to occurrence of more than one allele at gene's locus (position). Moreover, the rate of occurrence of such multiple alleles for a given gene must be at least 1 %. It may also be defined as occurrence of two or more alleles at a given gene locus with at least 1 % of frequency in a population.

Genetic polymorphism may be due to multiple reasons such as single nucleotide polymorphism (SNP), insertion or deletion of nucleotides, duplication of genes etc. Amongst these, the most important reason for genetic polymorphism is SNP.

SINGLE NUCLEOTIDE POLYMORPHISM (SNP)

These represent the most common and simplest form of DNA variations. About 90 % of total variations in the human genome are due to SNPs. SNP represent a single base pair difference in nucleotides in genome. SNP can be understood by a hypothetical assumption. Let us assume at any position, say 704, there is 'T' as a base pair in a genome in most of the population. However, in some persons there may be 'G' as a base pair at 704 position. Therefore, a single base pair difference creates variations in genes and such variations are termed as single nucleotide polymorphism. In human genome, about seven million SNPs have been found. However, all SNP are not functional i.e. all variations are not represented by change in expressions. SNPs can occur in protein coding regions or in non-protein coding regions also.

I. SNP in Protein Coding Region

SNP in protein coding region are more significant and have been classified into different types (**Table 13.1**):

1. **Silent SNPs:** Even in coding region, the presence of SNP does not produce any change in protein structure or expression. Such SNP are termed as silent SNPs. The silent SNPs mainly occur if there is change in nucleotide at 3rd position of codon (wobble position).

2. **Neutral SNPs:** In this type, there is change in amino acid sequence in proteins due to SNP. However, the change in amino acid sequences does not change the functions of protein. In other words, SNP does not produce change in the functions of proteins.

3. **Missense Mutation:** SNPs lead to change in the sequence of amino acids, which may produce proteins with altered functions.

4. **Nonsense Mutation:** In this case, SNP may produce a stop codon, which results in premature termination of the polypeptide chain. Thus, the proteins produced are different from the normal proteins.

TABLE 13.1 Different types of SNPs in protein coding regions

S. No	Types of SNP	Features
1.	Silent SNPs	• No change in protein structure • There is change in nucleotide at 3rd nucleotide of codon
2.	Neutral SNPs	• There is change in amino acid sequence in proteins • But there is no change in the functions of protein
3.	Missense Mutation	• There is change in protein structure and functions
4.	Nonsense Mutation	• There may be a stop codon, which prematurely terminates the polypeptide chain • Different proteins are formed

II. SNP in Promoter, Splice Sites and Untranslated Regions

SNPs in non coding regions such as promoters, splice sites and untranslated regions are also very significant. These may produce a number of changes in proteins by changing transcriptional regulation, mRNA stability, causing splicing defects, and translation efficiency.

PHARMACOGENETICS AND PHARMACOGENOMICS

These two terms are used interchangeably and indicate the influence of genetic makeup on the effects of drugs. However, more precisely, pharmacogenetics refers to how variation in one single gene may influence the response of a single drug. On the other hand, pharmacogenomics is a more broader term and it studies how all of the genes (genome) influence the responses to drugs.

POTENTIAL APPLICATIONS OF PHARMACOGENETICS/PHARMACOGENOMICS

Pharmacogenetics has opened the doors for 'personalized medicines' i.e. prescribing drugs on the basis of genetic constitution of a patient. This has been useful in main two area of patient care:

1. **Reduction in Side Effects:** It helps in improving the drug Safety and reduces the adverse effects of drugs in patients. There are a number of examples in this category, where a particular drug has to be avoided in patients with particular genotype. Some of the examples are given below:

    (i) Glucose-6-phosphate dehydrogenase (G6PD) deficiency is the most common example of pharmacogenetics in which patients deficient in this enzymes should not be prescribed drugs like quinolones, NSAIDS, sulfonamides etc. There is a risk of hemolytic anemia in such patients due to administration of these drugs.

    (ii) Irinotecan is an anticancer drug and is used in the treatment of colon cancer. However, some patients are not able to metabolize this drug due to deficiency of 'UGT1A1 enzyme'. This leads to severe and potentially life-threatening side effects. Therefore, irinotecan is avoided in patients with UGT1A1 deficiency.

    (iii) Children suffering from acute lymphoblastic leukemia are genetically tested for the presence of an enzyme 'thiopurine methyltransferase (TPMT)', which is responsible for metabolism of anticancer drugs. Therefore, such children with deficient TPMT are given low doses of anticancer drugs.

    (iv) The patients suffering from cancers (colorectal, breast, stomach) are also tested for 'dihydropyrimidine dehydrogenase (DPD)', which helps to metabolize fluorouracil. The patients deficient in this enzyme are given lower doses of 5-fluorouracil to avoid serious side effects.

2. **Selection of Appropriate Remedy:** It also helps in selecting an appropriate remedy for a particular set of patients. There are a number of conditions in which FDA has issued guidelines for pharmacogenetics testing before selecting a remedy **(Table 13.2)**.

TABLE 13.2 Some examples of clinically approved drugs for which pharmacogenetics testing is recommended to obtain satisfactory results in patients

S. No	Drug	Indication in Disease	Gene
1.	Cetuximab and panitumumab	Colon cancer	Negative for KRAS
2.	Trastuzumab	Breast cancer	Positive for HER2
3.	Crizotinib	Non-small-cell lung cancer	Positive ALK

(i) Cetuximab and panitumumab are monoclonal antibodies that target EGFR (Epithelial Growth Factor Receptors) expressed on the colon and head cancers to exhibit anticancer effects. However, these drugs are ineffective in certain patients due to KRAS mutations. KRAS is a membrane GTPase and important constituent of EGFR signaling pathways. FDA has labeled that these drugs are prescribed after genetic testing of 'KRAS gene' and should be prescribed in patients which have EGFR-expressing and KRAS negative colon cancer.

(ii) Trastuzumab is a recombinant humanized monoclonal antibody and it specifically targets the HER2 receptors. FDA recommends that this drug has to be prescribed in breast cancer patients in which HER2 is over-expressed. In case of normal HER2 expression, this drug is not effective in breast cancer.

(iii) Crizotinib is an ALK inhibitor and has been used to treat non-small-cell lung cancer. However, FDA has issued a prescription guideline that only patients with 'ALK positive' are prescribed this drug to mange advanced or metastatic non-small-cell lung cancer.

CHALLENGES TO PHARMACOGENOMICS

Despite the rapid progress made in the field of pharmacogenetics, there are a number of challenges in its practical use in clinical setup:

1. At present these types of tests are very expensive and all patients are not able to meet the expenses of these tests.

2. These types of tests are not available in all countries especially in poor and developing countries.

3. There are some privacy, ethical and legal issues associated with genetic testing.

GENETIC VARIATIONS IN

G-PROTEIN COUPLED RECEPTORS

INTRODUCTION AND GENERAL FEATURES

GTP-binding protein (G protein)-coupled receptors (GPCRs) represent one of the major classes of proteins in human genome. Moreover, these receptors are very important targets of commonly employed drugs. About 33 % of drugs available in market produce their therapeutic effects by acting on these G protein receptors. Considering their abundance and importance in the body, there is no surprise that there exist a large number of variants of these G proteins (polymorphism). These variations in G proteins account for difference in disease susceptibility as well as variations in drug responses in different set of people.

Structurally, G protein coupled receptors have common features. These receptors possess:

(a) seven hydrophobic transmembrane helices with three intracellular and three extracellular loops

(b) N-terminal domain in the extracellular region with a number of N-glycosylation sites. Drugs or ligands bind to these extracellular regions of receptors

(c) C-terminal domain in the intracellular domain. It has sites for phosphorylation.

The genetic variations have been reported in all the important structures of these receptors and these variations influence the response of drugs.

I. Genetic Variations in N-terminal Domain

N-terminal domain is present extracellularly and its length varies from receptor to receptor. It may have 154 amino acid residues in calcitonin receptors; while 36 amino acid residues are present in rhodopsin receptors. The genetic variations in this domain influence the response of drugs in a number of different ways:

1. **Changes in Receptor Binding Affinity:** Drugs generally bind to extracellular (N-terminal) domain of these receptors. There have been variations in the gene sequence in this domain, which influence the extent of drug binding to these receptors. Some of the examples of these variations are discussed below:

   (i) There have been *Cys23Ser* variants for 5-HT$_{2C}$ receptors in humans. *Cys23Ser* refers to substitution of cysteine (Cys) with serine (Ser) at 23rd position. The functional significance of these variations has been seen in schizophrenic patients treated with clozapine, ligand of 5-HT$_{2C}$ receptors. It has been reported that person with cysteine at codon 23 responded better to clozapine than patients with serine at this position.

   (ii) There have been genetic variations that influence N-glycosylation in G proteins. *Asn40Asp* variant of opioid receptor has been found in heroin addicts. This variant receptor possesses higher affinity for endogenous endorphins than wild-type (normal) receptors.

2. **Variations in Down-Regulation of Receptors:** The continuous or persistent binding of agonists/drugs to receptors produces down-regulation of G protein receptors. However, variations have been noted in down-regulation of receptors depending on the gene sequence. Some of the examples include the followings:

   (i) There have been variations in locus of β_2 receptors and main variants include *Arg16Gly* and *Gln27Glu*. These variants differ to the extent of receptor down-regulation in the presence of agonist or drug. There is faster down-regulation of receptors in *Arg16Gly* variants, but slower in *Gln27Glu* variants. The functional significance of *Arg16Gly* variant is that patients homozygous for *Gly16* develop faster down-regulation than patients homozygous for *Arg16*. Accordingly, the response to bronchodilator (β_2 agonist) therapy is comparatively less in patients homozygous for *Gly16*.

   (ii) The variants of *Gly22Ser* for 5-HT$_{1A}$ receptors show lesser receptor down-regulation and desensitization. The functional significance of this variation may be observed in patients treated with antidepressant drugs, selective serotonin reuptake inhibitors (SSRI). The therapeutic effects of these SSRI are dependent on down-regulation of these 5-HT$_{1A}$ receptors. Therefore, variation in down-regulation in patients may be reflected in variation in therapeutic effects in such patients.

II. Variations in Transmembrane Domains

Transmembrane domains of G protein receptors are composed of seven helices imbedded in the lipid bilayer of the plasma membrane. The variations in these domains may also produce variations in receptor expression, incidences of disease occurrence or drug response.

(i)   Substitution of proline residues at 242 or 505 or 540 positions with Alanine is associated with decrease in expression (35- to 100-fold) of M_3 muscarinic receptors.

(ii) The variants of *Cys109Arg* of endothelin B receptor have been linked with the development of Hirschsprung's disease, a congenital disease characterized by the absence of ganglion cells in the distal portion of the intestinal tract.

III. Variations in Intracellular Loop Domains

Intracellular domains are primarily responsible for cell signaling pathway. The following examples can give insight view of impact of variations of this domain.

(i)   The variants of *Pro310Ser* and *Ser311Cys* of dopamine 2 receptors have been identified. It is found that ligand binding affinity of *Ser311Cys* variant is less than *Pro310Ser* variant and normal (wild-type) receptors. Apart from binding affinity, difference in cell signaling magnitude has also been identified. Normal dopamine receptors inhibit forskolin-induced increase in cAMP levels by more than 90%. However, *Pro310Ser* and *Ser311Cys* variants inhibit cAMP levels by only 24% and 58%, respectively.

(ii) Substitutions of *'Arginine'* residue decreases cell signaling transduction pathways in response to M_1 muscarinic receptor activation.

(iii) Mutation of Arg143 in $\alpha 1$ -receptors is also known to produce defects in cell signaling transduction.

(iv) Three variants *Ala623Ile, Ala623Ser*, and Ala623Val result in constitutive expression of thyroid stimulating hormone (TSH) receptors, which is responsible for decreased TSH response.

IV. Variations in C-Terminal Domain

Intracellular C-terminal of G proteins is responsible for intracellular cell signaling and these contain Serine and/or threonine residues, which serve as a site of phosphorylation.

(i)   The variations in $P2Y_2$ receptors have been associated with variations in magnitude of cell signaling. There is less IP_3 (inositol triphosphate) accumulation in *Cys334* variant in comparison to *Arg334* variant.

(ii) There is a *Ser390Arg* variant of the endothelin B (ET_B) receptor in a Japanese patient, which is associated with Hirschsprung's disease. In this variant there is no change in binding affinity for endothelin in comparison to normal receptor. However, there was decrease in cell signaling as there was decrease in intracellular calcium level and decreased inhibition of adenylyl cyclase activity.

(iii) An increase in adenylyl cyclase activity has been noted in *Arg389* variant of β_1 receptors in comparison to *Gly389* variant.

(iv) The variation at C-terminal domain of the 5-HT$_{2A}$ receptor in the form of *Tyr452* variant decreases the response to clozapine due to inhibition of intracellular cell signaling.

V. Variations in Non-coding Regions

Variations have been noted in the promoter and 5' untranslated region (UTR) of G protein coupled receptors.

(i) Genetic variations in 5' promoter region of D4 receptors have been identified, particularly -*521C/T* polymorphism. It is found that *521T* allele has less transcriptional activity than -*521C* allele.

(ii) There have been variations noted in bradykinin B$_2$ receptors and these variations are associated with development of cardiomyopathy. In *412C/G, 704C/T* and *78C/T* variants, there is a decrease in binding affinity of transcriptional factor and it results in development of dilated cardiomyopathy.

REVIEW QUESTIONS

TWO MARKS QUESTIONS

1. What do you understand by Pharmacogenetics?
2. Define genetic polymorphism.
3. What are silent SNPs?
4. What are neutral SNPs?
5. Differentiate Pharmacogenetics and Pharmacogenomics.
6. What is significance of cloning of genes?
7. What is positional cloning?
8. What is functional cloning?

FIVE MARKS QUESTIONS

1. What do you understand by Single Nucleotide Polymorphism? What are its different types?
2. How do genetic variations in N-terminal domain of G proteins produce changes in drug response?
3. What are the different steps involved in positional cloning?
4. What is functional cloning? What are the steps involved in functional cloning?

TEN MARKS QUESTIONS

1. Discuss potential applications and challenges of pharmacogenetics in health care.
2. Discuss the influence of genetic changes in G proteins on drug response.

MULTIPLE CHOICE QUESTIONS

1. Pharmacogenetics studies the influence of genetic variations on
   - (a) Pharmacokinetics
   - (b) Pharmacodynamics
   - (c) Both a and b
   - (d) None of above
2. By definition, genetic polymorphism refers to occurrence of more than one allele at gene's locus at rate of occurrence of at least
   - (a) 1 %
   - (b) 2%
   - (c) 0.5 %
   - (d) No fixed value
3. The most common cause of genetic polymorphism is humans is
   - (a) Deletion of genes
   - (b) Duplication of genes
   - (c) Addition of genes
   - (d) SNP
4. In following SNP, there is no influence of genetic variation on protein structure:
   - (a) Neutral SNP
   - (b) Silent SNP
   - (c) Missense SNP
   - (d) None of above
5. In following SNP, there is no change in the function of proteins
   - (a) Neutral SNP
   - (b) Silent SNP
   - (c) Missense SNP
   - (d) Monsense SNP

6. In following SNP, there is premature termination of polypeptide
   - (a) Neutral SNP
   - (b) Silent SNP
   - (c) Missense SNP
   - (d) Nonsense SNP

7. In Glucose-6-phosphate dehydrogenase (G6PD) deficiency, there is increased risk of
   - (a) Bone marrow depression
   - (b) Agranulocytosis
   - (c) Hemolytic anemia
   - (d) Polycythemia

8. Trastuzumab, a recombinant monoclonal antibody, is prescribed in breast cancer patients
   - (a) With normal HER2 expression
   - (b) Reduced HER2 expression
   - (c) Increase in HER2 expression
   - (d) No relation with HER2

9. The Genetic Variations in N-terminal Domain of G proteins influences
   - (a) Binding affinity
   - (b) Intracellular signal transduction pathway
   - (c) Down-regulation of receptors
   - (d) Both a and c

10. The Variations in Intracellular Loop Domains of G proteins influences
   - (a) Binding affinity
   - (b) Intracellular signal transduction pathway
   - (c) Down-regulation of receptors
   - (d) Both a and c

CHAPTER 14

Polymorphisms Affecting Drug Metabolism and Drug Transporters

CHAPTER OUTLINE

Definition and General Features
Variations in Phase I Metabolism
Cytochrome P450 2D6
Cytochrome P450 2C19 (CYP2C19)
Cytochrome P450 2C9 (CYP2C9)
CYP3A4 and CYP3A5
Variations in Phase II Metabolism

N-Acetyltransferases
Thiopurine Methyltransferase (TPMT)
UDP Glucuronyltransferases (UGTs)

Genetic Variations in Drug Transporters
Definition and General Features
ABC Transporters
Solute Carrier (SLC) Transporters

DEFINITION AND GENERAL FEATURES

There have been large inter-individual variations during drug treatment, which are largely attributed to difference in genetic makeup. Amongst the different genetic factors, the polymorphism in drug metabolizing enzymes has been mostly studied. There are a large number of examples in clinical setup in which either the response to drug therapy is diminished or adverse effects are produced due to a given drug, mainly due to variations in drug metabolizing enzymes. There may be variations in enzymes of phase I and phase II metabolic pathway. In phase I metabolism, most of the drug metabolism reactions are carried by cytochrome P450 enzyme system and a large number of variants have been reported with these enzymes.

VARIATIONS IN PHASE I METABOLISM

1. **Cytochrome P450 2D6:** The heme-containing enzyme super-family is very large and represents a diverse group of enzymes. It is responsible for

the metabolism of about 25-30% of prescription drugs including tricyclic antidepressants, selective serotonin reuptake inhibitors, antiarrhythmic drugs, antipsychotic drugs and â blockers This enzyme has the largest phenotypic variations (more than 80 allelic variants) and classic cases of variations in metabolism of drugs such as 'sparteine' and 'debrisoquine' have been identified due to variations in this enzyme. The important allelic and phenotypic variants of this include the following **(Table 14.1)**:

TABLE 14.1 Different allelic and phenotypic variants of CYP2D6

S. No	Phenotype	Allelic variants
1.	Poor Metabolizers	*CYP2D6*3, CYP2D6*8, CYP2D6*36*
2.	Intermediate Metabolizers	*CYP2D6*9, CYP2D6*10, CYP2D6*17, CYP2D6*29, CYP2D6*41*
3.	Ultrarapid Metabolizers	*CYP2D6*1, CYP2D6*2, CYP2D6*35*

A. Poor Metabolizer Phenotype: These variants have poor metabolizing activity and no functional activity. These include *CYP2D6*3, CYP2D6*8, CYP2D6*36*.

B. Intermediate Metabolizer Phenotype: These variants have intermediate metabolizing activity and these include *CYP2D6*9, CYP2D6*10, CYP2D6*17, CYP2D6*29* and *CYP2D6*41*.

C. Extensive or Ultrarapid Metabolizer Phenotype: These variants have very rapid metabolizing activity and these include *CYP2D6*1, CYP2D6*2 and CYP2D6*35*.

The distribution of these allelic variants in different populations has also been identified. *CYP2D6*10* is more common in East Asians (38% to 50%); *CYP2D6*17 is* exclusively found in Africans population (21%); *CYP2D6*2 is* present in Caucasians (25 %) and Africans (31%).

There have some significant interactions noted in patients due to presence of these variants among populations.

A. Tamoxifen in Breast Cancer: Tamoxifen is metabolised by these enzymes to form endoxifen (4-hydroxy-*N*-desmethyltamoxifen), which is more potent estrogen receptor blocker. The anticancer property of tamoxifene has been largely attributed to this metabolite. It has been found that patients with poor metabolizer phenotype of CYP2D6 have lower levels of endoxifen and there are more chances of relapse of cancer in these persons.

B. Codeine in Postgestational Women as Analgesic: Codeine is prescribed in postgestational women for pain control due to childbirth because a very small quantity of codeine is excreted in breast milk. However, in ultrarapid CYP2D6 metabolizers, very high levels of morphine are detected in neonates, which is fatal. The high level of morphine in neonates is due to very rapid conversion of codeine to morphine, which is excreted in milk.

2. **Cytochrome P450 2C19 (CYP2C19):** The genes of these enzymes are located on the chromosome 10q24 and these enzymes metabolize diazepam, omeprazole, S-mephenytoin, and biguanides. About 30 allelic variants of *CYP2C19* have been identified. The important allelic and phenotypic variants of this include the followings **(Table 14.2)**:

TABLE 14.2 Different allelic and phenotypic variants of CYP2C19

S. No	Phenotype	Allelic variants
1.	Poor Metabolizers	*CYP2C19*2, CYP2C19*3, CYP2C19*4, CYP2C19*6, CYP2C19*7*
2.	Intermediate Metabolizers	*CYP2C19*5, CYP2C19*8*
3.	Ultrarapid Metabolizers	*CYP2C19*17*

A. ***Poor Metabolizer Phenotype:*** These variants have no functional activity and these include *CYP2C19*2*, *CYP2C19*3*, *CYP2C19*4*, *CYP2C19*6* and *CYP2C19*7*.

B. ***Intermediate Metabolizer Phenotype:*** These variants have reduced metabolizing activity and these include *CYP2C19*5* and *CYP2C19*8*.

C. ***Extensive or Ultrarapid Metabolizer Phenotype:*** These variants have very rapid metabolizing activity and these include *CYP2C19*17*.

Amongst these variants, CYP2C19*2 and CYP2C19*3 are the most common variants. CYP2C19*2 variant is mainly found in South Indians (30%) and CYP2C19*3 is mainly found in the Japanese people (13%).

Examples of Functional Significance

There have been some significant interactions noted in patients due to presence of these variants among populations.

A. ***Clopidogrel as Antiplatelet Drug:*** It is a prodrug, which is metabolized by CYP2C19 to form its active metabolite. However, in *CYP2C19*2 variants,* clopidogrel is not metabolized to form active metabolite and hence, the antiplatelet effect is not observed. In contrast, patients with *CYP2C19*17* alleles exhibit increased response and adverse effects (increased bleeding) due to increased pharmacological actions are observed.

B. *Omeprazole in Peptic Ulcers:* Omeprazole is also metabolized to form an active metabolite by CYP2C19. However, due to variants of this enzyme, there is difference in therapeutic response of omeprazole and its reduced effectiveness is found in poor metabolizers.

3. **Cytochrome P450 2C9 (CYP2C9):** This enzyme is responsible for the metabolism of drugs with narrow therapeutic index such as phenytoin and warfarin. The gene coding for CYP2C9 is located on chromosome 10q24.2. Apart from phenytoin and warfarin, this enzyme metabolizes other drugs (about 25% of clinically-available) including flurbiprofen, glipizide, tolbutamide. CYP2C9*1 is normal or wild type allele with normal enzymatic activity. However, CYP2C9*2 and CYP2C9*3 represent variants with highly-reduced enzymatic activities (poor metabolizers).

Examples of Functional Significance

There are some significant interactions noted in patients due to presence of these variants among populations.

A. *Phenytoin as Antiepileptic Drug:* CYP2C9 is an important enzyme for metabolism of phenytoin. Since this drug has narrow therapeutic index, therefore, decrease in CYP2C9 activity may increase the levels of phenytoin to produce toxicity.

B. *Warfarin as Anticoagulant:* Clinically available warfarin is a racemic mixture of the R and S enantiomers. However, S-isomer has high therapeutic activity than R-isomer (5 times more activity). S-warfarin is exclusively metabolized by CYP2C9 enzyme. Therefore, the metabolism of warfarin is near normal in CYP2C9*1 variants. However, the metabolism of S-warfarin is impaired in patients possessing CYP2C9*2 and CYP2C9*3 variants. Thus, these patients are more prone to bleeding in response to warfarin therapy.

4. **CYP3A4 and CYP3A5:** CYP3A4 is the most abundant enzyme in the liver and is responsible for metabolism of more than 50% of clinically-administered drugs such as immunosuppressants, anticancer drugs, macrolide antibiotics, opium, calcium channel blockers and statins. More than 26 variants of CYP3A4 are identified and these variants have different enzymatic activities. CYP3A4*2 and CYP3A4*3 variants are observed in Caucasian population. However, CYP3A4*18 variant is present in Chinese

people. Nevertheless, the clinical significance of these variants has not been identified till date. CYP3A5 is related to CYP3A4 and it has a broad overlap in substrate specificity with CYP3A4.

VARIATIONS IN PHASE II METABOLISM

1. **N-Acetyltransferases:** A classic clinical example of influence of variations in enzyme activity of N-acetyltransferases has been on antituberculosis agent, isoniazid. Indeed, the decreased metabolism of isoniazid in 'slow acetylators' (variants with decreased N-acetyltransferases activity) develop peripheral neuritis. However, this side effect does not appear in 'fast acetylators'. Similarly, slow acetylators are more prone to develop Systemic Lupus Erythematosus (SLE) in patients taking hydralazine.

2. **Thiopurine Methyltransferase (TPMT):** Different purine analogues such as 6-mercaptopurine and azathioprine have been used for the treatment of hematologic malignancies. These drugs are converted to thioguanine nucleotides, which are incorporated in DNA strands to produce DNA damage. These thioguanine nucleotides are metabolized in blood cells by enzyme TPMT. However, the patients with low TPMT activity have higher levels of thioguanine nucleotides in blood cells, leading to adverse effects like drug-induced neutropenia. On the other hand, patients with high TPMT activity have low levels of thioguanine nucleotides in blood cells, leading to decreased anticancer activity of purine analogues.

3. **UDP Glucuronyltransferases (UGTs):** These enzymes are very important part of phase II metabolism pathway. There have been variants of UGT and patients with absence of UGT activity tend to develop Gilbert syndrome, characterized by development of mild hyperbilirubinemia. Similarly, these variants also develop severe hematologic and gastrointestinal side effects in response to treatment with antineoplastic agent, irinotecan.

GENETIC VARIATIONS IN DRUG TRANSPORTERS

DEFINITION AND GENERAL FEATURES

Drug transporters are responsible for movement of drugs and metabolites into or out of cells. Thus, variations (polymorphisms) in genes encoding for drug transporters can significantly affect pharmacokinetics of drugs including absorption, distribution, and excretion. These processes in turn affect the effectiveness and safety of drugs. Drug transporters may be broadly classified into two classes, ABC and solute-carrier (SLC) transporters.

ABC TRANSPORTERS

ABC stands for ATP Binding Cassette and these transporters utilize ATP for the transport of drugs across the concentration gradient i.e., active gradient. The different members of this super-family of transporters are encoded by 49 genes. Furthermore, these transporters have been categorized in seven subfamilies from ABCA, ABCB, ABCC, ABCD, ABCE, ABCF and ABCG.

1. **ABCB1:** This gene is also termed as multidrug resistance 1 (MDR1) and it encodes a P-glycoprotein, which utilizes ATP to remove (efflux) various drugs from the cells. Since, this P-glycoprotein pump (efflux pump) removes drugs (such as anticancer drugs) outside the cells, therefore, cells becomes resistant to actions of drugs. Therefore, genes encoding these transporters are also termed as 'multidrug resistance genes'. There are a number of allelic variants for this ABCB1 gene. Amongst these variants, a single nucleotide polymorphism (SNP) at 3435C >T is very common. This variant is very commonly found in Asians (60%–72%) and Caucasians (34%–42%) population. However, this variant is uncommon in African people.

   These transporters are located on different sites in the body:

   (i) Surface of epithelial cells: These are widely present on the surface of epithelial cells of gastrointestinal tract. Thus, these mainly act to prevent the intestinal absorption of drugs.

   (ii) In Fetus: These transporter proteins prevent the entry of drugs in fetus from pregnant woman. Thus, these tend to protect fetus from harmful effects of drugs or foreign chemicals.

   (iii) Blood Brain Barrier: These are also located on blood brain barrier and efflux the drug from brain into periphery. Thus, these tend to protect the brain from drugs and xenobiotics.

   (iv) Kidney and Liver: These transporters operate to remove the drugs from kidney and from liver i.e. they enhance renal and hepatic excretion of drugs.

Functional Significance

Considering their wide spread distribution, it may be assumed that genetic polymorphism may significantly affect the efflux of drugs from the cells to alter their therapeutic response.

   (i) Overexpression of these genes in cancer cells makes the cells resistant to anticancer drugs.

(ii) The uncommon occurrence of 3435C >T variant in African people is correlated with decrease incidence of renal cell carcinoma in African people.

(iii) Since, many drugs employ ABCB1 transporter for their transportation; therefore, persons with allelic variants exhibit variable plasma levels of drugs e.g digoxin, cyclosporin, and fenofexadine etc.

2. **ABCC1 and ABCC2:** These two transporters are also important for transport and excretion of drugs such as anticancer drugs, toxic chemicals etc. For the transport of some molecules such as estrone sulfate, these transporters require the presence of glutathione co-transporters. There have been a number of variants (SNP) of these transporters such as V417I and G671V. G671V is a common variant in Caucasians (28%). V417I is a common variant in Asians (13%–19%), Africans (14%) and Caucasians (22%–26%). There variants have been associated with the development of drug resistance in patients suffering from cancer and AIDS.

3. **ABCG2:** This is also named as 'breast cancer resistance protein' (BCRP) or 'placenta-specific ABC protein' (ABCP). Nevertheless, this gene was first discovered in multidrug-resistant cell lines. Till date about 80 polymorphisms of ABCG2 gene have been detected. Amongst these variants, SNP C421A is widely studied and this variant has reduced transport activity. C421A variant is widely distributed in Asians (27%–35%) and Caucasians (9%–14%). Due to presence of this variant, the greater accumulation of anticancer drug, gefitinib has been seen in cells, which leads to greater side effects.

SOLUTE CARRIER (SLC) TRANSPORTERS

The members of this super-family of transporters are encoded by around 360 genes. Furthermore, the different members have been categorized in 46 subfamilies. Amongst all members, organic anion transporter (OAT), organic anion transporting polypeptides (OATP), and organic cation transporter (OCT) are more widely studied. The variants have been noted in these members due to polymorphisms in genes SLCO, SLC22, and SLC47.

1. **Organic Anion Transporting Polypeptides (OATPs):** This family of transporters is responsible for influx (cellular uptake) of endogenous as well as exogenous substances such as bile salts, hormones, antibiotics, cardiac glycosides, and anticancer agents. This family has 11 members including OATP1A2, OATP1B1, OATP1B3, OATP2B1, and OATPC. The various variants and their functional significance may be illustrated as follows:

(i) OATP1B1 transporter is encoded by SLCO1B1 and it is present on hepatocytes. It is essential for the hepatic uptake of simvastatin. However, 521T> C variant (SNP) of SLCO1B1 is associated with reduced OATP1B1 activity. Due to reduced activity of this transporter on hepatocytes, the hepatic uptake of simvastatin is reduced. It leads to an increase in levels of drug in blood, which is responsible for reduced efficacy as well as increase in toxicity.

(ii) The variants of OATPC i.e., OATPC*5 and OATPC*9 lead to decrease in transporter activity and it leads to reduced uptake of estrone sulfate.

2. **Organic Cation Transporter (OCT):** These transporters are encoded by SLC22A genes. There are three isoforms of this transporter family i.e. OCT1, OCT2, and OCT3. These transporters are primarily located on basolateral cell membrane of the renal proximal tubule. OCT2 270S variant has low transporter activity, while OCT2 270A variant has high transporter activity. Metformin, antidiabetic drug, is mainly excreted through kidney. Therefore, patients with OCT2 270A variant rapidly excrete metformin and decreased plasma levels of metformin are observed. On the other hand, patients with OCT2 270S variant have low transporter activity. Therefore, there is decrease in metformin excretion, leading to increase in its plasma levels.

REVIEW QUESTIONS

TWO MARKS QUESTIONS

1. How may variations in N-Acetyltransferases produce variations in response to drugs?

2. How may variations in Thiopurine Methyltransferase affect therapeutic response of drugs?

3. Enlist drugs whose responses are altered due to variations in Cytochrome P450 2D6?

4. How may persons be classified on the basis of variations in drug metabolizing enzymes?

5. What are ABC transporters?

6. What is the role of solute carrier transporters?

FIVE MARKS QUESTIONS

1. What is Cytochrome P450 2D6? How do variations in this enzyme alter response of drugs?
2. How do genetic variations in Cytochrome P450 2C19 account for variable responses?
3. What are solute carrier (SLC) transporters? What is their significance in altering the drug response due to genetic variations?

TEN MARKS QUESTIONS

1. How do variations in enzymes controlling phase I metabolism affect drug response?
2. How do variations in ABC transporters affect drug response?

MULTIPLE CHOICE QUESTIONS

1. In some persons, decrease in metformin levels is noted with its usual dose. It happens due to genetic variations in
   - (a) ABC transporters
   - (b) SLC transporters
   - (c) Cytochrome enzymes
   - (d) All the above
2. Multidrug resistance gene is related to
   - (a) ABC transporters
   - (b) SLC transporters
   - (c) Cytochrome enzymes
   - (d) All the above
3. ABC transporters use
   - (a) Active transport
   - (b) Passive transport
   - (c) Facilitated transport
   - (d) None of above
4. Gilbert syndrome, characterized by development of mild hyperbilirubinemia is due to deficiency of
   - (a) ABC transporters
   - (b) SLC transporters
   - (c) UDP Glucuronyltransferases
   - (d) N acetyl transferases

5. Isoniazid may lead to peripheral neuritis due to decrease in
   (a) ABC transporters
   (b) SLC transporters
   (c) UDP Glucuronyltransferases
   (d) N acetyl transferases

6. The metabolism of S-warfarin is normal in patients
   (a) CYP2C9*2   (b) CYP2C9*3
   (c) CYP2C9*1   (d) None of above

7. The effects of clopidogrel are not observed in following variants
   (a) CYP2C19*2   (b) CYP2C19*17
   (c) Both **a** and **b**   (d) None of above

CHAPTER 15

Proteomics Sciences

CHAPTER OUTLINE

Proteomics
Definition and General Features
Types of Proteomics
Techniques and Steps Involved in
Proteomics
Applications of Proteomics

Genomics
Definition and General Features
Genome Analysis
Different Areas of Genomics
Applications of Genomics

Metabolomics
Definition and General Features

Type of Metabolites
Techniques and Steps Involved in
Metabolomics
Applications of Metabolomics

Nutrigenomics
Definitions and General Features
Common Examples of Nutrigenomics
Potential Applications of Nutrigenomics

Functionomics
Definitions and General Features
Potential Applications

PROTEOMICS

DEFINITION AND GENERAL FEATURES

The word 'proteome' refers to the complete set of proteins in an individual and it is analogous to word genome which refers to complete set of inherited genes in an individual. Proteome is derived from genome by gene expression. Proteomics refers to large scale study of total proteins of an individual. In other words, proteomics also refers to identification and analysis of entire protein content. In comparison to genomics, proteomics is more complicated because genome remains almost constant in an organism. On the other hand, proteome differs from cell to cell and from time to time because expression of genes varies depending on cell and time.

TYPES OF PROTEOMICS

It may be broadly classified into three types **(Table 15.1)**:

TABLE 15.1 Different types of proteomics with key characteristics

S. No	Types of Proteomics	Features
1.	Functional Proteomics	• Elucidate the functions of proteins· Characterize enzyme activities, significance of protein-protein, protein-DNA/RNA interactions
2.	Structural Proteomics	• Characterize the 3D structures of proteins • Identify potential proteins-protein interacting and drug binding sites· Identify post-translational modifications of the proteins
3.	Expression Proteomics	• Analyze protein expression· Identify the differences in protein expression in normal and diseased cell

1. **Functional Proteomics:** The major goal of functional proteomics is to elucidate the biological functions of proteins. It includes identifying protein functions, characterization of enzyme activities, significance of protein-protein, protein-DNA/RNA interactions. This type of proteomics is performed by large-scale measurement of enzymatic activities of kinase, phosphatase, proteases or other protein modifying enzymes. Alternatively, identifying epigenetic modifications at proteins may also be used to study functional proteomics.

2. **Structural Proteomics:** The major goal of structural proteomics is to characterize the three-dimensional structures of proteins. It helps in understanding the target sites of proteins, where drugs bind. It also helps to elucidate the potential proteins-protein interacting sites. The identification of post-translational modifications of the proteins also constitutes structural proteomics. The different types of post-translational modifications in proteins include phosphorylation, ubiquitination, methylation, acetylation, glycosylation, oxidation and nitrosylation. This type of proteomics is generally done using X-ray crystallography and NMR spectroscopy.

3. **Expression Proteomics:** It is also termed as differential proteomics and its objective to identify or analyze protein expression in an organism. Its major application is to identify the differences in protein expression in normal and diseased cell/tissue. The identification of differences in protein expression in a disease condition projects that protein as potential drug target.

Expression proteomics is generally done using 2D-gel electrophoresis and mass spectrometry.

TECHNIQUES AND STEPS INVOLVED IN PROTEOMICS

Proteomics involves some basic steps and these include the followings **(Figure 15.1)**:

I. Protein Extraction and Purification

This is the initial step and it involves extraction of proteins from tissues. It is followed by purification of proteins and removal of non-protein portions. The purification of proteins may be achieved using density gradient centrifugation, size exclusion chromatography or affinity chromatography etc.

II. Separation of Proteins

In a subsequent step, extracted and purified proteins are separated depending on their size, shape or charge. The separation techniques may include following:

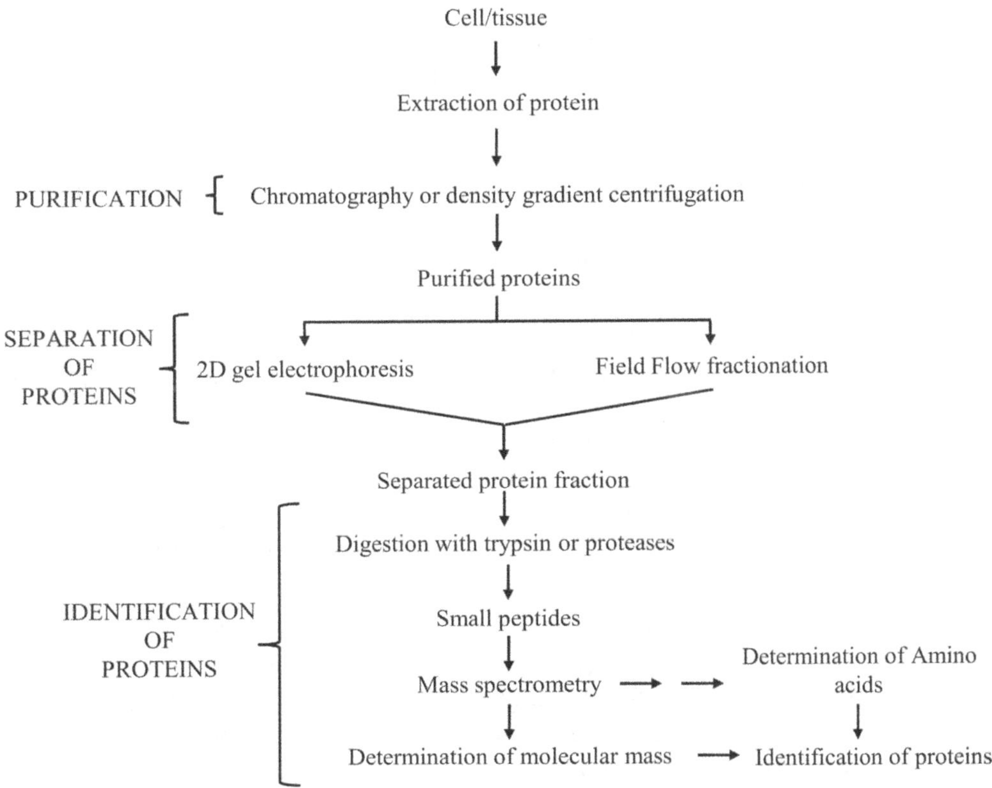

FIGURE 15.1 Steps and techniques involved in proteomics

1. **Two Dimensional-Gel Electrophoresis:** This is very commonly employed technique for protein separation as it can distinguish up to 10,000 proteins. In this type of electrophoresis, proteins are separated based on their charges in one dimension. Thereafter, gel is turned 90 degrees from its initial position and proteins are separated on the basis of difference in their size. Since the separation occurs in second dimension, therefore, this technique is termed as 2D-gel electrophoresis. Mostly, polyacrylamide gel (PAGE) is employed; therefore, this process is also termed as 2D-PAGE. The steps involved in separation of proteins involve the followings:

    (i) *Isoelectric Focusing (First Dimension Separation):* It is first stage or first dimensional protein separation on the basis of difference in isoelectric points (pI). Proteins are different from one another depending on the isoelectric point and no two proteins have same isoelectric point. Isoelectric point of a protein is a pH, where overall charge on proteins becomes zero. In this technique, a pH gradient is created in a gel, protein sample is loaded and electric current is applied. Proteins migrate towards cathode or anode depending on their charge. However, protein stop moving at the point of gel, where pH is equals pI of a protein. Because proteins move till there is charge on them and when charge becomes zero, they top moving. Thus, different proteins stop at different points on a gel and in this way, these proteins are separated from one another. Therefore, the first dimension separation of proteins is done on the basis of their charges.

    (ii) *Second Dimension Separation:* After first dimension separation, electric current is applied perpendicular to the original orientation of electrodes. Proteins start migrating in second direction in the gel depending on their size and shape.

    (iii) *Isolation of separated proteins:* Following 2D electrophoresis, the separated proteins bands are visualized by staining methods **(described in gel electrophoresis chapter)**. In differential expression proteomics, the protein maps (separated pattern of proteins) of healthy and diseased tissues are compared to analyze the difference in expression of proteins. Moreover, gel area containing protein bands are cut and proteins are isolated from gel pieces to identify the nature of proteins by mass spectrometry.

2. **Field Flow Fractionation (FFF):** It is a separative technique in which a sample protein is pumped through a long and narrow channel and field (electric, gravitational, magnetic, thermal or centrifugal) is applied perpendicular to the direction of flow. This application of field separates different proteins in a sample, depending on their different mobilities under the force exerted by the field.

III. Identification of Proteins

1. **Immunoassays:** These constitute one of the mostly commonly employed methods to analyze proteins. The basis of immunoassays is detection of protein (antigen or antibody) by formation of specific immune complex (antigen-antibody complex). ELISA **(Discussed in ELISA and Microarray Chapter)** and western blotting are more commonly employed immunoassays. In western blotting, protein mixture is separated in gel electrophoresis. Thereafter, separated proteins are transferred to a membrane and transferred proteins are analyzed by specific binding with antibodies.

2. **Protein Chips and Microarrays:** The major advantage of using protein chips and micro arrays is that thousands of protein may be detected in a short span of time **(Discussed in ELISA and Microarray Chapter).**

3. **Mass Spectrometry:** It is a method that helps in precise measurement of molecular weight of a substance including proteins. It is required that for mass spectrometry, substances have to be gaseous phase. Therefore, the use of mass spectrometry for protein analysis was possible with the advent of 'matrix assisted laser detection of desorption/ionization' (MALDI) and 'electrospray ionization' (ESI). The different steps in mass spectrometry include the followings:

   (i)   The proteins are digested with the help of proteolytic enzymes such as trypsin to form smaller peptides. Thereafter, the molecular weights of peptides are measured using mass spectrometry.

   (ii) It is followed by analysis of protein molecules by MALDI-based peptide mass fingerprinting.

   (iii) The spectra of molecular weights obtained from mass spectrometry are compared with theoretical spectra calculated from protein sequences from available databases. In other words, the sequence of amino acids determined from mass spectrometry is compared with available database to validate the structure of proteins.

APPLICATIONS OF PROTEOMICS

1. The major use of proteomics is to understand the structure and function of different proteins. Furthermore, it also helps in understanding protein-protein interactions in an individual.

2. Proteomics studies is of great help in pathophysiology of diseases as it helps in detecting defects in protein structure, function or expression pattern in association with diseases.

3. Proteomics may be useful in creating 'biomarkers'. Biomarker is a characteristic molecule that is objectively measured and evaluated a disease

indicator. Proteomics is very useful in identifying biomarkers that may be used to diagnose disease.

4. Proteomics is very important in drug development because most of times proteins are employed as drug targets. Identifying the correlation between development of disease and alteration in protein helps scientists to develop new drugs.

GENOMICS

DEFINITION AND GENERAL FEATURES

Genomics is the interdisciplinary branch of science dealing with study of structure and functions of genomes. A genome refers to complete set of genes in an organism. It studies the expression of genes to produce proteins along with sequencing and analysis of genome **(Table 15.2)**. The entire genome of humans was decoded in 2003 as 'Human Genome Project'. As per its report, about 22,300 protein-coding genes have been identified in human beings.

TABLE 15.2 Key Differences between genome and genetics

S. No	Genomics	Genetics
1.	It deals with collective study of all genes of an organism i.e genes genome	It deals with study of individual genes genome
2.	It deals with study of expression of genes along with sequencing and analysis of genome	It deals with inheritance of characters

GENOME ANALYSIS

Genome analysis involves three steps **(Figure 15.2)**:

(a) Sequencing of DNA

(b) Assembly of gene sequences to create a representation of the original chromosome,

(c) Annotation and analysis of representation of chromosome

1. **Sequencing of DNA (Gene Sequencing):** The details of gene sequencing are discussed in separate chapter **(Gene Sequencing Chapter, Unit I).**

2. **Assembly of Gene Sequences:** In gene sequencing, small DNA portions are studied at a time, about 20 to 1000 base pair long. However, chromosomes are much bigger units. Therefore, DNA sequences of all short pieces of

DNA are merged or aligned or assembled to reconstruct the sequence of whole chromosome. This process of aligning and merging fragment of DNA to create a representation of original chromosome is called as assembly of genes sequences.

3. **Annotation:** This is also an important step of gene analysis and it involves attaching the biological information to DNA sequences. In other words, the biological role of different DNA sequences is determined. In involves identifying portions of DNA which do not encode proteins and which actually encode proteins.

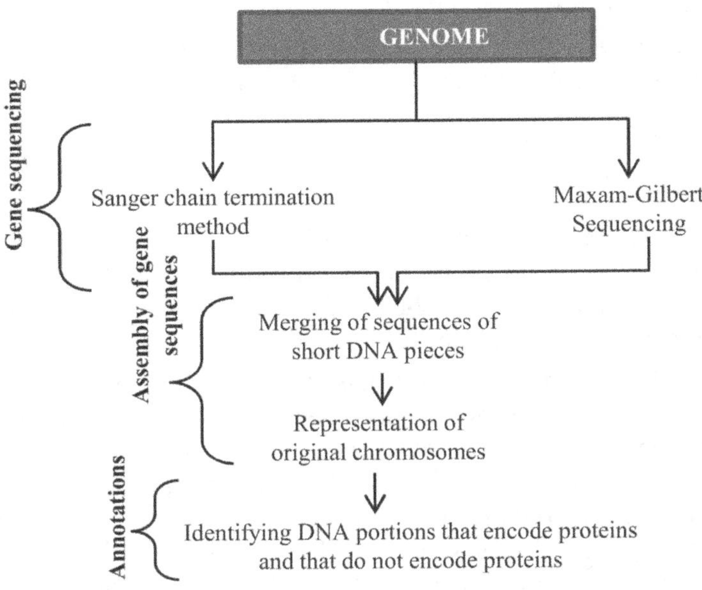

FIGURE 15.2 Three key steps involved in gene analysis

DIFFERENT AREAS OF GENOMICS

1. **Functional Genomics:** The main aim of this type of genomics to describe the functions of genes and their interactions. It includes study of gene functions, gene transcription, translation and protein interactions. The expression levels of RNA and proteins are measured to understand the biological function of the genes. It also studies the complex interactions between genotypes.

2. **Structural Genomics:** It studies the three dimensional structures of proteins encoded by gene. Indeed, using high throughput technology, structures of proteins are determined using experimental and modeling approaches. Structural genomics aims to reveal the structure of every protein encoded by genome.

3. **Epigenomics:** It refers to study of all epigenetic changes in genome. Epigenetic modifications refer to all those modifications that lead to alteration in protein expression without any change in DNA sequence. Two major types of epigenetic modifications include histone acetylation/deacetylation and DNA methylation/demethylation.

4. **Metagenomics:** Metagenomics refers to the study of the metagenome. The term metagenome is used to refer to a collective genome of microorganisms obtained from an environmental sample. This type of genomics is also termed as 'environmental' or 'community genomics'. The main aim of this type of genomics is to understand the microbial diversity and ecology a specific environment.

5. **Comparative Genomics:** It refers to comparative differences in genomes of different species such as humans, rodents, monkeys etc.

APPLICATIONS OF GENOMICS

1. **Genomic Medicine:** It refers to new medical discipline in which genomic information of the patient is used for diagnosis or therapeutic decision-making in clinics. This is an emerging field of medicine and research is underway to fully explore its potential in clinics.

  (i) *Genome Based Diagnosis:* FDA has approved about 5 human genetic tests, and more than 100 nucleic acid-based tests for microbial pathogens. Gene sequencing is used to investigate outbreaks of infectious diseases such as Ebola virus, drug-resistant Staphylococcus aureas and Klebsiella pneumoniae, bacterial meningoencephalitis. Gene sequencing also used to diagnose genetic diseases such as sickle cell anemia and cystic fibrosis. The presence of biomarkers of cancers in the blood is detected by doing DNA sequencing of fragments released by tumors in the blood.

  (ii) *Personalized Medicine (Pharmacogenomics):* It is the application of genomics in medicine in which genetic makeup of patient is studied and a drug is given according to the genotype of that patient. In other words, a single drug cannot produce similar effects in all humans due to difference in genetic makeup. Thus, the response of a drug varies from one person to another. Therefore, a decision of giving a particular drug to patient is guided by genetic makeup of that individual.

2. **Creation of Synthetic Species:** The applications of genomics have expanded in the field of biotechnology to produce partially synthetic species of bacteria. For example, the genome of *Mycoplasma genitalium* has been used a template to synthesize new bacterium *Mycoplasma laboratorium*, which is distinct from original bacteria.

3. **Conversation of Species:** Environmentalists have employed genomics to conserve extinct species.

METABOLOMICS

DEFINITION AND GENERAL FEATURES

The term 'metabolome' refers to all metabolites in a cell, tissue, organ or organism, which are the end products of cellular and chemical processes. It includes all metabolites such as metabolic intermediates, hormones, signaling molecules, and secondary metabolites present in biological tissues. The scientific study of metabolome is termed as 'metabolomics'. Therefore, metabolomics may also be defined as the scientific study of chemical processes involving metabolites. It involves study of biological fluids to analyze the changes in metabolites and correlate with the disease development. Indeed, the picture of biological fluid can give an indication about the health of an individual. The development of advanced form of analytical techniques such as gas chromatography-mass spectrometry (GC-MS) helped in measuring metabolites in human urine or tissue extracts and metabolic profile could be created. Later, NMR spectroscopy also helped in identifying and measuring different metabolites in the body fluids. Under the Human Metabolome Project, the team of Dr. David Wishart of the University of Alberta, Canada, completed the first draft of the human metabolome in 2017 and it included database of approximately 2500 metabolites, 1200 drugs and 3500 food components.

There is another term 'metabonomics' which is defined as quantitative measurement of the metabolic response of an individual to pathophysiological stimuli or genetic modification. In other words, it is concerned with changes in metabolites in the body in response to environmental stimuli such as infectious agents, toxins or genetic manipulations **(Table 15.3).** Metabolomics is very complex as the levels and nature of metabolites keep on changing very rapidly. Mostly, metabolic profiling is done using biofluids such as blood or urine, which are easily obtained from body.

TABLE 15.3 Differences between metabolomics and metabonomics

S. No	Metabolomics	Metabonomics
1.	The major emphasis is on metabolic profiling at a cellular or organ level and is concerned with normal endogenous metabolism	The major emphasis is on quantitative changes in metabolic profile in diseases condition or due to external stimuli
2.	The metabolic profiling is done using mass spectrometry-based techniques	The metabolic profiling is done using NMR

TYPE OF METABOLITES

Metabolites are intermediate products of any metabolism and in metabolomics, metabolites is generally a small size molecule with size less than 1 kDa except for albumin and lipoproteins, which are large sized metabolites. In metabolome, there is a complex network of enzymatically controlled metabolic reactions. In these reactions, metabolites formed as end product of one reaction becomes reactant of another metabolic reaction. In humans, metabolites may be:

1. **Endogenous metabolites:** These are formed inside the body and these include glucose, hormones etc.

2. **Exogenous metabolites:** These are foreign in nature and enter in the body from outside e.g. drugs. These are also termed as xenometabolites. The study of such extracellular (foreign) metabolites is termed as   'exometabolomics'.

In plants, metabolites are classified as primary or secondary metabolites

1. **Primary Metabolites:** These are produced by plants and these are required for growth, differentiation and reproduction.

2. **Secondary Metabolites:** It is also produced by plants. However, these are not as essential for plants as primary metabolites. These are generally isolated by humans for the commercial use e.g. drugs, dyes etc.

TECHNIQUES AND STEPS INVOLVED IN METABOLOMICS

There are two main steps in metabolomics, separation of metabolites and detection of metabolites **(Figure 15.3)**.

1. **Separation of Metabolites:** Samples containing metabolites are very complex; therefore, it is essential to separate these metabolites before their analysis. However, NMR based detection methods do not require separation steps. However, for mass spectrometry based detection methods, it is essential to separate these metabolites from complex mixture.

   There are different methods that may be used for separation and these include:

   (i) *Gas Chromatography (GC):* It is widely used technique for this purpose and it is used in association with mass spectrometry (MS); therefore the combined technique is termed as GC-MS. It has very high resolution. However, it is important to understand that metabolites have to be in gaseous (volatile) state for their separation. Therefore, metabolites are chemically modified (derivatization) to make gaseous.

   (ii) *High Performance Liquid Chromatography (HPLC):* It is also used in association with mass spectrometry and combination is termed as LC-MS. It has the advantage that metabolites may be separated in liquid phase also (unlike GC). However, it has less resolution in comparison to gas chromatography.

(iii) *Capillary Electrophoresis*: It is useful for charged metabolites and suitable for wider range of metabolites than gas chromatography.

2. Detection (Analysis) Methods

(i) Nuclear Magnetic Resonance (NMR): It is very useful technique as it does not require the separation of metabolties before analysis/detection. Furthermore, all metabolites may be measure simultaneously. Therefore, NMR may also be termed as universal detector.

(ii) Mass Spectrometry (MS): It is used along with GC, HPLC or capillary electrophoresis to analyze metabolites. In this technique, metabolites are fragmented and from fragmentation pattern, structures of metabolites are elucidated.

In mass spectrometry, metabolites are provided a charge and transferred to the gas phase. There are different methods to provide charge and these include 'electron ionization (EI)', atmospheric-pressure chemical ionization (APCI), and electrospray ionization (ESI). There is development of different technologies in MS to measure a large number of metabolites in a complex mixture of biofluid. These include Nanostructure-Initiator MS (NIMS), MALDI and Secondary ion mass spectrometry (SIMS).

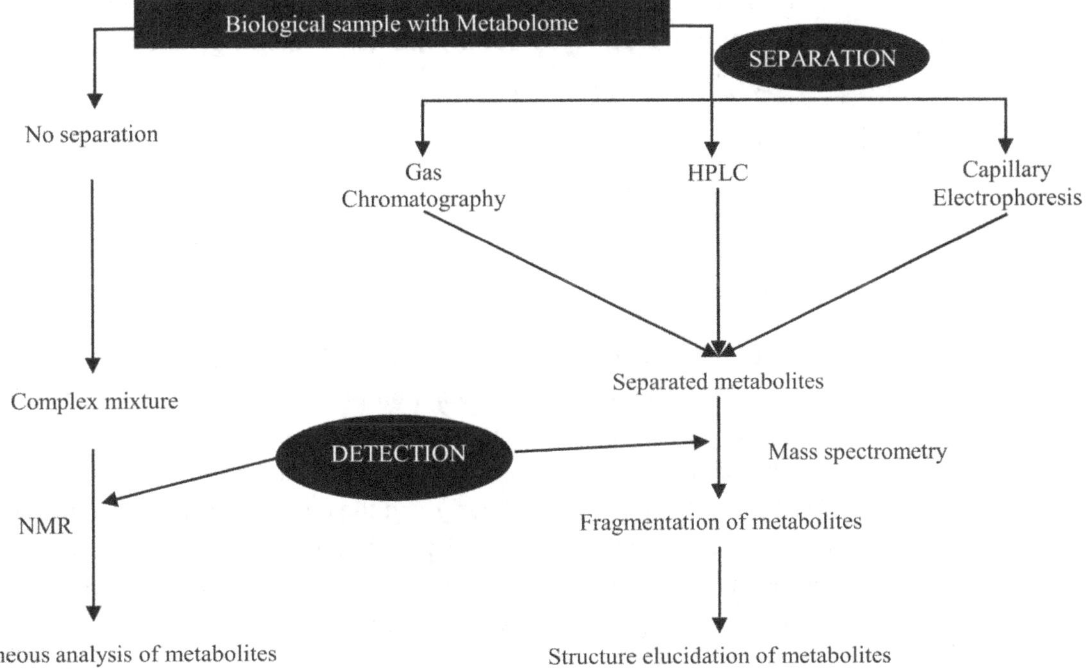

FIGURE 15.3 Techniques and steps involved in Metabolomics

APPLICATIONS OF METABOLOMICS

It is one of emerging field with a large number of potential applications. These include:

1. **Disease Diagnosis:** One of the important applications of identifying metabolites in biofluids is that these can define the state of a person i.e. healthy, diseased or prone to disease. For example, an increase in glucose (in diabetes mellitus) is metabolic change and appearance of proteins in urine (diabetic nephropathy) is an indicative of disease. Accordingly, metabolic profile of a person may be used to define the health of a person.

2. **Toxicity assessment:** Metabolic profiling may be used to detect the physiological changes induced by toxic chemicals. Thus, toxicity potential of any chemical such as new drug may be assessed by generating metabolic profile in the presence of chemical, whose toxicity is to be evaluated.

3. **In Functional genomics:** Metabolomics may be used to determine the phenotype changes due to genetic alteration. Any change in DNA or genome is represented by alteration in metabolites. Thus, alteration in genomics is represented in the form of alteration metabolic profile.

4. **Environmental metabolomics:** Metabolomics is also used to understand the functional interactions between living organisms with environment. Thus, it may provide valuable information regarding function and health of organisms.

NUTRIGENOMICS

DEFINITIONS AND GENERAL FEATURES

It is the branch of genomics, which studies the influence of genetic variation on nutrition and influence of nutrients on genes. In this branch, a correlation is made between gene expression and metabolism of nutrients. It has been the advancement in nutritional sciences by incorporation of genomics with nutrition. Accordingly, nutrigenomics has given the concept of 'personalized nutrition' i.e., giving nutrition of persons depending on its genotype. A term 'nutriome' has been introduced which refers to ideal combination of micronutrients and their doses that promotes stability to genome and DNA.

COMMON EXAMPLES OF NUTRIGENOMICS

There are a number of examples which exhibit the relationship between genes and nutrition.

1. **Lactose Intolerance:** Some persons are not able to tolerate lactose (present in milk) because these lack genes responsible for production of enzyme lactase in the small intestine. Therefore, it is recommended to avoid milk in persons with 'lactose intolerance'.

2. **Phenylketonuria:** Phenylketonuria, an inborn error of metabolism, is another example of nutrigenomics. Due to genetic variation, some persons lack phenylalanine hydroxylase, which leads to decrease in phenylalanine metabolism and its accumulation may produce neurological damage.

3. **Caffeine:** Caffeine is metabolized by cytochrome P450 1A2 (CYP1A2) enzyme, and polymorphism of this gene determines the metabolism of caffeine. There are two types of individuals, 'rapid' caffeine metabolizers and 'slow' caffeine metabolizers depending on the composition of CYP1A2 gene. The large intake of caffeine in 'slow' caffeine metabolizers increases the risk of myocardial infarction.

POTENTIAL APPLICATIONS OF NUTRIGENOMICS

1. **Obesity:** It is the most commonly studied topic in nutrigenomics. It has been identified that there are certain genes which are linked with the development of obesity such as FTO, APO B, MC4R, SH2B1 and MTCH2. Nutrigenomics has been used to take preventive measures to treatment or mange obesity.

2. **Cancer:** Nutrigenomics has also been studied in the field of oncology. It has been shown that deficiency of certain micronutrients induces DNA damage (as by carcinogens) and thus, incorporation of such nutrients in diet may prevent DNA damage and prevent cancer development.

3. **Anti-ageing:** Lack of nutrients is associated with accumulation of free radicals and killing of cells in the form of ageing. Identification of nutrients that prevent free radical accumulation may prevent premature ageing of cells.

4. **Prevention of Diseases:** As explained above, there are certain diseases that may occur due to improper metabolism of nutrients such as lactose intolerance and phenylketonuria. The spectrum of such diseases is increasing and advancement in nutrigenomics may help in identifying more diseases resulting due to lack or improper metabolism

FUNCTIONOMICS

DEFINITIONS AND GENERAL FEATURES

It is an emerging field of science and deals with creating a unique profile of vital functions of an individual. It may also be called as fingerprinting of vital functions of an individual. A unique profile depicting all vital functions of an individual is created in functionomics and it may be used to predict the future aspects of health, diseases and lifespan of that individual. It is also termed as 'functional genomics', in which a blueprint of genomics is translated into blue print of vital functions to predict health, diseases and life expectancy.

POTENTIAL APPLICATIONS

Using functionomics, the four main vital functions are studied involving arterial function, fitness, metabolism and the autonomous nervous system. By using these vital functions, it is possible to compare a person (under investigation) with a normal or ideal person of same age and gender. It is also possible to determine the rate of ageing (whether it is slow or fast). Research has shown that these vital functions may be controlled to slow down ageing, enhance fitness, quality of life and prevent chronic diseases such as diabetes, cancers and dementia etc.

REVIEW QUESTIONS

TWO MARKS QUESTIONS

1. Define proteome and proteomics?
2. What are the methods used to separate proteins for proteomics?
3. What is isoelectric focusing? What is its use in proteomics?
4. What do you mean by Two Dimensional-Gel Electrophoresis?
5. What are the potential applications of proteomics?
6. Differentiate genomics and genetics.
7. What is epigenomics?
8. What are personalized medicines?
9. What is metabolome and metabolomics?
10. Define functionomics

FIVE MARKS QUESTIONS

1. What is proteomics? What are its different types?
2. How are proteins identified in proteomics?
3. What are the key steps involved in genomics?
4. What are the techniques and steps involved in metabolomics?
5. What are the applications of metabolomics?

TEN MARKS QUESTIONS

1. Write a note on techniques and steps involved in proteomics?
2. What is genomics? What are its different types? What are its potential applications?
3. Write a note on nutrigenomics.

MULTIPLE CHOICE QUESTIONS

---

1. A complete set of proteins in an individual is termed as
   (a) Genome
   (b) Proteome
   (c) Metabolome
   (d) None of above
2. Which of following is variable?
   (a) Genome
   (b) Proteome
   (c) Both a and b
   (d) None of above
3. Post-translational modifications of the proteins are identified in:
   (a) Functional proteomics
   (b) Structural proteomics
   (c) Expression proteomics
   (d) None of above
4. 2D electrophoresis is employed in proteomics to
   (a) Isolate proteins
   (b) Separate proteins
   (c) Identify proteins
   (d) All the above
5. Mass Spectrometry is employed in proteomics to
   (a) Isolate proteins
   (b) Separate proteins
   (c) Identify proteins
   (d) All the above
6. Which of following is involved in genome analysis?
   (a) Sequencing of DNA
   (b) Assembly of gene sequences
   (c) Annotation and analysis
   (d) All the above

7. Epigenetic changes in genome are determined using
    (a) Functional genomics   (b) Structural genomics
    (c) Epigenomic   (d) Metagenomics

8. Microbial diversity and ecology a specific environment is studied using
    (a) Functional genomics   (b) Structural genomics
    (c) Epigenomic   (d) Mtagenomics

9. In metabolomics, separation is not required in the following
    (a) NMR   (b) Mass spectrometry
    (c) Gas chromatography   (d) None of above

10. Lactose Intolerance and Phenylketonuria are studied under
    (a) Proteomics   (b) Genomics
    (c) Metabolomics   (d) Nutrigenomics

UNIT - 4

Immunotherapeutics, Cell Culture and Biosimilars (Immunotherapeutic Agents and Biosimilars)

16. Immunotherapeutics and Biosimilars 255

17. Animal Cell Culture 269

18. Assays and Flow Cytometry (Principles and Applications 291

Immunotherapeutics and Biosimilars

CHAPTER OUTLINE

Immunotherapeutic Agents
Definition and General Features
Types of Immunotherapeutic
Agents in Clinical Practice
Monoclonal Antibodies
Production of Monoclonal Antibodies
Humanization of Antibodies
Types of Monoclonal Antibodies
Fusion Proteins

Recombinant Cytokines
Soluble Cytokine Receptors
Cellular Therapy

Biosimilars
Definitions and General Features
Common Biologics in Medicine
Approval to Market Biosimilars
Examples of Approved Biosimilars

IMMUNOTHERAPEUTIC AGENTS

DEFINITION AND GENERAL FEATURES

Immunotherapeutic are the agents that are used to either activate or suppress the immune response and the therapy is termed as immunotherapy. It is also termed as 'biologic therapy' or 'biotherapy'. Recently, immunotherapy has been particularly used for the management of different types of cancers. Immunotherapy works by different mechanisms and these may include:

(i) Non specific activation of body's immune system to fight against pathogen or cancer

(ii) Specific activation of immune cells to attack and kill cancer cells specifically

(iii) Supplementation of body immune system by exogenous delivery of immune specific protein products

TYPES OF IMMUNOTHERAPEUTIC AGENTS IN CLINICAL PRACTICE

There are different types of immunotherapeutic products that are used in clinics and these include the followings:

1. Monoclonal Antibodies
2. Fusion proteins
3. Recombinant cytokines
4. Soluble Cytokine Receptors
5. Cellular therapies

1. **Monoclonal Antibodies:** These are the antibodies, which bind to the same epitope of an antigen. In other words, these antibodies have monovalent affinity for a single epitope. Epitope is the part of antigen, which is responsible for activation of immune response. These antibodies are made by immune cells, which are clones of a unique parent cell. In contrast, polyclonal antibodies have polyvalent affinity and these bind to different epitopes of same antigen or different antigens. Moreover, these are produced by different types of immune cells (plasma cells) **(Table 16.1).**

TABLE 16.1 Key differences between monoclonal antibodies and polyclonal antibodies

S.No	Monoclonal Antibodies	Polyclonal Antibodies
1.	These have monovalent affinity	These possess polyvalent affinity
2.	These bind to same epitope of an antigen	These bind to different epitopes of same antigen or different antigens
3.	These are produced by clones of immune cells of unique parent cells	These are produced by different types of immune cells

Production of Monoclonal Antibodies: Monoclonal antibodies are produced by 'Hybridoma Technology'. In this technology, two different types of somatic cells i.e. antibodies secreting 'Plasma cells (B cells)' and cancerous cells 'Myeloma cells' are fused to form 'hybridoma cells'. The B cells are isolated from mice after antigenic stimulation. The hybridoma cells possess the useful properties of both parents i.e. antibody secreting property of B cells and immortality of myeloma cells **(Figure 16.1).** Thus, hybridoma cells are immortal and secrete antibodies. These cells are grown in culture media (as animal cells) and antibodies are collected, purified and commercially used.

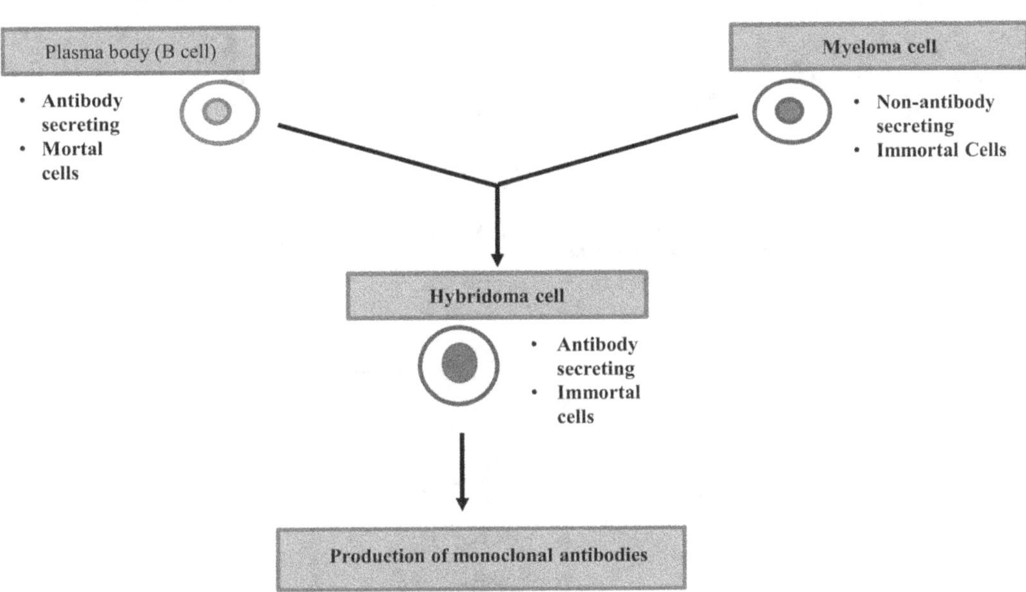

FIGURE 16.1 Principle of formation of hybridoma cells for the production of monoclonal antibodies

Humanization of Antibodies: Since monoclonal antibodies are produced from using mouse B cells; therefore, murine antibodies may trigger/activate the host immune response in humans to produce adverse effects. The process of removing mouse antigenic portions from the monoclonal antibody and replacing with human variants is termed as 'humanization of antibodies'. Such antibodies with similarity to human antibodies are termed as 'humanized antibodies'. Recombinant DNA technology is used to make monoclonal antibodies as humanized and the main purpose of humanization is to reduce untoward side effects of murine and chimeric antibodies.

In this humanization process, the DNA of mouse antibody is merged with DNA of human immunoglobulin. The resultant DNA is added in a cloning vector and DNA-cloning vector construct is added in a mammalian cell (host cell). In the host cells, replication of DNA-cloning vector takes place, which is followed by antibody (protein) production. For creating chimeric antibodies, DNA of whole variable region of mouse antibody is merged with DNA of human constant region of antibody **(Figure 16.2)**. However for humanized antibodies, only some portions of variable region (antigen binding hypervariable regions) of mouse antibody are used and rest of antibody is composed of DNA of human antibody **(Figure 16.3)**. Fully human monoclonal antibodies are produced

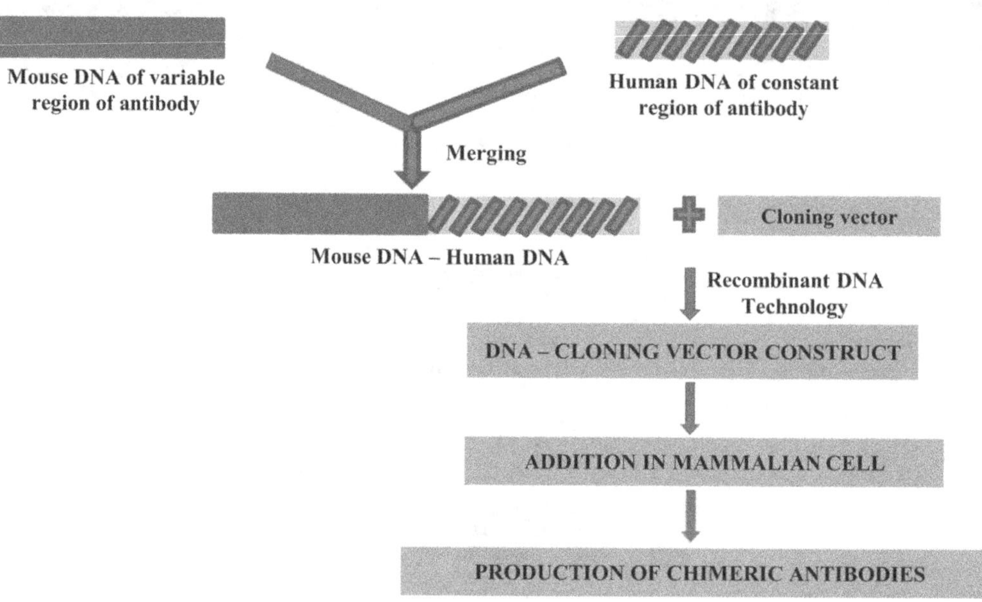

FIGURE 16.2 Basic steps involved in production of chimeric antibodies using recombinant DNA technology

in transgenic mice. These mice contain human immunoglobulin genes and from these mice, B cells are isolated. These mice produce fully human monoclonal antibodies. The major advantage of humanized and full human monoclonal antibodies is reduced immunogenicity. These antibodies do not produce hypersensitivity and adverse effects in patients. ***Types of Monoclonal Antibodies:*** Indeed, monoclonal antibodies are of different types depending on the origin. These may be murine, chimeric, humanized and fully human antibodies.

1. *Murine Monoclonal Antibodies:* In hybridoma technology, B cells are of murine (mouse) origin. Thus, monoclonal antibodies produced during hybridoma technology are termed as 'murine monoclonal antibodies'. These antibodies serve as foreign proteins in humans and immune system is activated against these antibodies. Indeed, antibodies are produced against these mouse monoclonal antibodies, which are termed as HAMA (Human Anti-mouse antibodies) response. This is manifested in the form of development of hypersensitivity reaction (type III).

2. *Chimeric Monoclonal Antibodies:* In order to overcome the activation of immune response against monoclonal antibodies, scientists

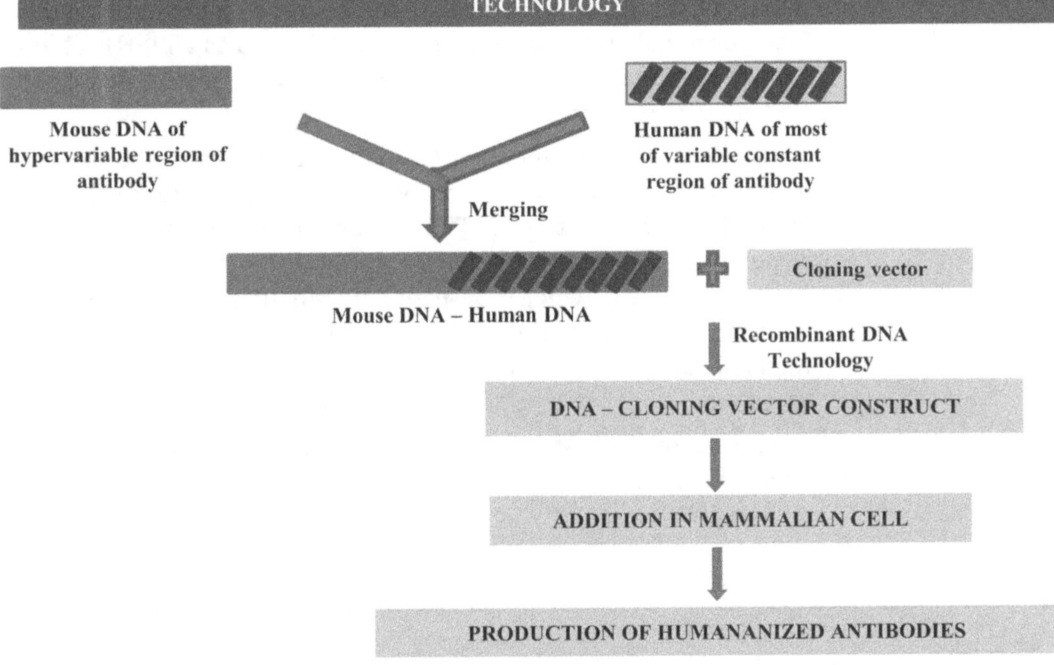

FIGURE 16.3 Basic steps involved in production of humanized monoclonal antibodies using recombinant DNA technology

employed recombinant DNA technology to replace mouse Fc portion of antibody with human portion. This led to creation of chimeric antibodies with portions of both humans and mice. Thus, these chimeric antibodies have variable portions of mouse type and constant portions of human type. Although, the immune activation is relatively less with chimeric antibodies, yet it activates immune response and produces undesirable side effects in humans. These are named using suffix 'xi' along with 'mab'. The examples of chimeric antibodies include basiliximab as anti–IL-2 receptor and rituximab as anti–B cell (CD20).

3. *Humanized Monoclonal Antibodies:* To further reduce the incidences of hypersensitivity due to activation of immune response, scientists further replaced antigenic portions (proteins) of antibodies with human portions. In other words in humanized antibodies, the protein sequences are modified to enhance their similarity to human antibodies. This process of removing mouse antigenic portions and replacing with human variants is termed as 'humanization of antibodies'. In these antibodies, only hyper-variable portions of mouse antibody are retained and rest of antibody is of human type. The

examples of humanized antibodies include bevacizumab as anti–VEGF-A; certolizumab as anti–TNF-alpha; daclizumab as anti–IL-2 receptor; omalizumab as anti-IgE; Trastuzumab as anti–HER2 and alemtuzumab as anti–B cell (CD52). These are named using suffix 'zu' along with 'mab'.

4. *Fully Human Monoclonal Antibodies:* Fully human monoclonal antibodies do not contain any portion of mouse antibody and the whole antibody is of human type. Thus, these antibodies do not produce hypersensitivity reactions. These antibodies are produced using transgenic mice in which mouse immunoglobulin genes are replaced with human immunoglobulin genes. An example of fully human monoclonal antibody includes adalimumab as anti-TNF-alpha. These are named using suffix 'u' along with 'mab'.

Therapeutic uses of Monoclonal Antibodies: Therapeutic uses of monoclonal antibodies may be summarized in **Table 16.2.**

TABLE 16.2 Therapeutic uses of monoclonal antibodies in clinics. RA: Rheimatois Arthritis, IBD: Inflammatory Bowel Disease

S. No	Monoclonal Antibodies	Type	Target	Therapeutic uses
1.	Adalimumab	Fully Human	Anti–TNF-alpha	Moderate to severe RA, psoriasis, moderate to severe drug resistant IBD
2.	Certolizumab	Humanized		
3.	Golimumab	Fully Human		
4.	Infliximab	Chimeric		
5.	Omalizumab	Humanized	Anti-IgE	Bronchial Asthma
6.	Pertuzumab	Humanized	Anti-HER2	HER2 positive metastatic breast cancer
7.	Trastuzumab			
8.	Bevacizumab	Humanized	Anti-VEGF-A	Metastatic colorectal cancer
9.	Ramucirumab	Fully Human	Anti–VEGF cancer,	Metastatic colorectal receptor-2 non–small cell lung cancer, gastric or gastroesophageal junction adenocarcinoma
10.	Ranibizumab	Humanized	Anti-VEGF	Macular degeneration, Diabetic retinopathy
11.	Siltuximab	Chimeric	Anti–IL-6	Moderate to severe RA
12.	Tocilizumab	Humanized	Anti–IL-6 receptors	Moderate to severe RA
13.	Basiliximab	Chimeric	Anti-IL-2	Prevention of acute transplantation rejection

2. Fusion Proteins: Fusion proteins are made by joining two or more different genes that encode for separate proteins. In other words, two or more genes encoding for different proteins are joined (fused) to form a chimeric gene. Later on, this chimeric gene is expressed in a host cell to form fusion proteins. These fusion proteins are also termed as 'chimeric or hybrid proteins'. These fusion proteins are made by recombinant DNA technology. The basic purpose of making fusion proteins is to incorporate the desirable properties of two more proteins in a single protein molecule. A large number of fusion proteins have been made to modulate the immune response. The examples and therapeutic uses of fusion proteins are explained below:

1. Etanercept is a fusion protein and acts as TNF-α blocker. It is created by fusion of genes encoding for tumor necrosis factor receptor and Fc segment of IgG antibody. It acts as decoy receptor and binds to TNF-α in systemic circulation, thus, the levels of TNF-α circulating in the blood are reduced. It is approved for the management of rheumatoid arthritis, psoriatic arthritis and ankylosing spondylitis.

2. Aflibercept is another fusion protein and acts as VEGF (vascular endothelial growth factor) blocker. It is created by fusion of genes encoding for VEGF receptors and Fc portion of IgG. It is approved for the treatment of macular degeneration and metastatic colorectal cancer.

3. Rilonacept is developed as a fusion protein to trap IL-1 (interleukin 1 inhibitor). It is created by fusing genes encoding for interleukin-1 receptor and Fc region human IgG1. It is an 'orphan drug' and has been used for the treatment of familial cold auto-inflammatory syndrome and neonatal onset multisystem inflammatory disease.

3. Recombinant Cytokines: Cytokines are small proteins that play a key role in cell communication and cell signaling, particularly in immune cells. These cytokines include chemokines, interferons, interleukins, lymphokines, and TNF-α, which are released by immune cells such as macrophages, lymphocytes, and non-immune cells such as endothelial cells and fibroblasts. Cytokines are endogenous in nature and stimulate the functioning of immune system. Accordingly, these cytokine proteins have been made by recombinant DNA technology and these recombinant cytokine are clinically used to stimulate the immune response. The examples of these recombinant cytokines include the followings:

1. Interferons

   (i) Interferon α is used for the management of hepatitis B, hepatitis C, AIDS-related Kaposi sarcoma, hairy cell leukemia, chronic myelogenous leukemia and metastatic melanoma

    (ii)   Interferon beta-1a and interferon beta-1b are clinically employed for the management of multiple sclerosis

    (iii)   Interferon gamma is used as immuno-stimulatory agent and is used to control chronic granulomatous infections.

2. Interleukins

    (i)   IL-2 is clinically employed to stimulate the immune system and is approved for the management of metastatic renal cell carcinoma and metastatic melanoma

    (ii)   IL-11 acts as 'thrombopoietic growth factor' and increases the synthesis of platelets. Therefore, it has been approved to prevent the occurrence of thrombocytopenia following chemotherapy

3. Colony Stimulating Factors

    (i)   G-CSF (Granulocyte-Colony Stimulating Factor) helps to stimulate the production of granulocytes and has been approved to prevent or reverse neutropenia following chemotherapy.

    (ii)   GM-CSF (Granulocyte Macrophage-Colony Stimulating Factor) helps to stimulate the synthesis of granulocytes and macrophages. It is also approved to prevent or reverse neutropenia following chemotherapy.

SOLUBLE CYTOKINE RECEPTORS

There has been a development of molecules that may act as cytokine receptors. These agents bind to circulating cytokines and prevent the binding of cytokines to their actual receptors located on immune cells. Thus, these act to prevent the activation of immune system. An example in this category includes 'Anakinra' which has been approved for the treatment of rheumatoid arthritis. It is made by recombinant DNA technology and it is very similar to human interleukin 1 receptor protein. Thus, it binds to circulating IL-1 to prevent its biological actions.

CELLULAR THERAPY

It is a novel therapy in which immune cells are isolated by a process called as 'leukapheresis' and later, activated by incubating with antigen and colony stimulating factor. The activated immune cells are returned to humans to attack on antigen. Indeed, the purpose is to enhance or amplify the inadequate natural immune response. Generally, this has been done to treat cancer. An example in this category includes 'Sipuleucel-T', which is approved for the treatment of prostatic cancer. In this case, dendritic cells (antigen-presenting cells) are isolated using leukapheresis procedure. Later, these cells are incubated with the antigen 'prostatic acid phosphatase' and GM-CSF, which helps the dendritic cells to mature. This process leads to activation of dendritic cells and these activated cells are reinfused into the patient. These cells act on prostate antigens and reduce the growth of prostatic cancer.

BIOSIMILARS

DEFINITIONS AND GENERAL FEATURES

A biosimilar is a biological product that is very similar to a reference (standard) biological product and there are no clinically meaningful differences in terms of safety, purity, and potency. Indeed, a biosimilar is a biological product and is an identical copy of an original product that is manufactured by a different company. These are officially approved versions of originally patented biological products. After the expiry of a patent of original biological molecule, another company can manufacture that biological product. Accordingly, biological product produced by another company after the expiry of patent of an original biological product is called as biosimilar. The term 'biosimilar' is analogous to term 'generic' for traditional drugs.

COMMON BIOLOGICS IN MEDICINE

Biologics (biological product) are the products produced or isolated from the biological source. The biological products include a vaccines, blood and blood components, gene therapy, tissues, and recombinant therapeutic proteins such as hormones (insulin, growth hormones), cytokines, clotting factors, monoclonal antibodies etc. These may be composed of sugars, proteins, or nucleic acids or combinations of these substances. Since biological products exhibit high molecular complexity in comparison to traditional drugs; therefore, biosimilars may not be simply regarded as 'generic'. In comparison to generics, these biologics are quite sensitive to changes in manufacturing processes.

APPROVAL TO MARKET BIOSIMILARS

Every biological product displays variability, even within different batches of the same product. Accordingly, there is variability in biological products due to change in manufacturing unit and processes. Drug approving authorities such as Food and Drug Administration (FDA) require that biological products manufactured by an industry is very similar in nature and composition to an earlier approved biological in terms of safety and efficacy. Accordingly, analytical studies showing similarity of biological product with the reference product; animal studies showing efficacy and toxicity; clinical studies showing pharmacokinetics and pharmacodynamics are to be conducted and documented.

EXAMPLES OF APPROVED BIOSIMILARS

1. **Zarxio as a Biosimilar to Neupogen:** Neupogen was earlier clinically approved biological to increase the number of granulocytes in cancer patients following chemotherapy. Neupogen is the trade name and it contains 'filgrastim', which is a recombinant granulocyte colony-stimulating factor (G-CSF). After patent expiry, Sandoz's got approval for Zarxio, which also has filgrastim. However, in order to differentiate two biosimilars, nomenclature differences were introduced as per licensing requirement. In this case, Sandoz's filgrastim is written as 'filgrastim-sndz' in order to differentiate from originally approved filgrastim. Therefore, filgrastim-sndz is biosimilar to filgrastim. It is mandatory to add four words after the name of drug. Those four words are arbitrary and have not any significance in terms of meanings.

2. **Inflectra is biosimilar to Remicade:** Inflectra having 'infliximab-dyyb' was another biosimilar approved in the U.S to Remicade having 'infliximab'. Infliximab is a chimeric monoclonal antibody and it specifically targets tumor necrosis factor alpha (TNF-α). These may be used in rheumatoid arthritis, Crohn's disease, ankylosing spondylitis, ulcerative colitis, and psoriasis. The arbitrary four words 'dyyb' are used to differentiate 'infliximab-dyyb' from originally approved 'infliximab'.

3. **Erelzi is a Biosimilar to Enbrel**: In 2016 the third biosimilar i.e. Sandoz's Erelzi (etanercept-szzs) was FDA-approved. Erelzi is biosimilar to Amgen's Enbrel (etanercept). Etanercept is a fusion protein produced by recombinant DNA technology. It is made by fusion of TNF-α receptor with the constant end of the IgG antibody. As a fusion protein, it binds to circulating TNF-α and neutralizes its effects. It is also used in rheumatoid arthritis, Crohn's disease, ankylosing spondylitis, ulcerative colitis, and psoriasis. The arbitrary four words 'szzs' are used to differentiate 'etanercept-szzs' from originally approved ' etanercept'.

4. **Amjevita is a Biosimilar for Humira:** Amgen's Amjevita (adalimumab-atto) is another biosimilar to humira (adalimumab). Adalimumab was the first fully human monoclonal antibody approved by FDA. It is an anti-

TNF-α monoclonal antibody and has similar clinical indications as that of etanercept. The arbitrary four words ' atto' are used to differentiate ' adalimumab-atto' from originally approved ' adalimumab'.

5. **Renflexis is a Biosimilar to Remicade :** First, Inflectra (infliximab-dyyb) was approved as biosimilar to Remicade (infliximab). Later, FDA approved Renflexis (infliximab-abda) as biosimilar to Remicade (infliximab).

REVIEW QUESTIONS

TWO MARKS QUESTIONS

1. What do you understand by humanized monoclonal antibodies?
2. What is the purpose of humanization of monoclonal antibodies?
3. What do you understand by cellular therapy?
4. What do you understand by soluble cytokine receptors? What are their uses?
5. Give examples of fusion proteins.
6. What are fully human monoclonal antibodies?
7. What do you mean by chimeric monoclonal antibody?
8. What is hybridoma technology?
9. Differentiate monoclonal and polyclonal antibodies.
10. What are Human Anti-mouse antibodies?
11. What do you mean by biosimilars?
12. What are biologics? Give Examples.
13. What is the difference between generic and biosimilars?
14. What are the regulatory tests to be cleared for approval of biosimilars?

FIVE MARKS QUESTIONS

1. What do you understand by humanization of antibodies? How is it done?
2. Write therapeutic applications of monoclonal antibodies.
3. What are recombinant cytokines? What are their therapeutic uses?
4. What are fusion proteins? Give examples along with their clinical uses.
5. What are biosimilars? Give examples of common biosimilars approved for clinical use?

TEN MARKS QUESTIONS

1. Write a note on immunotherapeutic agents?

2. What are monoclonal antibodies? How are these produced? What are its different types? Write their therapeutic uses.

MULTIPLE CHOICE QUESTIONS

1. Monoclonal antibodies bind to
   - (a) Single epitope
   - (b) Multiple epitopes
   - (c) Single antigen
   - (d) None of above

2. Adalimumab is
   - (a) Murine
   - (b) Chimeric
   - (c) Humanized
   - (d) Fully human

3. Omalizumab is
   - (a) Murine
   - (b) Chimeric
   - (c) Humanized
   - (d) Fully human

4. Basiliximab is
   - (a) Murine
   - (b) Chimeric
   - (c) Humanized
   - (d) Fully human

5. Etanercept is
   - (a) Monoclonal antibody
   - (b) Fusion protein
   - (c) Cellular therapy
   - (d) Recombinant cytokine

6. GM-CSF is
   - (a) Monoclonal antibody
   - (b) Fusion protein
   - (c) Cellular therapy
   - (d) Recombinant cytokine

7. Recombinant cytokines are generally used to
   - (a) Activate immune system
   - (b) Suppress immune system
   - (c) Do not modulate immune system
   - (d) None of above

8. Which of followings is biologic?
   - (a) Monoclonal antibody
   - (b) Vaccine
   - (c) Gene therapy
   - (d) All the above

9. Which of following tests are required for the approval of biosimilar?
   - (a) Analytical tests
   - (b) Preclinical testing
   - (c) Clinical testing
   - (d) All the above

10. Which of following is biosimilar?
    - (a) Etanercept-szzs
    - (b) Etanercept
    - (c) Amjevita
    - (d) Inflectra

Animal Cell Culture

CHAPTER OUTLINE

Brief History of Animal Cell Culture
Type of Animal Cells

Culture Systems for Cell Growth
Anchorage dependent Culture System
Anchorage Independent Culture System

Types of Cell Cultures
Primary Cell Culture
Secondary Cell Culture
Transformed Cell Culture

Culture Media Counting the Cells in Animal Cell Culture
Haemocytometer
Coulter Counter

Pattern of Cell Growth

Storage of Cells

Characterization of Cell Line
Monitoring Cell lines for Genetic Stability
Karyotyping
Isozymes
Fluorescent labeled Antibodies
Monitoring Cell Lines for Cell contamination

Applications of Animal Cell Culture

BRIEF HISTORY OF ANIMAL CELL CULTURE

Tissue culture generally refers to the process of growth of cells, tissues or organs obtained from suitable animal or plant donor in an artificial environment. The artificial environment is provided in the form of suitable growth media, which supplies the necessary nutrients required for growth of the tissue. Depending on the donor being used, the cell culture may be either 'plant tissue culture' or 'animal cell culture'. When complete organs or portions of organs are used for the process, it is called 'organ culture'. On the other hand, cell culture refers to the process, where the desired cells are isolated from the related organ and maintained in the culture media as cells.

The first successful animal cell culture was conducted by Ross Harrison in 1907. He used the 'Hanging Drop Technique' to observe the growth of frog embryo in the clotted lymph fluid (as culture media). Over a few weeks, he observed the growth of nerve cells in the culture media. However, he faced the problem of 'bacterial contamination', which quickly outpaced the growth of animal tissue and bacterial cells replaced the animal cells. This problem of bacterial contamination was partially overcome in 1912 by Alexis Carrel, who maintained aseptic conditions throughout the process using Carrel's flask **(Figure 17.1)** for the cell growth.

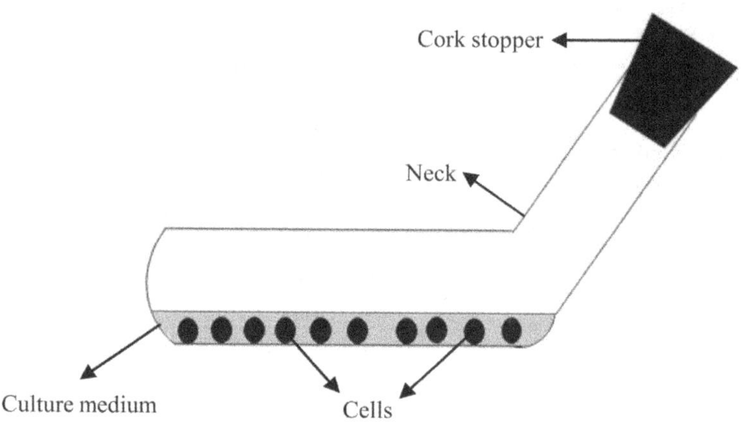

FIGURE 17.1 Carrel's flask

Several further developments in the animal cell culture made it a successful tool for scientists in late 1940s. In the era of antibiotics, streptomycin and penicillin were used to keep the cell cultures free of bacterial growth. This allowed hassle-free usage of biological fluids and embryonic extracts for carrying cell culture in the laboratories. Further into the development, the biological fluids (used conventionally for cell growth) were replaced by chemical nutrient media. The problems faced with biological fluids, such as, inconsistency in different batches, chances of contamination, and complicated sterilization methods were eliminated with chemical nutrient media. In 1949, the cell culture technique was taken into large scale to grow poliovirus. For this, the poliovirus was grown on the embryonic cells obtained from humans. Further in 1950, the polio vaccine was commercialized for vaccination of at large scale.

TYPE OF ANIMAL CELLS

There are different types of animal cells, employed in animal cell culture.

1. Epithelial Tissue

(a) It envelops the organs, blood vessels and forms the lining of the cavities. For example, skin, lining of gastrointestinal tract, glands, etc.

(b) For cell culture, these cells can grow only on a substrate which can provide them a site for attachment. Hence, they are also known as anchorage-dependent cells (discussed below).

(c) They form mono-layers.

(d) Under the microscope these appear like cobble-stone.

2. Connective Tissue

(a) It is found in bone, cartilage, CNS and several fibrous tissues.

(b) Fibroblasts make up the fibers and matrix of the connective tissue.

(c) These cells also require substrate for growth and these are also termed as anchorage-dependent cells.

(d) These are spherical in shape, when isolated and become spindle shaped on attaching to the substrate.

3. Muscle Tissue

(a) It consists of tubules stacked together to form proteins responsible for structural functions, namely, actin and myosin.

(b) Myoblasts undergo different stages of differentiation to form myotubes, which may be used to study the different stages of differentiation.

4. Nervous Tissue

(a) Its function is to transmit the electrical signals throughout the body.

(b) Embryonic tissue may be employed to study the growth of nervous tissue.

CULTURE SYSTEMS FOR CELL GROWTH AND BASIC EQUIPMENTS USED IN CELL CULTURE LABORATORY

Culture systems are important for the growth and maintenance of animal cells. Depending on whether the growth of cells in a culture medium requires a substrate for attachment, or it can exist as a suspension in the culture medium, the culture systems are of following two types:

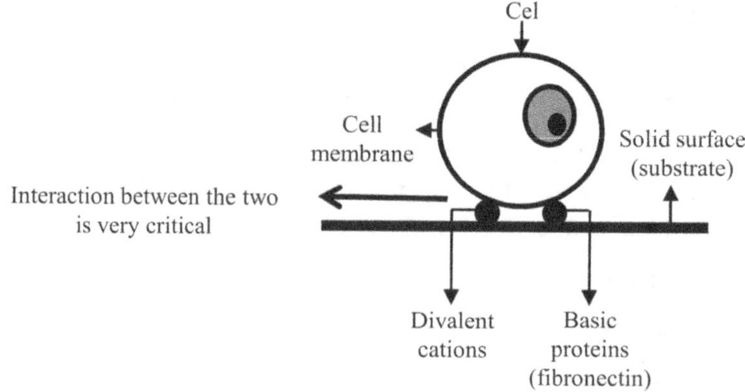

FIGURE 17.2 Anchorage dependent cell culture system

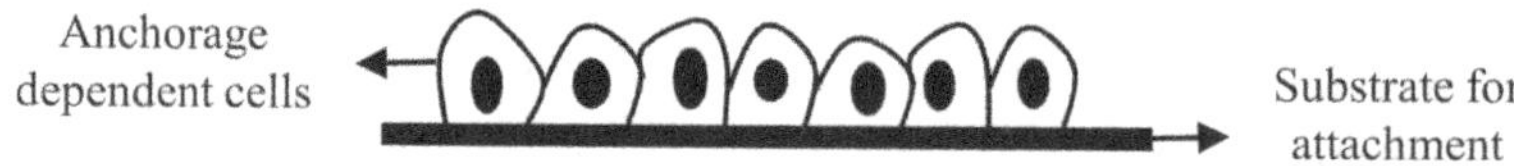

FIGURE 17.3 Epithelial cells as anchorage dependent cells

ANCHORAGE DEPENDENT CULTURE SYSTEM AND EQUIPMENTS

These culture systems require a substrate for attachment of cells. Without attaching to the substrate (a solid surface), the cells are unable to grow. It is also known as 'Monolayer culture system' because cells can grow in a single layer only. The substrate is generally made of glass or treated plastic and these include, T-flasks, roller bottles and multiple well plates. The substrate may also be coated with attachment factors including fibronectin, collagen, laminin and gelatin **(Figure 17.2)**. This helps in easy attachment of the cells to the substrate and proper growth of the cells. Moreover, anchorage dependent cells should be preferably grown on the porous substrates to allow their growth in a polarized environment. These cells may also be grown in suspension by using glass beads, polyacrylamide, dextran molecules and plastic beads, which provide a solid support for their growth. The choice of substrate depends on number of cells, cost and the culture environment. However, one of the major disadvantages of these types of cells is that it can only form one layer of cells i.e., monolayer of cells. Multi-layers of cells cannot be obtained. Epithelial cells, connective tissue cells, muscular cells and nervous tissue cells are anchorage dependent cells and all these cells require substrate to grow.

ANCHORAGE INDEPENDENT CULTURE SYSTEM AND EQUIPMENTS

The cells used in this type of culture system do not require any substrate for attachment. They can grow freely in the culture medium in the floating form. Hence, it is also referred to as 'suspension culture systems'. The cells in anchorage independent culture system may either be grown in constantly agitated vessels, so as to keep the cells suspended consistently in the medium. They may also be grown in stationary culture containers, such as T-flask or bottles **(Figure 17.4)** in which the cells are not agitated. Spinner flasks rotated magnetically or shaken Erlenmeyer flasks are used as constantly agitated vessels. The cell lines which are used in 'anchorage independent' or 'suspension culture systems' include cells of blood and lymph.

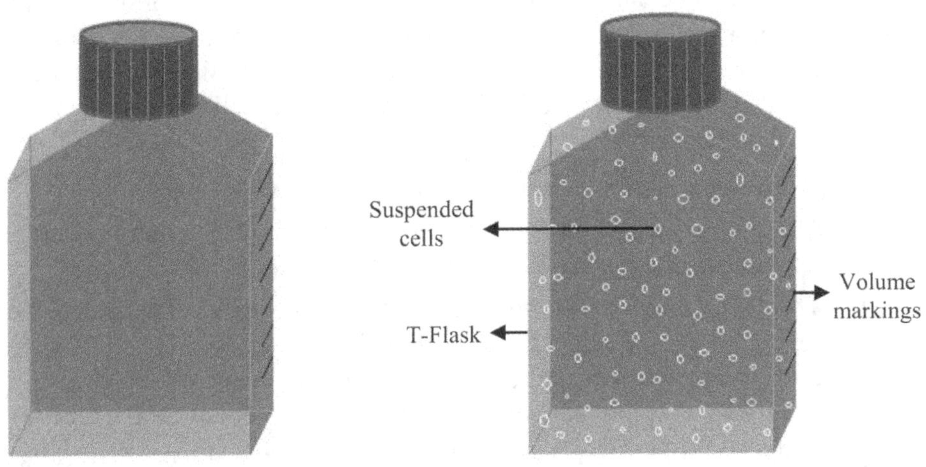

FIGURE 17.4 T-Flask used for growth of anchorage independent culture systems

OTHER EQUIPMENTS IN CELL CULTURE

Apart from equipment mentioned for the growth of anchorage dependent and anchorage independent cells, there is requirement of other basic equipments and these include:

1. ***Laminar Flow Hood or Cell Culture Hood Or Biosafety Cabinet:*** It is required for carrying aseptic culturing of cells. HEPA filters are provided in the laminar flow to prevent contamination.

2. ***CO_2 Incubator:*** The purpose of incubators is to provide the appropriate environment for cell growth.

3. Hemocytometer and Coulter counter (described below)

4. Liquid nitrogen or Cryostorage container (for storage of cells, described below)

5. Others such as centrifuge, refrigerators, sterilizers (autoclaves), water bath, microscope

FINITE (NORMAL) VS CONTINUOUS (TRANSFORMED) CELL LINES

There are mainly two types of cells, cells with finite life span and cells with infinite life span, continuous cell lines. Finite cell lines stop dividing after a certain amount of time. On the other hand, the cells of continuous cell lines continue to divide and hence, these are known as 'immortal cells'. These cells of continuous cell lines are also called as 'transformed cells' and these are formed by inducing changes in the finite cell lines using transforming agents including certain drugs, radiations or viruses. These transforming agents transform normal cells to form immortal or continuous cell lines. Hence, these cells are called transformed cells. These transformed cells grow faster and hence, are easier to grow.

There are following characteristics of 'Normal cells':

(a)   The cells have diploid chromosome pattern and this genetic pattern is retained during the process of sub-culturing.

(b)   There is inhibition on the growth of cells after formation of the monolayer for anchorage dependent cells. For anchorage independent cells, there is inhibition of growth after an increase in the density of the culture. It signifies that growth of cells is taking place in a controlled manner.

(c)   There is finite life span and cell growth is followed by death of cells after some time. Approximately after 50 generations of human embryonic cells, there is death of these cells **(Figure 17.5)**. The cells obtained from embryo have a greater growth capacity in comparison to cells isolated from adult tissue.

(d)   These cells do not show formation of tumors and hence, these are non malignant.

The following are characteristics of transformed cells:

(a)   Transformed cells have mutated genetic makeup.

(b)   These do not show controlled cell growth and their growth is not dependent on anchorage or density.

(c)   These are immortal cells and hence, these continue to divide indefinitely.

(d)   These are malignant cells and hence, can lead to tumor formation.

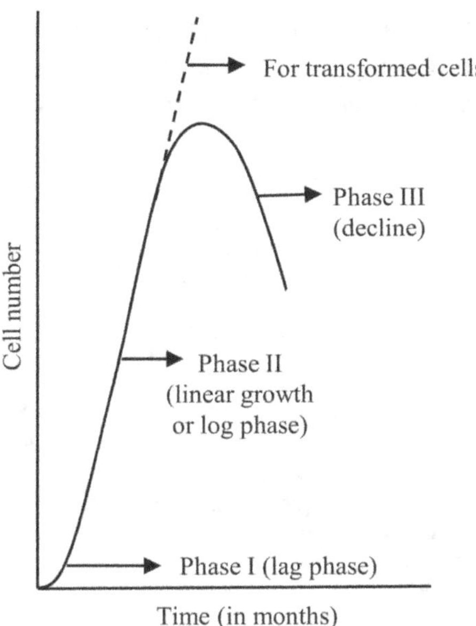

FIGURE 17.5 Growth curve depicting growth of human embryonic cells and transformed cells

Hybridomas (hybrid cells) are examples of transformed cells, which are used in animal cell culture. These cells are obtained by fusing cells from two different types of cells i.e., lymphocytes and myeloma cell. Lymphocytes are used for their capability of producing antibodies, while myeloma cells have capability of unlimited division (immortal). The resultant hybrid cells exhibit the characteristics of both parent cells and thus, hybridoma cells are immortal and produce antibodies.

TYPES OF CELL CULTURES

Cell cultures have been divided into the following three main types:

1. **Primary cell cultures:** A primary culture is made by inoculating cells obtained from animal or human tissue directly in a suitable growth medium. The tissue isolated from the animal or human body is excised into very small fragments with the help of scissors and forceps. These fragments are placed in a sterile medium and the tissue fragments are disaggregated into individual cells by treating them with proteolytic enzyme, trypsin. One can easily selective grow certain types of cells by carefully choosing the composition of the growth medium **(Figure 17.6)**. For establishing a primary culture of blood cells, the suspension may be subjected to density gradient centrifugation to separate the different components of blood.

The gradients necessary for the separation of different blood components are established by using 'Ficoll' and 'Percoll' media. This method has been widely used for separation of lymphocytes **(Figure 17.6)**.

In case where anchorage dependent cells obtained from the animal or human tissue being used:

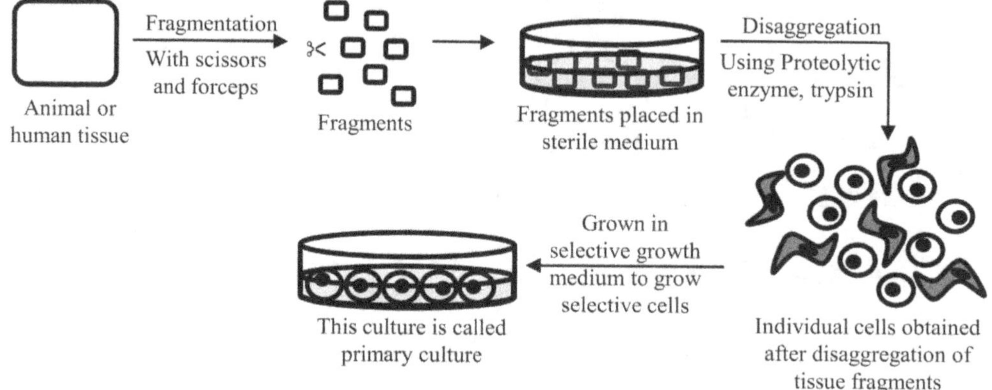

In case where blood (non-anchorage dependent) is the animal or human tissue being used:

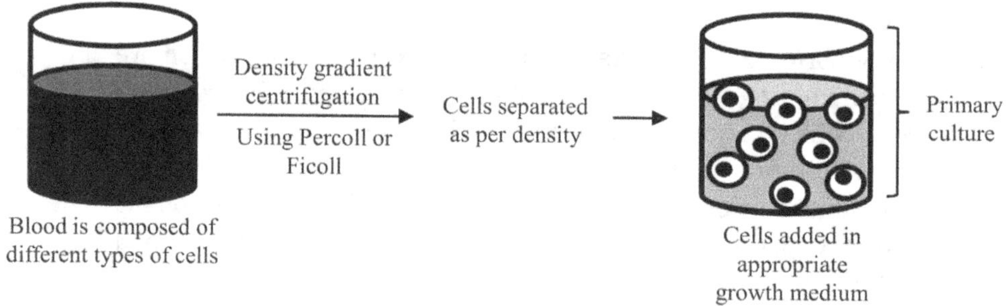

FIGURE 17.6 Steps involved in the formation of primary culture

2. **Secondary cell cultures:** A secondary cell culture is obtained by sub-culturing of the primary cell culture. For sub-culturing cells of suspension culture, the primary culture is diluted with fresh growth media to obtain the secondary cell culture, for example with lymphocytes. For sub-culturing anchorage dependent cells, some of the cells of the primary culture are removed and inoculated in a fresh culture medium **(Figure 17.7)**. In relation to sub-culturing, a term 'passage number' is used. The passage number refers to the number of times sub-culturing has been done, after original isolation of cells from the primary culture. Split ratio is the ratio which tells us about the number of new culture produced after each sub-culturing. This split ratio forms a basis of relationship between the passage number and generation number and is given in the following equation **(Equation 17.1)**.

Generation number = Passage number × split ratio/2…   …..(17.1)

In case where anchorage dependent cells obtained from the animal or human tissue being used:

For anchorage dependent cells:

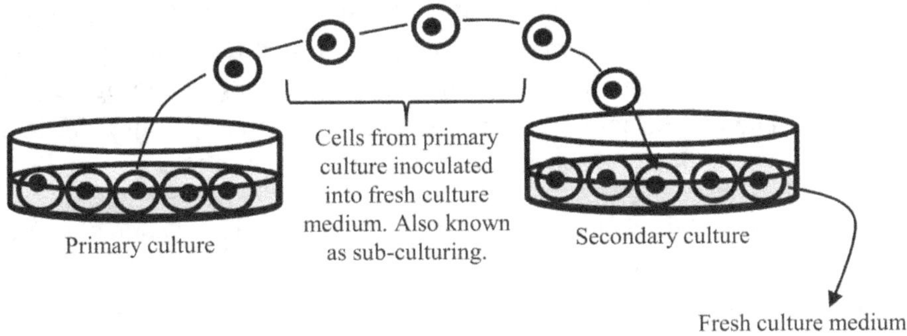

For non-anchorage dependent cells:

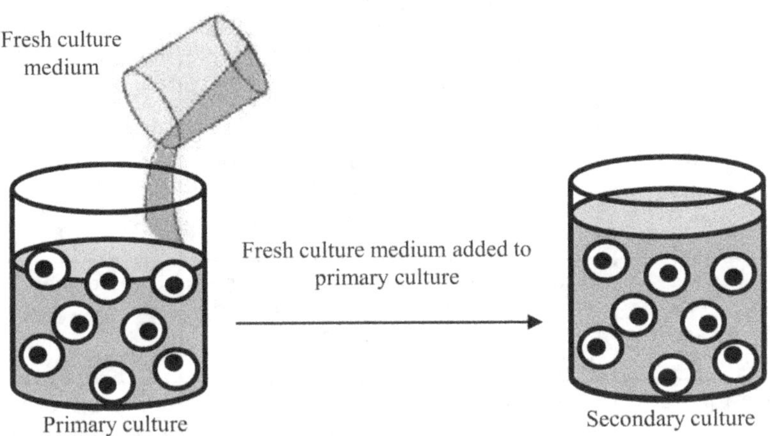

FIGURE 17.7 Procedure for formation of secondary culture

3. **Transformed cell cultures:** The transformed cells refer to those cells, which have acquired the ability of growing continually and these cells exhibit immortality. These cells grow infinitely and hence, may also be said to have become immortal **(Figure 17.5)**. This occurs through transformation of the normal cells either by the use of drugs, radiations or viruses. In this process of transformation, the cells lose their sensitivity to the growth controlling stimuli and hence, these cells become devoid of growth regulation. In other words, transformed cell cultures become independent of anchorage dependence and density inhibition (as discussed previously). Moreover, changes in the pattern of chromosomes in the nucleus of such cells are also observed as a result of transformation. HeLa cell lines are the examples of transformed cells and these are obtained from a cervical cancer.

Despite the fact that transformed cells show infinite and rapid growth, their use in production of biological products on a large scale has been a matter of debate. The main concern of the scientists regarding the use of transformed cells for biological production is that these cells may possibly transfer tumor forming characters in biological products. Therefore, there is a restricted use of these cell cultures for large scale production of products to be used clinically.

TABLE 17.1 Difference between different characteristics of primary, secondary and transformed cell cultures

Characteristics	Primary cell cultures	Secondary cell cultures	Transformed cell cultures
Formation	By inoculation of cells obtained from the tissues into suitable culture medium (Figure 17.6).	By inoculation of cells taken from primary cell culture into fresh culture medium or by dilution of primary culture with fresh culture medium (Figure17.7).	Transformed cells are inoculated into the suitable culture medium.
Type of cells used	Both anchorage dependent and non-anchorage dependent	Both anchorage dependent and non-anchorage dependent	Transformed cells
Growth pattern	Normal growth pattern (Figure 17.5)	Normal growth pattern (Figure 17.5)	Infinite growth, immortal (Figure 17.5)
Life span	Finite	Finite	Infinite
Characters of normal cells	Maintained	Maintained	Not Maintained
Malignancy	Absent	Absent	May be present
Use in large scale production	Yes	Yes	Restricted use (due to possible tumor formation)

CULTURE MEDIA

In late 1940s, the scientists used biological fluids as culture media for providing nutrients necessary for the cells to grow. The originally used and favored culture media was 'Cockerel plasma' mixed with extracts of embryo. However, it was more vulnerable to bacterial contamination and there was no uniformity across different batches. Therefore, to overcome the problems related to biological culture media, chemically defined media was used. Eagle's Minimum Essential Medium (EMEM) was formulated by Eagle in 1955. It was specifically used for growth of HeLa cells and mouse L cells. Thereafter, several modifications in EMEM led to the formulation of various media for animal cell culture. Dulbecco's minimum essential media (DMEM by Dulbecco) and Glasgow's minimum essential media (GMEM by Glasgow) are two of the EMEM's modified versions of culture media. These culture media are generally composed of amino acids, growth factors, vitamins, carbohydrates and salts.

1. Carbohydrates are used as a source of energy for the cells. One of the most commonly used carbohydrates is glucose. Moreover amino acids, especially glutamine may also serve as a source of energy.

2. Various salts are added in varying amounts in order to keep the media isotonic. This prevents osmotic imbalance of the media. Generally, bicarbonate and carbon dioxide (5-10%) are used as a buffer system for the culture media.

3. The vitamins and hormones are added as per the requirements of the cells to be grown. They serve as co-factors. The concentration of vitamins and hormones is comparatively low in comparison to other components.

4. Other than the above components, most of the cultures are also supplemented with 10% v/v blood serum. It is required for maintaining growth of cells. The most common source of serum is either bovine or equine. A very effective and common source is 'fetal calf serum' because it has very high content of embryonic growth factors. However, inclusion of serum has certain limitations. It decreases batch to batch uniformity, increases the cost of culturing (fetal calf serum is costly), and it may also increase the chances of contamination of the media.

5. Therefore, to prevent these limitations, formulations with 'low content of serum' or 'serum free cultures' are employed. Certain other ingredients are added in media to replace the serum. An example of such medium includes 'HITES medium' and it is composed of hydrocortisone, insulin, transferrin, estrogen and selenite. Growth factors obtained from endocrine glands or epidermal or fibroblast growth factors may be used to completely substitute serum in the culture medium.

COUNTING THE CELLS IN ANIMAL CELL CULTURE

Cell counting is very an important component in animal cell culture and samples are taken from culture media after every 24 hours to count the number of cells. The cells are counted by the following two methods. The purpose of counting the cells is to determine the growth of cells in the culture.

1. **Haemocytometer:** A predetermined volume of the sample is used to count the number of cells by examining it under the microscope. The sample is loaded onto the haemocytometer (a slide with grids on it). The maximum amount of sample volume that can be loaded is $0.1\,\mu L$. To differentiate between viable and non viable cells, dye such as tryptan blue (0.2%) is used. The non viable cells are stained blue, while viable cells do not get stained. This is because viable cells are not permeable, but non-viable cells become permeable and allow the entry of the dye inside the cell **(Figure 17.8)**. On the other hand, using mixture of citric acid (0.1 mol/L) and crystal violet (0.1%), the nuclei of cells can be stained purple and be counted. For anchorage dependent cells, which remain firmly attached to the solid substrate, the nuclei counting technique is the preferred one **(Figure 17.9)**.

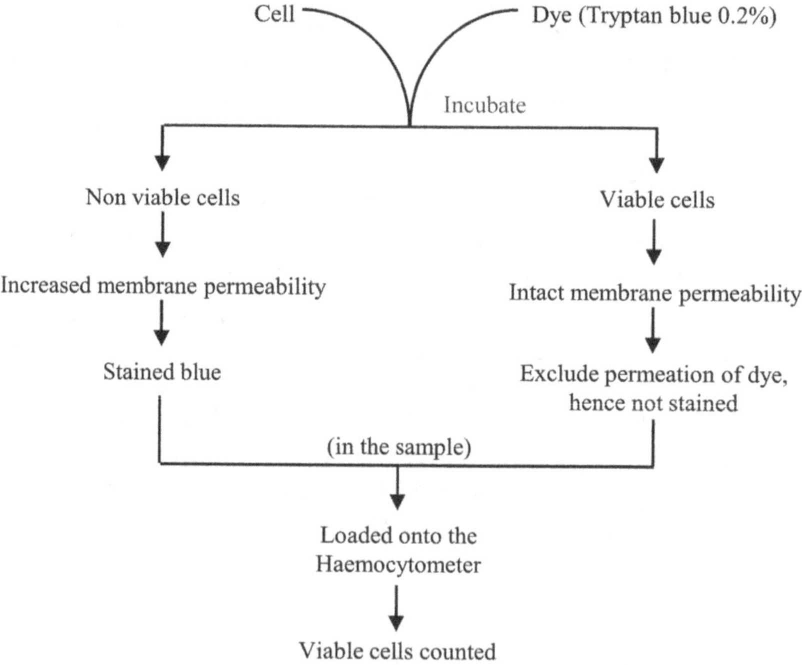

FIGURE 17.8 Cell counting using haemocytometer, wherein viable cells (non-stained) and non-viable cells (stained) are counted on a slide using a microscope.

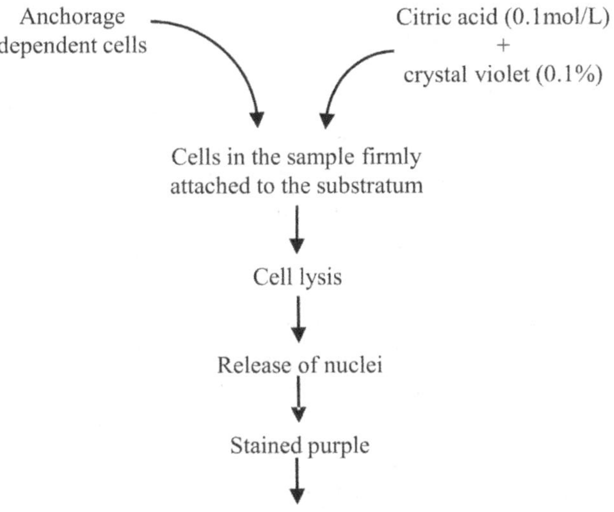

FIGURE 17.9 Counting of anchorage dependent cells using Haemocytometer

2. **Coulter Counter:** It is an electronic device, which works on the principle of counting the cells in a pre-determined volume of sample by allowing it to pass between two electrodes. By passage of the cells, the flow of current between the electrodes is impeded, which results in voltage change and a signal is recorded electronically **(Figure 17.10)**. An advantage of method is that it takes very less time to analyze the whole sample. However, it is disadvantageous in that it counts all the cells present in the sample, whether viable or non-viable. Also, to insure correct results, the sample must be free of any clumps of cells, otherwise wrong results will be obtained.

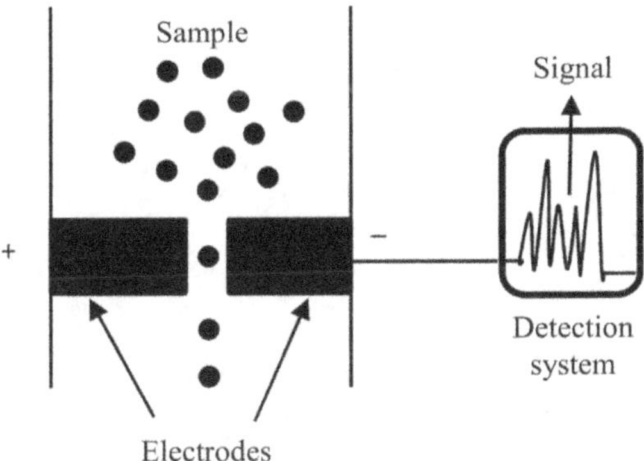

FIGURE 17.10 The principle of coulter counter

PATTERN OF CELL GROWTH

The pattern of growth in animal cells culture is same as that of the microorganisms and it follows the 'S shaped pattern'. The minimal volume of cell inoculum required for early growth of the cells is approximately 10^5cells/mL. Initially, there is 'lag phase' during which the growth takes place at a very slow rate. During this phase, cells slowly release growth factors and this phase ends, when enough of growth factors accumulate in culture media. The length of the lag phase generally depends on the state of cells, during their inoculation. The cells obtained from an exponentially growing culture exhibit a very short lag phase, but those cells which have been stored earlier or are taken from a stationary culture have a longer lag phase. In order to accelerate growth, 'feeder layer of cells' or 'conditioned media' is added. Feeder layer of cells refers to irradiated cells which are incapable of growing, but are metabolically active. These feeder cells do not multiply; however, these release growth factors in the media to facilitate growth of the cells. Conditioned media is obtained from exponentially growing cell culture.

The next phase is known as the 'log phase' or 'exponential growth phase', during which there is very fast growth of cells and cells increase their number in an exponential manner. Within 15-25 hours, the number of cells in the media gets double and this time is termed as 'doubling time'. This phase is followed by 'stationary phase' during which the number of cells become almost constant. At this stage, the nutrients in the media are exhausted or the metabolites responsible for inhibition of cell growth accumulate to bring the cell growth to a halt. The cell number is generally around $1\text{-}2 \times 10^6$ cells/mL in this phase **(Figure 17.11)**.

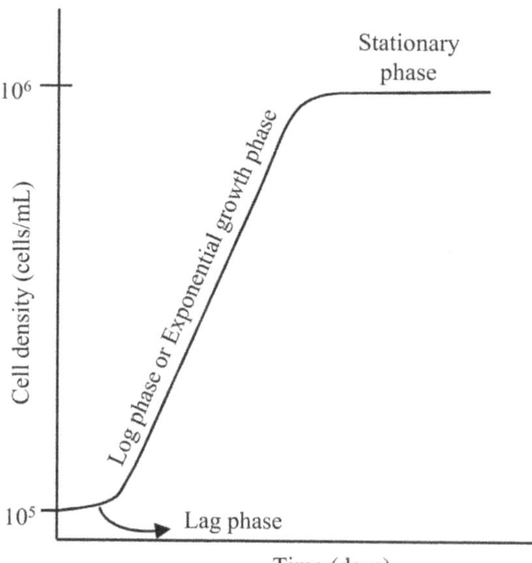

FIGURE 17.11 Growth curve for cells

The anchorage dependent cells usually show a growth, till the substratum is available. These cannot grow in multi-layers. It means, once the monolayer on the substratum is formed, the cells cannot grow any further. Therefore, specially designed apparatus are used to have more surface area. Normal cell densities obtained with anchorage dependent cells is within 5×10^5 cells/cm². However, with Roux bottle having high surface are with range of 200 cm², the number of cells produced is expected to be around 10^8 cells/cm².

STORAGE OF CELLS

Storing the cells at low temperatures can help keep them viable for long periods. The cells at a volume of approximately 10^7cells/mL are stored in the frozen form in small plastic ampoules. The medium in which the cells are stored are generally included with cryopreservatives such as 10% glycerol or dimethylsulfoxide (DMSO). The cell suspension is frozen at –70°C for few hours or at –196°C for long period of time using liquid nitrogen.

CHARACTERIZATION (MONITORING) OF CELL LINES

It is important to characterize cell lines periodically to check the genetic stability and possible contamination.

1. **Monitoring of Cell Lines for Genetic Stability:** On repeated sub-culturing, there is a tendency that cell lines may undergo genetic changes. Moreover, the cell lines may get contaminated or cross contaminated with some other cells. For example, HeLa cells grow faster than most of the cells, so if cell culture gets contaminated by HeLa cells, HeLa will outnumber the originally intended cells. Hence, characterization of the cell lines is necessary to ensure the growth of normal and desired cell lines. The methods used for characterization of cell lines are:

A. *Karyotyping:* Using this method, a change in the chromosomes or any damage inflicted to the chromosomes can be analyzed. Karyotype refers to the distribution of chromosomes, which is a characteristic feature of every species. The steps involved in karyotyping include:

(a) The growth of cells is optimized

(b) The cells are blocked in the mitosis stage by addition of colchicine or colcemid, which act as mitotic inhibitor. These halt the cell division and cells are arrested in metaphase.

(c) The separation between chromosomes is maximized by putting hypotonic solution, which causes swelling of cells

(d) Fixative agent, methanol:acetic acid (3:1 v/v) is added.

(e) Cells are smeared on the slide and allowed to dry

(f) Suitable dye such as Giemsa or acetic orcein is used to stain the chromosomes

(g) The chromosomes are then counted under the microscope. A photomicrograph may also be taken

The Karyotype of cultured cells is obtained and saved. Later on, karotype of subsequent generations is obtained and compared with the original karotype, which helps in identifying any change in genetic sequence during sub-culturing.

B. *Obtaining Pattern of Isozymes (Zymography):* The pattern analysis of isozymes for certain enzymes can be used to establish the identity of cell lines. All isozymes of a given enzyme are separated using gel electrophoresis and zymogram (banding pattern) is obtained. Zymogram is a characteristic feature of every cell line. Generally, glucose-6-phosphate dehydrogenase, lactate dehydrogenase, and nucleoside phosphorylase are employed to obtain zymogram.

C. *Fluorescent labeled antibodies:* Fluorescent labeled antibody, which is specific to the antigens present on the cell membrane can be used to identify a cell line. For example, fluorescein isothiocyanate is a fluorescent dye, which is attached to antibody **(Figure 17.12)**. Under microscope, the cells with fluorochrome on their surface show fluorescence and can thus be identified.

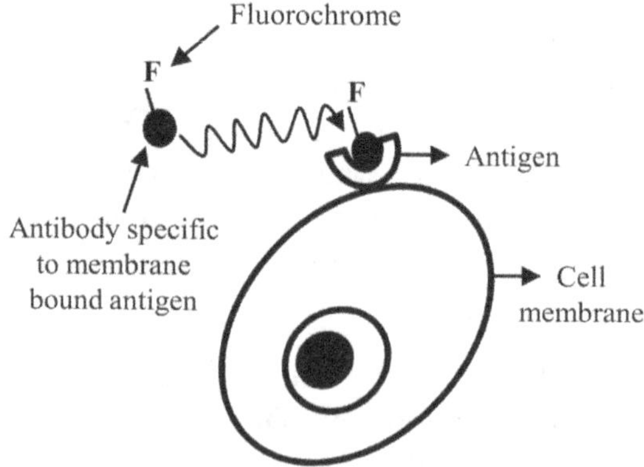

FIGURE 17.12 Fluorescent labeling using antibodies

2. **Monitoring cell lines for cell contamination:** Cell cultures are at a risk of getting contaminated with both chemical substances as well as microorganisms.

A. *Chemical Contamination*: It is comparatively more difficult to detect due to invisibility of the chemicals in the cultures. The most common sources of chemical contamination include endotoxins, plasticizers, metal ions, chemical disinfectants, etc.

B. *Biological Contamination*: The animal culture media are highly susceptible to biological contaminants (microorganisms) such as yeast, bacteria and fungi. However, these contaminations are easy to identify because of visible effects produced by these microorganisms, which include changes in the turbidity and pH of the culture. However, mycoplasma and viruses are exceptions as contamination due to these are difficult to identify and eradicate. Mycoplasma are about 0.3–0.5 μm in size and these have the ability to grow inside the cytoplasm of the animal cell. The contamination with mycoplasma is difficult to identify, moreover, after it gets established it becomes difficult to eradicate it from the cell culture. To detect the presence of mycoplasma in the culture, a fluorochrome called 'bisbenzamide' is added. It works by intercalating with the DNA of the mycoplasma and under the UV light it gives off fluorescence. Hence, it stains mycoplasma infected cells. To remove mycoplasma from the cell culture, they are treated with a mixture of antibiotics, kanamycin and tylocine.

Precautions and Prevention

Microorganisms have a capability of multiplying at a rate faster than that of the cells in the medium. Therefore, cell lines need to be cultured and handled under good aseptic conditions. The laminar flow cabinet fitted with HEPA filters should be employed for carrying aseptic operations. Moreover, the sterility of the solutions and the media should be ensured by incubating them at a temperature suitable for the growth of bacteria and fungus. This helps in identifying if the media is contaminated or not. To decrease the chances of contamination, antibiotics may be added in the media (**Figure 17.13**).

APPLICATIONS OF ANIMAL CELL CULTURE

Over the years, after vast development in animal cell culture, it has become one of the important tools in the field of medicine. Currently, it has been employed in following ways:

1. **Basic Sciences:** Culturing the animal cells has made it possible for the learners and researchers to understand the basic cell biology and related biochemistry, the response of cells to disease causing agents, the

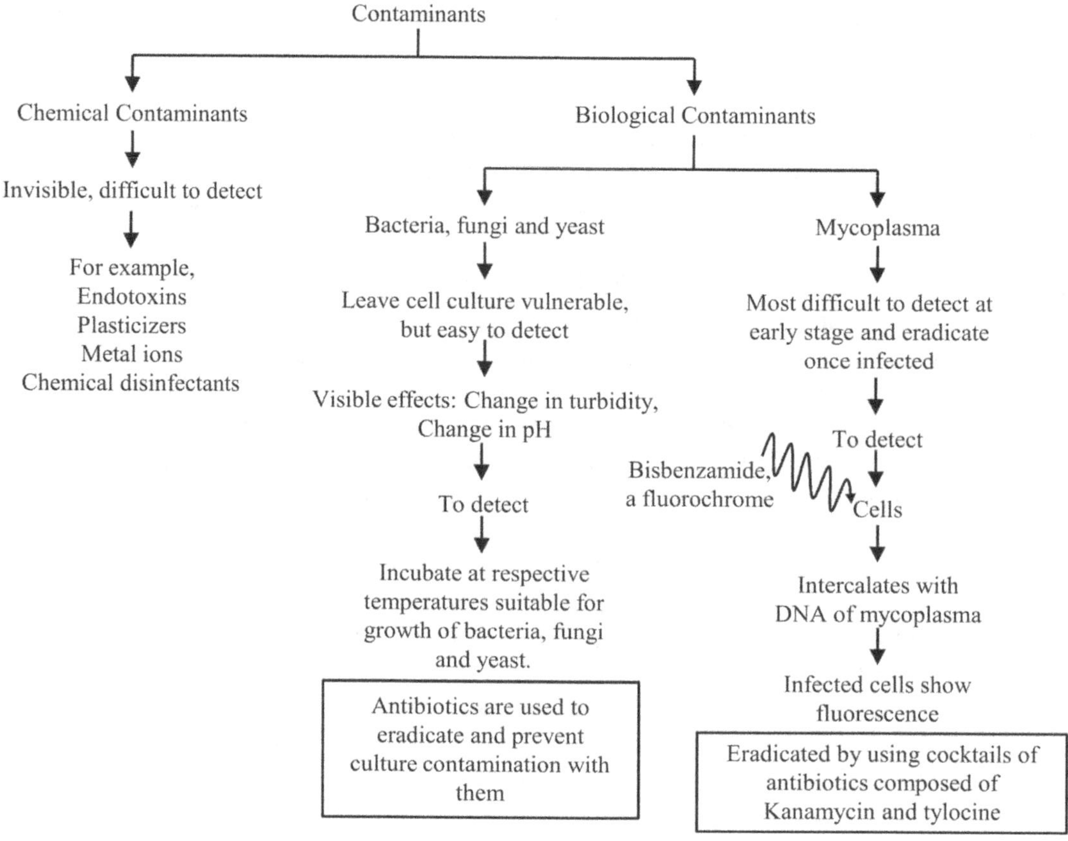

FIGURE 17.13 Source of contamination, their detection and eradication

mechanism by which the drugs affects the cells, the factors responsible for ageing, and how the cells obtain nutrition.

2. **Cancer Research:** Cell culture technique has enabled us to grow both cancer as well as normal cells. Hence, the differences between the normal and cancer cells can be easily studied. Also, normal cells can be converted into cancerous cells by treating them with viruses, chemicals, and radiations. Therefore, it can be very helpful in understanding the mechanisms responsible for inducing mutations or cancer development. Moreover, the effect of anti-cancer drugs can also be studied in-vitro using cancer cells.

3. **Testing the toxicity of drugs:** Instead of testing new drugs for toxicity *in vivo* alone, it is preferable to test them *in vitro* using cell culture as well. Many drugs, chemicals and cosmetics can be tested for their toxic effect by noting their effects on the growth and survival of different types of cells, for example liver and kidney derived cell cultures.

4. **Virology:** The study of replication of viruses in cell cultures has been one of the earliest applications of cell culture. It has been very helpful in production of vaccines, such as polio, rabies, chicken pox, hepatitis B and measles. Also, viruses can be detected, isolated, and the mechanism of their growth and infecting other cells can be understood with the help of cell culture.

5. **Manufacturing Biologics from Cells:** Cells have been genetically engineered so that they can produce medicinally important proteins (biologics). On large scale, these biologics are produced with the help of cell culture. For example: production of monoclonal antibodies, insulin, hormones, etc.

6. **Organogenesis:** Embryonic and adult stem cells can also be grown *in vitro* so as to provide as a replacement for damaged organs and tissues. Currently, artificial skin is produced in the laboratories by this technique for the treatment of burns and ulcers. Moreover, efforts are also being made to prepare organs, such as, liver, kidney and pancreas in the laboratories so as to provide treatment of certain diseases.

7. **Genetic Counseling:** Fetal diseases are diagnosed much earlier with the help of a diagnostic technique called 'amniocentesis'. It involves withdrawing some fetal cells present in the amniotic fluid and culturing them to identify any abnormalities in the chromosomes.

8. **Genetic Engineering:** It has now become possible to modify the characteristics of cultured cells by adding new desired genetic material in them. It is an important way by which the researchers can study the effects that are imposed by inducing some specific genetic changes in the cells. Moreover, it can also be used to produce the desired proteins on large scale by culturing the cells of interest.

9. **Gene Therapy:** Genetic engineering of cells has led to opening possibilities of treating some gene related diseases. The patients with altered/ faulty/ missing genes may be treated by removing the faulty gene and replacing it with the correct gene. The cells after being modified are then cultured followed by injecting them back in the patient.

10. **Screening and Development of New Drugs:** This is very important application in new drug discovery in pharmaceutical industry. Cell based assays have gained importance in the pharmaceutical industry over time. These are routinely used for high throughput screening of new drugs. Earlier 96 well plates were used for carrying out these tests, but now 384 and 1536 well plates are being put to use due to increase in the use of this test for drugs.

REVIEW QUESTIONS

TWO MARKS QUESTIONS

1. Draw a pattern of animal cell growth in culture media.
2. What is the importance of animal cell culture in new drug discovery?
3. What is HITES media?
4. What is carrel flask?
5. What is hanging drop technique?
6. What are the advantages of serum free cultures?
7. How is coulter counter used for cell counting?
8. What are anchorage and anchorage independent cells?
9. What is cryopreservation and how animal cells are cryopreserved?
10. How can mycoplasma be detected and removed from animal cell culture?

FIVE MARKS QUESTIONS

1. What are the differences between normal and transformed cells?
2. Write a note on culture media employed for animal cell culture?
3. What are different methods of counting cells number in cell culture?
4. What are primary, secondary cell cultures and transformed cell lines?
5. Explain methods of for monitoring the cell lines for genetic stability.

TEN MARKS QUESTIONS

1. What are the different methods of monitoring cultured animal cells?
2. What are the applications of animal cell culture?

MULTIPLE CHOICE QUESTIONS

1. Which of following shows anchorage independent growth?
   (a) Epithelial cells   (b) Lymphocytes
   (c) Smooth cells   (d) All the above

2. Which of following is advantage of serum free culture media?
    (a) Consistency   (b) Cheap
    (c) Less contamination   (d) All the above

3. In trypan blue test, viable cells are
    (a) Stained   (b) Non stained
    (c) Gives fluorescence   (d) Gives chemilumniscence

4. Which of following is not a limitation of coulter counter method?
    (a) Speed
    (b) Differentiation between viable and nonviable cells
    (c) Counting cells in aggregates
    (d) Useful for anchorage dependent cells

5. Which of following is used for stability of genetic monitoring?
    (a) Karyotyping
    (b) Zymogram
    (c) Fluorescent labeled antibodies
    (d) All the above

CHAPTER 18

Assays and Flow Cytometry
(Princciples and Applications)

CHAPTER OUTLINE

Cell Viability Assays
Definitions and General Features
Tetrazolium Reduction Assays
Resazurin Reduction Assay
Propidium Iodide Based Cell Viability Assay
Protease Activity Based Viability Assay
ATP Assay
Evans Blue and Trypan Blue Test
Applications

Calcium Influx Assays
Chemiluminescence Method
Fluorescence Method
Applications

Glucose Uptake Assays
Definitions and General Features
Measurement of Glucose uptake using Radiolabeled 3-o-methylglucose
Measurement of Gucose uptake using Radio-labeled 2-deoxyglucose
Measurement of Glucose uptake by Detecting Intensity of Fluorescence
Application

Flow Cytometry
Definition and General Features
Principle
Working
Applications

CELL VIABILITY ASSAYS

DEFINITIONS AND GENERAL FEATURES

Cell viability assays are used to estimate/determine the number of viable (live) cells in a cell culture, tissues or multi-well plates. In other words, these tests are used to identify the number of living cells in a total number of cells. These assays are generally performed to

(i)   measure cell proliferation in animal cell culture or others

(ii)   evaluate the cytotoxic effects of test compounds

1. **Tetrazolium Reduction Assays:** Among a variety of tetrazolium compounds used to detect viable cells, the most commonly used compounds include MTT, MTS, XTT, and WST-1. These compounds fall into two basic categories:

(i) Chemicals that penetrate in the viable cells e.g. MTT. These are directly converted into colored formazan inside the cells.

(ii) Negatively charged chemicals that do not penetrate in the cells e.g. MTS, XTT, and WST-1. These require additional electron acceptor that may help in reducing tetrazolium to colored formazan product.

MTT Based Cell Viability Assay: MTT refers to 3-(4,5-dimethylthiazol-2-yl)-2,5-diphenyltetrazolium and it is one the most commonly employed cell viability test. MTT is dissolved in a physiological solution, added to cells in a culture (at a final concentration of 0.2 - 0.5 mg/ml) and incubated for about 4 hours at 37°C. Inside the viable cells, MTT is reduced to intensely colored formazan by NADH and intensity of color (measured at 570 nm) is directly proportional to number of viable cells. However, due to absence of NADH in dead cells, MTT is not reduced in dead cells and such cells do not give any color **(Figure 18.1)**.

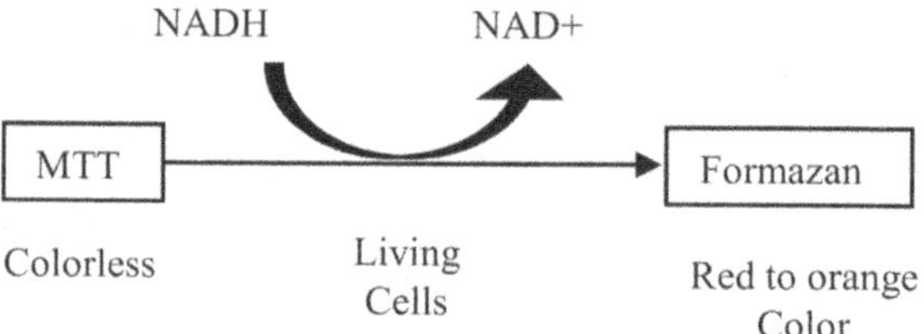

FIGURE 18.1 Principle of reduction of colorless MTT to form red-orange colored formazan in living cells in the presence of NADH

The conversion of MTT to formazan and amount of colored signal is dependent on number of factors such as time of incubation, concentration of MTT, number of viable cells and metabolic activity of cells. Therefore, these parameters must be taken into consideration for interpreting the results.

MTS, XTT, and WST Based Cell Viability Assay: These are recently developed tetrazolium reagents that may also be reduced to formazan products in the presence of viable cells. However, these reagents (cannot penetrate and enter inside the cells) are used in combination with electron acceptor reagents such as phenazine methyl sulfate (PMS) or phenazine ethyl sulfate (PES). Phenazine methyl sulfate penetrates the viable cells and get reduced in the cytoplasm by accepting electrons. After reduction, the reduced form of phenazine methyl sulfate moves outside the cell, where they convert tetrazolium salts to soluble colored formazan products **(Figure 18.2)**.

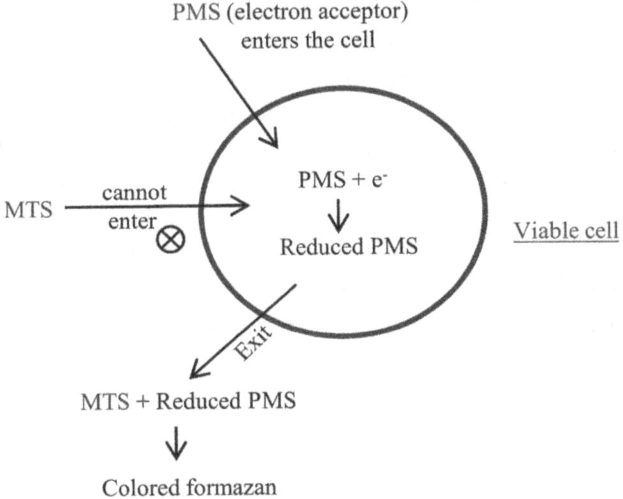

FIGURE 18.2 Principle of reduction of MTS in association with PMS to form colored formazan

2. **Resazurin Reduction Assay (Alamar Blue):** Resazurin reduction assay is a fluorescent assay and this assay has been used to check cell viability in a number of cell proliferation and cytotoxicity assays. Resazurin (7-hydroxy-3H-phenoxazin-3-one-10-oxide) is a blue dye and it gets reduced to highly fluorescent compound resorufin (pink in color) in the presence of mitochondrial enzymes. This conversion can take place only in the viable cells with active metabolism. On the other hand, dead cells are unable to reduce the dye to give fluorescence. This assay involves the addition of 20 µL resazurin (0.15 mg/mL) to 100 µL cell suspensions and incubation of 1 to 4 hours. Thereafter, fluorescence is checked at an excitation wavelength of 560 nm and 590 nm for emission. This assay method has a number of advantages including speed, reliability, sensitivity and cost.

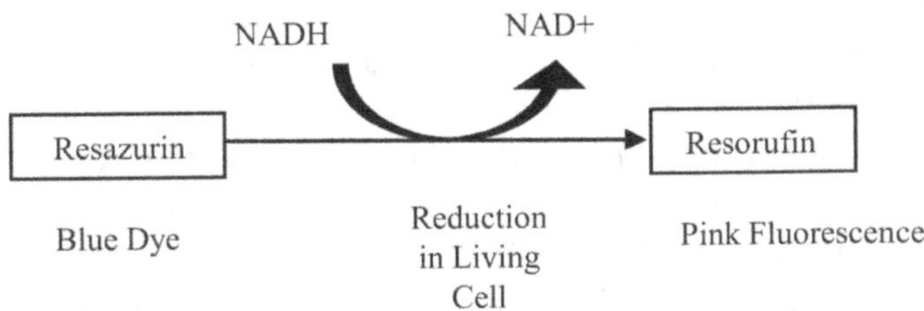

FIGURE 18.3 Principle of reduction of blue colored dye Resazurin to pink fluorescence emitting resorufin in living cells

3. **Propidium Iodide Based Cell Viability Assay:** Propidium iodide assay is also a fluorescence-based method to assess the cell viability. It is a dye, which cannot penetrate the living cells i.e. it is impermeable and cannot cross the membrane of viable cells. However, in dead cells, there is an increase in permeability of cell membrane due to its rupturing. Therefore, this dye can enter inside the cells to bind and intercalate with DNA. The intercalated complex of DNA-propidium iodide gives fluorescence, which is measured using excitation wavelength of 488 nm and emission wavelength of 617 nm. Thus, living cells do not emit fluorescence, while dead cells give fluorescence with propidium iodide **(Figure 18.4)**.

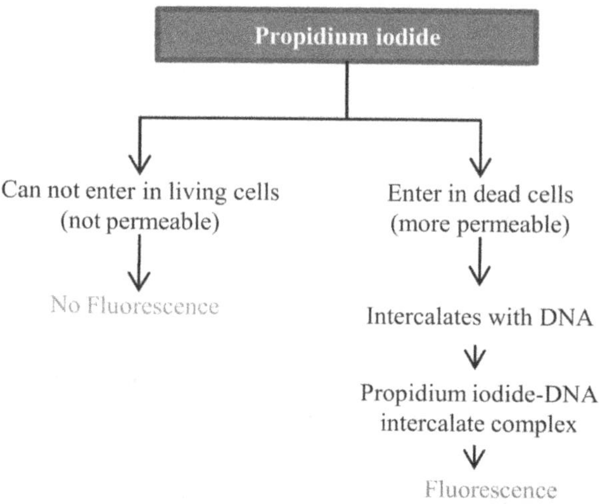

FIGURE 18.4 Differentiation of dead cells (more permeable) and living cells (less permeable) using propidium iodide

4. **Protease Activity Based Viability Assay:** In this assay, measurement of cellular protease activity within a live cell serves as a marker of cell viability. A cell permeable fluorogenic protease substrate, GF-AFC (glycylphenylalanyl-aminofluorocoumarin), is used to detect protease activity of living cells. The GF-AFC penetrates the live cells, where aminopeptidases present in cytoplasm removes amino acids to release aminofluorocoumarin (AFC). AFC in free form gives fluorescence, which is directly proportional to the number of viable cells **(Figure 18.5)**. On the contrary, dead cells do not possess (or lose) protease activity and thus, GF-AFC remains inside the dead cells in bound form. Due to absence of free AFC in dead cells, there is no fluorescent signal. Cell culture and an equal volume of GF-AFC substrate is added in a well and incubated for 30 minutes to 3 hours. Thereafter, fluorescence is measured at 380-400 nm excitation and 505 nm emission wavelengths.

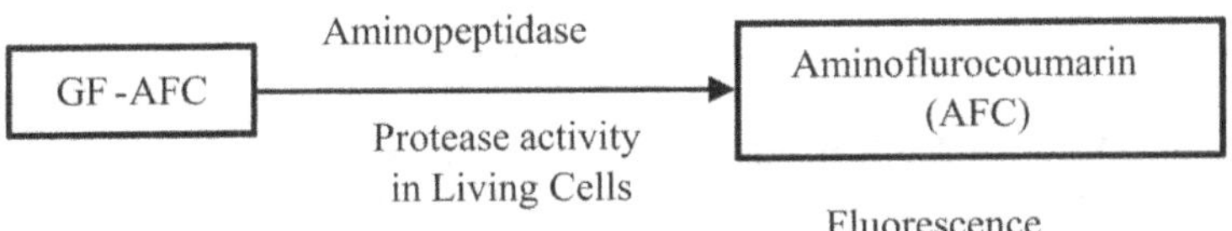

FIGURE 18.5 Conversion of GF-AFC to fluorescence emitting AFC in living cells due to the presence of protease activity. However, dead cells are unable to perform this conversion as they lose protease activity.

5. **ATP Assay:** ATP has been widely accepted as a useful marker of cell viability. In dead cells, there is loss of plasma membrane integrity and mitochondrial dysfunction. Therefore, dead cells lose the capability to synthesize ATP. Moreover, activation of ATPases inside the cells depletes remaining ATP. Thus, dead and viable cells are differentiated on the basis of ATP content. In this method, ATP detection reagent is added, which gives luminescent (light) signal. ATP detection reagent contains the followings:

(i) A detergent to lyse the cells and release ATP from cells.

(ii) ATPase inhibitors to prevent degradation of ATP. Thus, ATP released from the lysed cells is stabilized.

(iii) Luciferin as a substrate and luciferase as an enzyme to catalyze the reaction of ATP and luciferin. It produces a light, which remains stable for hours **(Figure 18.6)**.

(iv) It is one of the fastest and most sensitive cell viability assay methods.

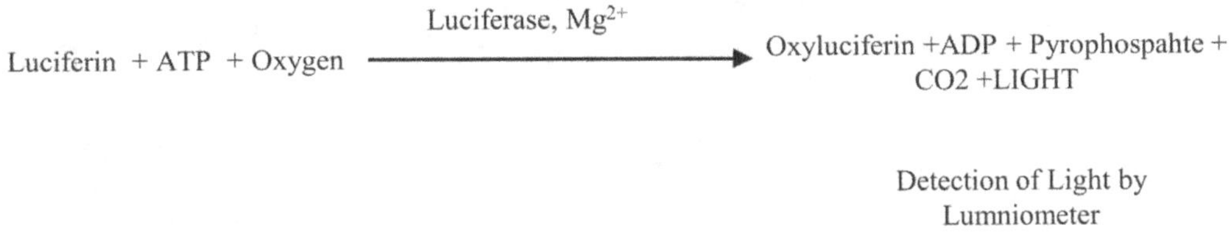

FIGURE 18.6 ATP reacts with luciferin in the presence of oxygen and luciferase to yield light as signal, which is detected by lumniometer.

6. **Evans Blue and Trypan Blue Test:** Evans blue and trypan blue are grouped under 'dye exclusion tests' and these are also commonly used to count the number of viable cells in cell culture. This test is based on the principle that dead cells are permeable due to loss of membrane integrity, while living cells are non-permeable. Due to increase in cell permeability of dead cells, these dyes can enter the cells and make cells blue in color. On the other hand, living and viable cells remain colorless. In this assay, cell suspension is mixed with trypan blue or Evan blue. Thereafter, a drop of cell suspension is transferred to a hemocytometer, and visualized under microscope to count the blue (dead cells).

APPLICATIONS OF CELL VIABILITY ASSAYS

1. These assays are very important in animal cell cultures and the numbers of viable cells are routinely checked during cell culturing.

2. These tests are very important in toxicological studies, where the toxicological effects of new drugs, cosmetics or other agents on cells can be determined in the form of mortality of cells. These tests can be used to determine LD_{50} of chemicals or drugs.

CALCIUM INFLUX ASSAYS

Calcium plays an important role in cell signaling systems; therefore, it is important to measure intracellular calcium levels. There are a number of methods to measure intracellular calcium ions and these include the followings:

1. **Chemiluminescence Method:** Aequorin is a calcium-sensitive bioluminescent protein obtained from the jellyfish *Aequorea victoria* and this has been extensively used as a calcium indicator. The aequorin forms a complex with calcium ions and emits light (chemiluminescence). The luminescence intensity is directly proportional to the Ca^{2+} concentration **(Figure 18.7)**. It is a very sensitive method of calcium measurement.

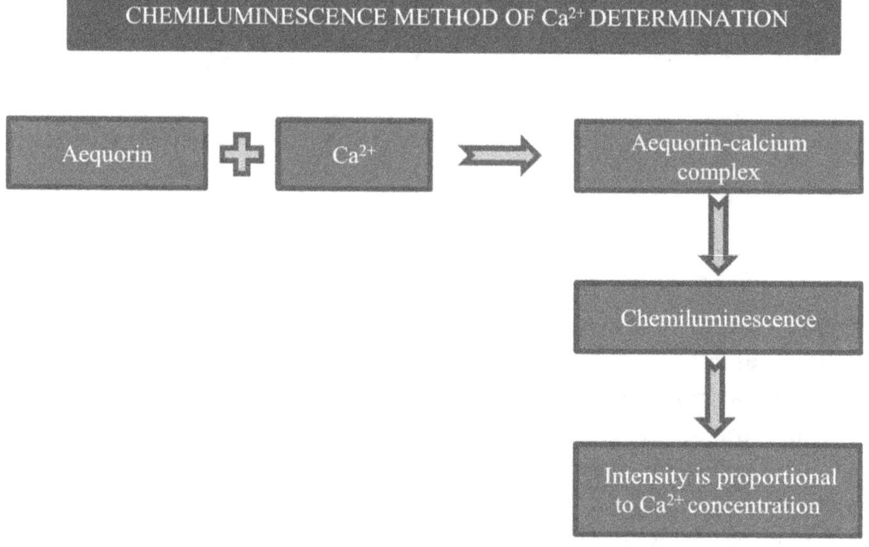

FIGURE 18.7 Principle of calcium determination with Aequorin using chemilumniscence

2. **Fluorescence Method:** To measure intracellular Ca^{2+} concentration, fluorescent indicators are also very frequently used. The various indicators used for this purpose include the followings:

(i) ***Indo-1 AM:*** Indo1-AM is very frequently used for measuring cellular calcium levels. Chemically, it is in acetyloxymethyl ester and it is cell permeable. This moiety enters the cells and it is cleaved by intracellular esterases to remove acetyl groups and make indo-1 from indo-1AM. Indo-1 is not cell permeable and it remains confined inside the cell. Inside the cell, indo-1 combines with calcium ions and this complex emits fluorescence under UV light at ~420nm. The intensity of fluorescence is directly proportional to calcium concentration **(Figure 18.8)**. It is also important to know that indo-1 *per se* (in unbound form) also emits fluorescence; however at different wavelength ~510nm. Therefore, the ratio of fluorescence intensity at these two wavelengths indicates the changes in intracellular calcium concentration.

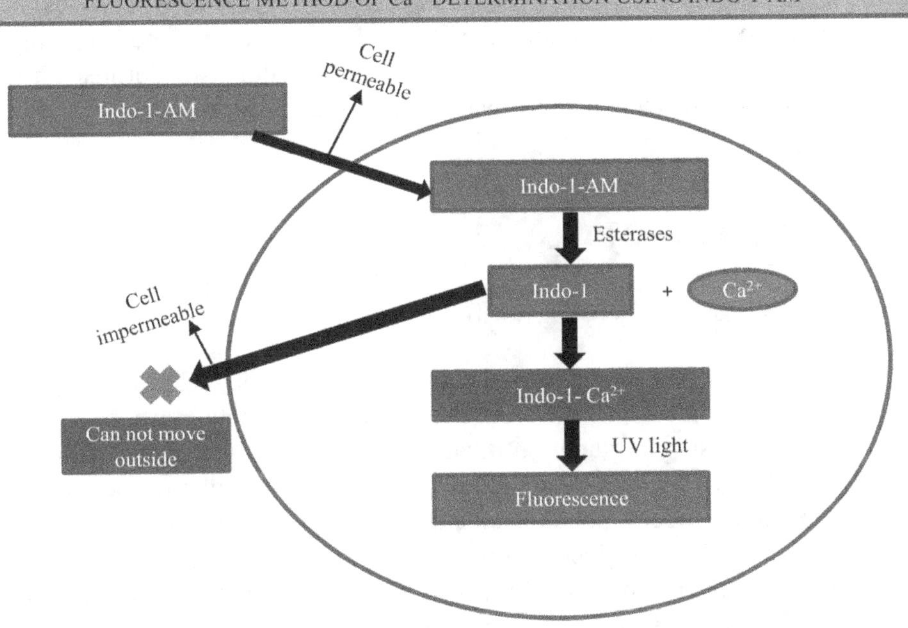

FIGURE 18.8 Principle of calcium determination with Indo-1-AM using fluorescence method

(ii) ***Fura 2 Ester:*** The basic principle of calcium determination using Fura 2 ester is similar to Indo-1 AM. Fura-2-acetoxymethyl ester (fura-2 AM) is cell permeable and enters inside the cells. Inside the cell, cellular esterases hydrolyse fura-2 AM to remove ester (acetoxymethyl group). Fura 2 is cell impermeable and it cannot move out. Fura 2 combines with Ca^{2+} to form a complex, which gives fluorescence at 335 nm (excitation wavelength) and 510 nm (emission wavelength). The intensity of fluorescence is directly proportional to calcium concentration. Moreover, *per se* fura-2 AM (unbound form) also gives fluorescence at 363 nm (excitation wavelength) and 510 nm (emission wavelength). In both states, the emission maximum is about 510 nm.

(iii) Others: There other fluorescence indicators used to measure calcium ion concentration and these include fluo-3 AM and fluo-4 AM. The principle of calcium determination is similar to Fura- 2 AM and indo-1 AM based methods. Fluo-3 is non-fluorescent compound; however, after forming a complex with Ca^{2+}, fluorescence is obtained, which is proportional to calcium concentration. Fluo-4 is an improved version of Fluo-3 and it gives brighter fluorescence.

APPLICATION OF CALCIUM ASSAYS

Since, calcium is an important cell signaling molecule, therefore, estimation of changes in the intracellular calcium levels helps to delineate the signal transduction mechanisms of various pharmacological agents.

GLUCOSE UPTAKE ASSAYS

DEFINITIONS AND GENERAL FEATURES

Glucose is the main source of energy in organisms, including humans and the uptake of glucose by different tissues such as skeletal muscles and liver is an important step in glucose utilization. Generally, glucose is transported across membranes by two different mechanisms i.e., Na^+ glucose co-transporter and Na^+ independent glucose transporter glycoproteins (GLUT). In mammalian cells, families of glucose transporters (GLUT) are located on the liver and muscles and perform this function. On the liver cells, GLUT2 is predominant, while GLUT4 is more predominant on the skeletal muscles. Glucose transporters facilitate the movement of glucose across the plasma membrane down its chemical gradient. Glucose uptake assays are done using radiolabeled glucose or radiolabeled glucose analogs such as 2-deoxyglucose (2-DG) and 3-O-methyl-D-glucose (3-MG). The different methods employed for measuring glucose uptake are as follows:

MEASUREMENT OF GLUCOSE UPTAKE USING RADIOLABELED 3-*O*-METHYLGLUCOSE

The glucose uptake activity in cultured cells is commonly analyzed using radioactive hexose e.g. 3-methyl glucose (3-MG). It is a non-phosphorylatable glucose analog and it accurately measures the rate of glucose transport as there is no interference from glucose-metabolizing steps. As the cells take-up radio-labeled glucose, there is an increase in radioactivity in cells. Therefore, the appearance of radioactivity is directly proportional to glucose up taken by cells.

The advantages of this method include better signal-to-noise ratio, high specificity, need of very short incubation time and no interference from glucose metabolism. However, the major limitation is use of radioactive substrate and need of special precautions to deal with radioactive substances. Therefore, this method may not be routinely used in laboratory.

MEASUREMENT OF GLUCOSE UPTAKE USING RADIO-LABELED 2-DEOXYGLUCOSE

The measurement of 2-deoxyglucose (2-DG) in the cells is also a reliable method to estimate the amount of glucose up-taken. The method is based on the fact that glucose and 2-deoxyglucose are taken up by the cells in the same manner. Therefore, the amount of 2-dexoyglucose up-taken by the cells represents the amount of glucose up-taken by the cells. As 2-DG enters inside the cells, it is phosphorylated to form 2-DG-6 phosphate, which accumulates in the cells. The accumulation of 2-DG-6 phosphate takes place because it is not further metabolized inside the cells. This assay is particularly useful to assess the extent of glucose uptake by glucose transporters, GLUT1 and GLUT4.

MEASUREMENT OF GLUCOSE UPTAKE BY DETECTING INTENSITY OF FLUORESCENCE

To overcome the problems related to radiolabeled analogs such as high cost, requirement of specialized equipment and training, non-radio-labeled forms of deoxyglucose are employed. Therefore, a rapid, inexpensive, and reproducible nonradioactive microplate assay for analyzing glucose uptake has been devised. The principle is that as deoxyglucose enters inside the cells, it is allowed to react with substrate that gives fluorescence. The intensity of fluorescence is directly proportional to amount of deoxyglucose present inside the cells.

In this assay, deoxyglucose is phosphorylated to deoxyglucose-6 phosphate. Thereafter, enzyme glucose-6-phosphate dehydrogenase (G6PDH) catalyzes the conversion of deoxyglucose-6 phosphate to 2-deoxy-6-phosphogluconate and concurrently, there is conversion of $NADP^+$ to NADPH. Resazurin is employed as a substrate, which is acted upon by diaphorase to form fluorescence emitting resorufin. The intensity of fluorescence is directly proportional to amount of deoxyglucose **(Figure 18.9).**

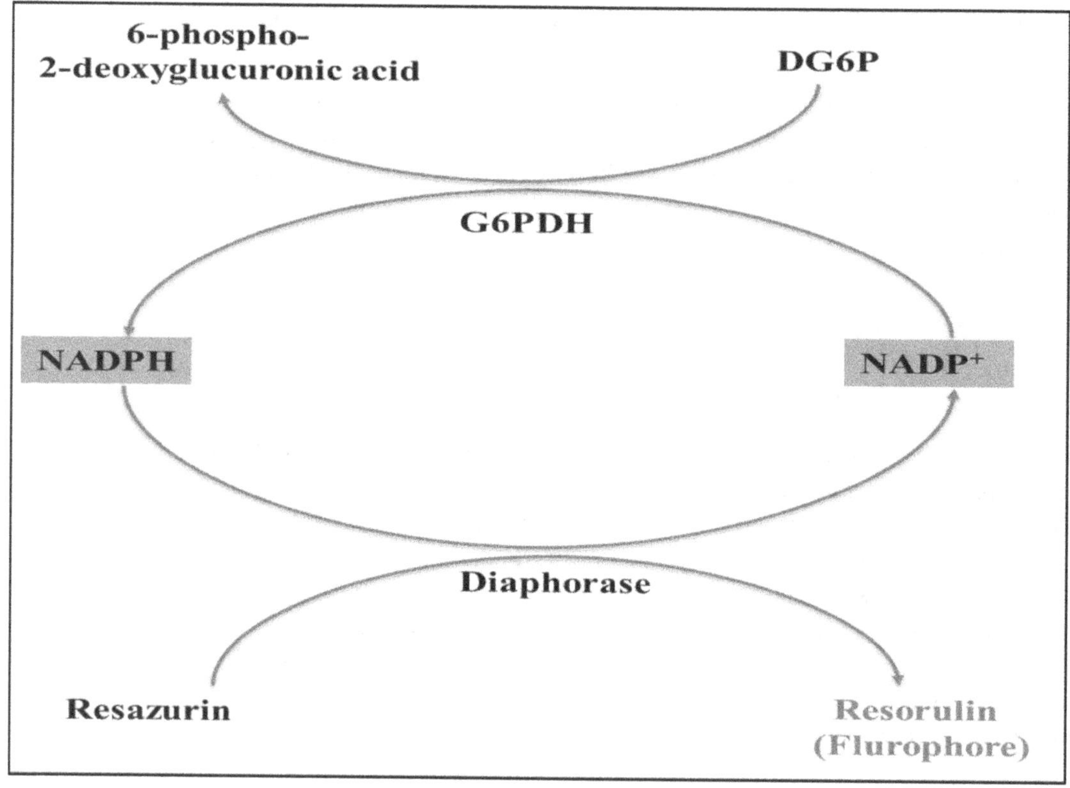

FIGURE 18.9 Principle involved in measuring glucose uptake by measuring the intensity of fluorescence

APPLICATION OF GLUCOSE UPTAKE ASSAYS

The major application of glucose uptake assay is study the phenomenon of insulin resistance. These tests are very commonly employed for screening anti-diabetic agents, which produce beneficial effects in diabetes by decreasing insulin resistance.

FLOW CYTOMETRY

DEFINITION AND GENERAL FEATURES

Flow cytometry is a quantitative technique of single cell analysis. A flow cytometer is an instrument, which is used to identify cells on the basis of amount of scattered light or emission of fluorescence, when the cell are allowed to pass through a laser beam. Based on the principle of flow cytometry, Fluorescence-activated cell sorter (FACS) has been designed, which is used to separate cells from thousands of other cells. In other words, FACS is used to separate heterogeneous population of cells on the basis of amount of light scattered or fluorescence emitted. Flow cytometer was developed in 1970's and it is one of the essential instruments in biologic sciences and clinical laboratories. Earlier flow cytometers were large and were available in limited centers. However, modern day flow cytometers are smaller, cheap and user-friendly. These features have led to its widespread use in different fields related to biological sciences.

PRINCIPLE

Flow cytometer is used to characterize single cell on the basis of its optical and fluorescence characteristics.

(i) As the light is allowed to fall on the cell, there is scattering of light, which is detected using optical detectors. Depending on the extent and direction of scattering, physical properties of cell such as cell size and internal complexities can be determined **(Figure 18.10)**.

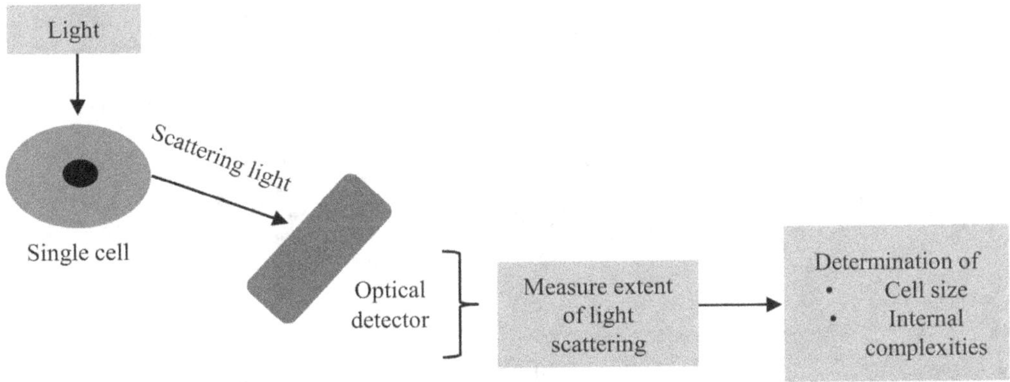

FIGURE 18.10 Principle of flow cytometer on the basis of light scattering

(ii) Alternatively, fluorescent dyes are allowed to bind with cell. These dyes may be specific for internal structure such as nucleus or external structure such as antigens on cell surface. Accordingly, these cells emit fluorescence on passing through light and several characteristics of cells may be noted on the basis of intensity of fluorescence. The fluorescence is detected using fluorescence detectors. For example, propidium iodide specifically bind/intercalate with DNA and amount of fluorescence is directly proportional to amount of DNA. Thus, fluorescence intensity can be used to analyze gain or loss of DNA in a cell (DNA content aneuploidy) **(Figure 18.11A)**. Similarly, antibody linked fluorescent dyes are used to bind specifically to cell surface antigens and depending on presence or absence of fluorescence, the presence or absence of surface antigens is determined **(Figure 18.11B)**. This process of identifying and analyzing cell surface antigen is termed as "immunophenotyping ".

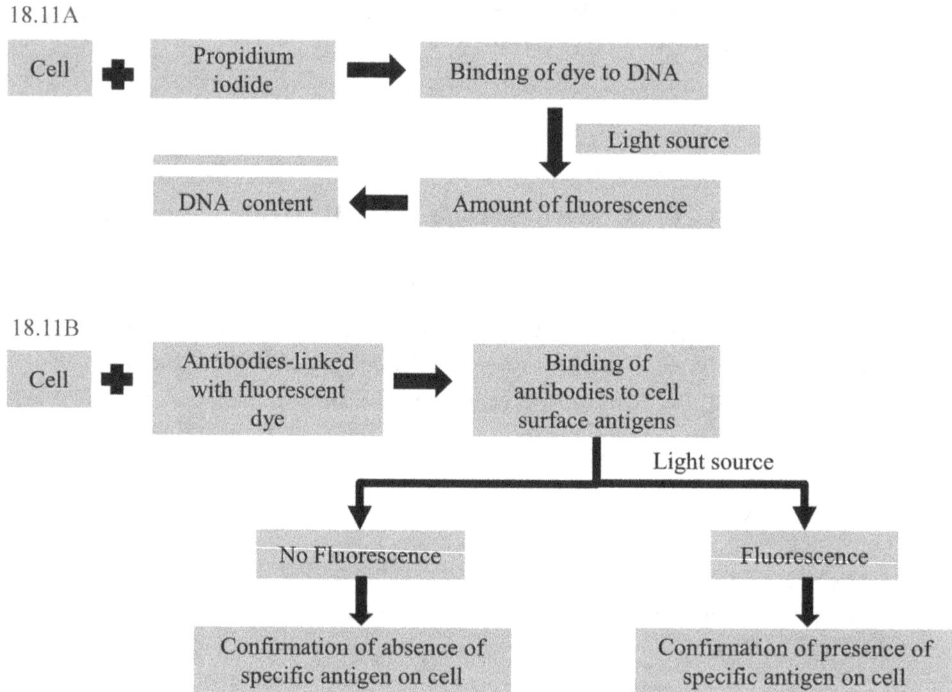

FIGURE 18.11 Principle of Flow Cytometer on the Basis of Fluorescent Properties of Cell. Determination of DNA content (18.11A) or immunophenotyping by determining the presence or absence of surface antigens on cells (18.11B).

WORKING

The different steps involved in flow cytometry are explained below:

1. It is important to note that flow cytometry may be performed only for cell suspension. In other words, cells should be separate from one another as this technique deals with a single cell analysis.

2. Accordingly, this technique is more difficult to perform on cultured cells because in these cases, cells are bound to one another through extracellular matrix. Therefore, samples must be treated with proteases to degrade the extracellular-matrix proteins and make cells free from one another.

3. A cell suspension is allowed to react with a fluorescent dye-linked with antibody or a fluorescent dye that binds to DNA.

4. Thereafter, cell suspension is mixed with isotonic 'sheath fluid'. The sheath fluid surrounds the cell suspension and helps in maintaining laminar flow inside the flow cytometer.

5. Indeed, the suspension is forced through a nozzle, which forms tiny droplets containing a single cell.

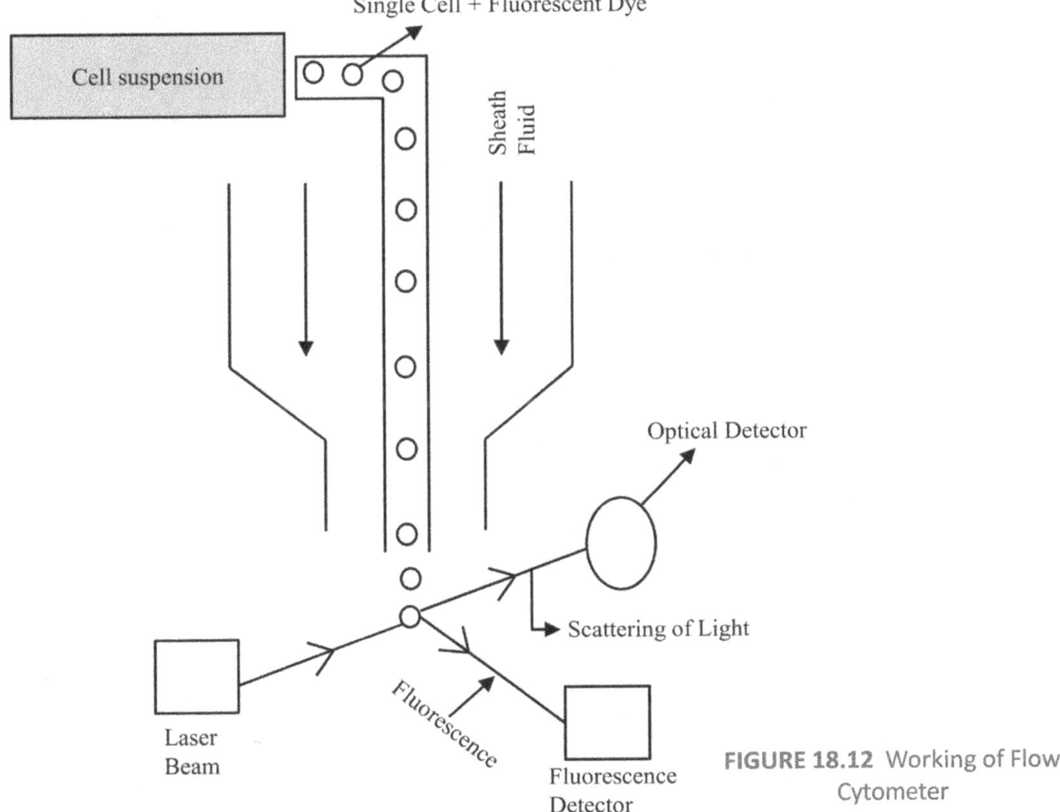

FIGURE 18.12 Working of Flow Cytometer

6. The cell suspension moves in downward direction in such a manner that a single cell passes at a time through a focused laser beam.

7. At the interrogation point, a laser light strikes to the cell and light is scattered in different directions, which is detected using optical detectors.

8. Moreover, due to binding of fluorescent dyes with the cells, fluorescent light is also emitted, which is detected using fluorescent detectors **(Figure 18.12)**.

9. In FACS, in which cell sorting is done, each droplet (having a single cell) is given an electric charge proportional to the amount of fluorescence. Thus, different cells acquire different charges depending on the fluorescence. These cells with different charges are separated by allowing to pass through electrodes. These cells are deflected differently depending on the charge and thus, different cells are collected **(Figure 18.13)**.

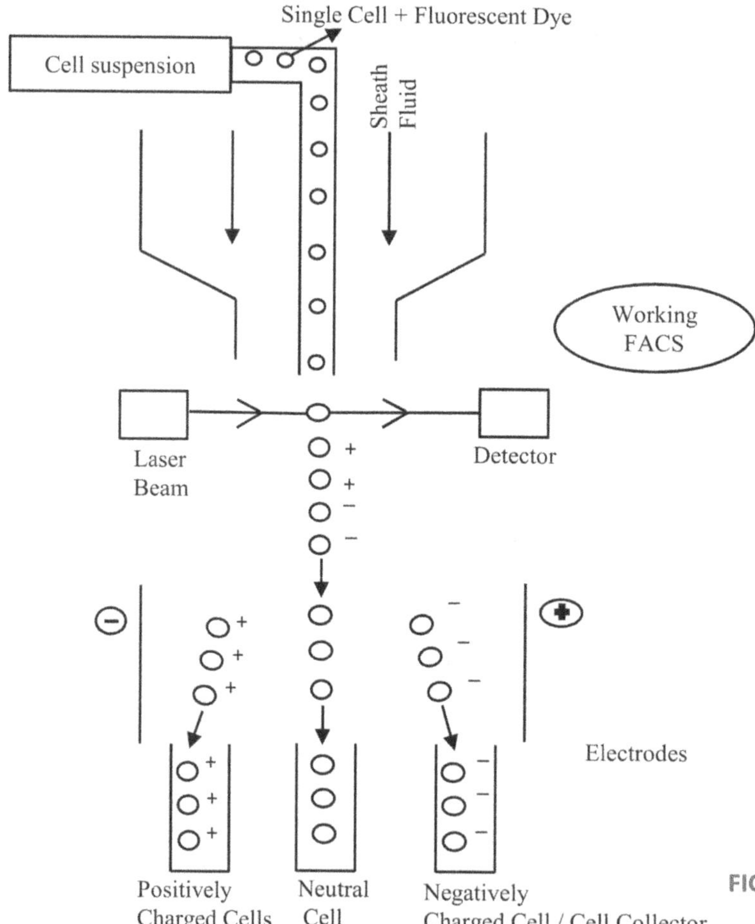

FIGURE 18.13 Working of FACS, in which cells are sorted depending on their charge.

APPLICATIONS

Flow cytometers have been very frequently used in laboratories for various purposes and these include the followings:

1. **Cell Sorting:** It is an important application of flow cytometry in which FACS is used to sort (separate) cells in a short span of time. e.g. separation of different lymphocytes from the blood.

2. **Immunophenotyping:** This technique is very commonly used to identify the presence of surface antigens on cells, particularly on lymphocytes. Identification of such antigens helps in diagnosis and classification of different blood cancers such as acute leukemias, non-Hodgkin lymphoma etc. The identification of such antigens is also important because treatment strategy is also dependent on antigenic parameters.

3. **Detection of Minimal Residual Disease:** It is a routine technique to detect minimal residual disease, which refers to presence of malignant cells after the treatment. After treatment, their number is significantly reduced so that these cannot be detected by conventional morphologic methods. These residual malignant cells may cause relapse in patients. PCR is another technique which may be used for detecting residual malignant cells and it is more sensitive method than flow cytometry.

4. **DNA Content Analysis to Detect Ploidy:** Flow cytometry may be used to detect abnormal DNA content in a cell, which is termed as "DNA content aneuploidy". DNA aneuploidy leads to cancer development and it has been associated with a large number of cancers. The DNA content is determined by allowing 'propidium iodide' to bind with DNA, which intercalates with DNA helical structure. The amount of fluorescence emitted is directly proportional to amount of DNA in a cell **(Figure 11A)**.

5. **Reticulocytes and Platelet Count:** Flow cytometry is very common technique in hematology and is used to measure the number of reticulocytes as well as platelets in the blood. Reticulocytes are immediate precursor cells of RBC and their number may be used as an index of RBC synthesis. Their number is increased during hemolytic anemia such as thalassemia, sickle cell anemia. Moreover, their number may be used to analyze the regenerative capability of bone marrow after chemotherapy or bone marrow transplantation. Platelets play an important role in hemostasis and their reduced number is correlated with development of bleeding disorders.

REVIEW QUESTIONS

TWO MARKS QUESTIONS

1. What are most commonly employed compounds in tetrazolium reduction based cell viability assays?
2. What is the basic principle of tetrazolium based cell viability assays?
3. What is the principle of resazurin reduction cell viability assay?
4. What is the principle of propidium iodide based cell viability assay?
5. How may calcium be measured using chemilumniscence method?
6. Write two applications of flow cytometry?
7. What is flow cytometer?
8. What is the application of glucose uptake assay?
9. Write applications of cell viability assays?
10. What is the application of calcium assay?

FIVE MARKS QUESTIONS

1. Explain protease activity based viability assay?
2. Explain ATP based cell viability assay?
3. What do you understand by Evans Blue test for assessing cell viability?
4. What are other similar types of dyes that may substitute Evan blue?
5. What are fluorescence based calcium assay methods?
6. Write a short note on glucose uptake assays.

TEN MARKS QUESTIONS

1. Write a note on different types of cell viability assays.
2. Write a note on calcium assays methods.
3. Explain glucose uptake assay methods.
4. What are flow cytometers? What is its principle and applications?

MULTIPLE CHOICE QUESTIONS

1. Which of following does not give fluorescence with calcium?
    (a) Fura 2
    (b) Fluo-3
    (c) Aequori
    (d) Fluo-4

2. Which of following gives chemilumniscence with calcium
    (a) Fura 2
    (b) Fluo-3
    (c) Aequorin
    (d) Fluo-4

3. In trypan blue test, viable cells are
    (a) Stained
    (b) Non stained
    (c) Gives fluorescence
    (d) Gives chemilumniscence

4. The emission of light in ATP viability test show
    (a) Dead cells
    (b) Injured cells
    (c) Live cells
    (d) It is not a test for viability

5. Intercalated complex of DNA-propidium iodide gives fluorescence and emission of fluorescence is an indication of
    (a) Dead cells
    (b) Injured cells
    (c) Live cells
    (d) It is not a test for viability

6. Flow cytometry is used to
    (a) Measure calcium levels
    (b) To assess cell viability
    (c) To characterize cell type
    (d) To measure glucose uptake

7. The signal noted in glucose uptake assay after adding resazurin and deoxyglucose in cells is
    (a) Radioactivity
    (b) Color
    (c) Light
    (d) Fluorescence

8. Which of following is an application of flow cytometry?
    (a) Cell sorting
    (b) Immunophenotyping
    (c) DNA content
    (d) All the above

UNIT - 5

Cell Signaling

19. Receptors and Secondary Messengers 311

20. Intracellular Signaling Pathways 333

Receptors and Secondary Messengers

CHAPTER OUTLINE

Receptors

Classification Of Receptor Family
G-Protein Coupled Receptors
Ligand Gated Ion Channels
(Ionotropic Receptors)
Receptor Tyrosine Kinase
(Enzyme-Linked Receptor)
Nuclear Receptors
G-Protein Coupled Receptors
Structural Features of
G-Protein Coupled Receptors
Signal Transduction
G-Protein Coupled Effector Systems

Second Messengers
Inositol Trisphosphate (IP_3)
Biosynthesis inside the Cells
IP_3 Signaling Pathway
Diacylglycerol (DAG)

Signaling Pathway
Clinical Uses of Protein Kinase
C Modulators

Nitric Oxide
Introduction and Brief History
Synthesis of NO by Nitric Oxide Synthase
Key Targets of NO
Physiological Functions of NO
Pathophysiological Role of NO
Clinical Uses of Drugs Modulating
Nitric Oxide

Calcium Signaling
Introduction and Historical Development
Channels and Proteins Modulating
Calcium Levels inside the Cytoplasm
Calcium as Secondary and Tertiary
Messenger
Intracellular Signaling Cascade

RECEPTORS

Receptors are the protein structures, which bind with drugs, hormones or neurotransmitters to produce biological actions. The receptors may be present on the cell membrane, cytoplasm or in nucleus. Mostly, receptors are present on the surface of cell membrane. The molecules which bind to receptors are termed as ligands. The ligand binding with receptors leads to signal transduction. Signal transduction (cell signaling) is the transmission of physical or chemical signals from a cell's exterior to cell's interior through a series of molecular events.

CLASSIFICATION OF RECEPTOR FAMILY

Receptors have been classified into different types, depending on structure and functions.

1. **G-Protein Coupled Receptors:** These are the mostly widely expressed receptors in the body (Discussed Below).

2. **Ligand Gated Ion Channels (Ionotropic Receptors):** These receptors generally enclose an ion channel and binding of a ligand to external surface of these receptors leads to opening of ion channel. Due to opening of these ion channels, there is inward/outward movement of ions such as Na^+, K^+, Ca^{2+} or Cl^- leading to change in membrane potential, either depolarization or hyperpolarization. These receptors have a heteromeric structure and each subunit consists of an extracellular ligand-binding domain and a transmembrane domain. The transmembrane domain includes four transmembrane alpha helices. The ligand-binding cavities are located at the interface between the subunits.

Nicotinic acetylcholine receptor is a prototype of this receptor and it consists of a pentamer of protein subunits (2α, β, γ and δ). Acetylcholine binds to this receptor at the interface of each alpha subunit. The binding of acetylcholine is followed by alteration in configuration of receptor and opens the ion channels. The opening is followed by inward movement of Na^+ ions down the electrochemical gradient into the cell. The net inward movement of Na^+ (positive ions) leads to depolarization of the postsynaptic membrane and initiates an action potential. The other ligand gated ion channels are enlisted in **Table 19.1**.

TABLE 19.1 Examples of Ligand Gated Ion Channels

S.No	Name of Receptor	Actions	Ligands
1.	Nicotinic	Inflow of Na^+ ions (excitation) (agonist)	Acetylcholine Hexamethonium, Decamethonium (Antagonists)
2.	AMPA receptor	Inflow of Na^+ and Ca^{2+} ions (agonist)	Glutamate (excitation)
3.	NMDA	Inflow of Na^+ and Ca^{2+} ions (excitation)	Glutamate (agonist)
4.	$GABA_A$ receptor	Inward Movement of Cl^- ions (inhibition)	GABA
5.	5-HT	Excitation a well as inhibition depending on receptor subtype and location	Serotonin
6.	Glycine Receptors	Inward Movement of Cl^- ions (Inhibitory)	Glycine

3. Receptor Tyrosine Kinase (Enzyme-Linked Receptor): These receptors are also present on the cell surface and a large number of cytokines, growth factors (e.g. vascular endothelial growth factors) and hormones including insulin produce their actions through these receptors. These receptors have generally three main components:

(i) ***Extracellular domain:*** This domain faces extracellular space and it possesses a ligand binding site. Thus, a ligand binds to this site to initiate cell signaling cascade.

(ii) ***Transmembrane helix:*** There is a single transmembrane alpha helix, which links extracellular domain to intracellular domain.

(iii) **Intracellular Domain:** This structural part of receptor faces towards cytoplasm and it possesses enzymatic function. Generally, the enzyme is tyrosine kinase which leads to phosphorylation of tyrosine residues of its own structure i.e. it leads to autophosphorylation.

Signal Transduction: The binding of ligand to extracellular domain leads to dimerization of receptors. It means, two structural units of receptors couple with each other. In certain cases if dimer of receptors is already present, ligand binding stabilizes the dimer form of receptors. Dimerization leads to activation of tyrosine kinase activity of receptors and it induces autophosphorylation of tyrosine residues of its own structure. Thereafter, intracellular signaling proteins bind to the phosphorylated form of intracellular domain of receptors **(Figure 19.1)**.

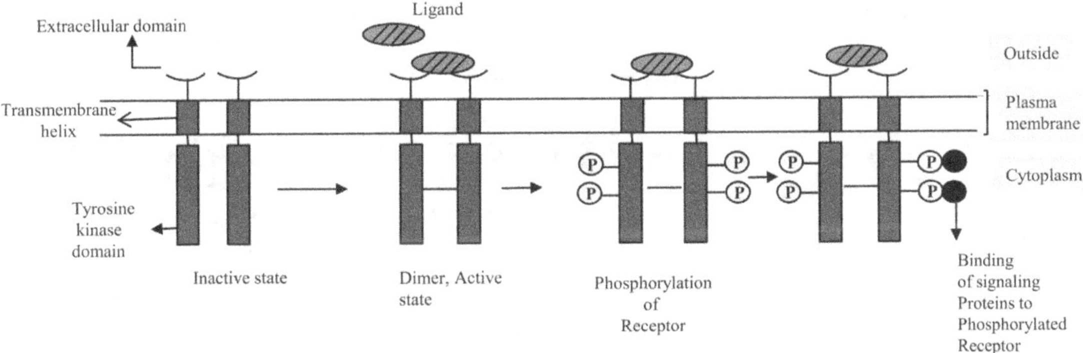

FIGURE 19.1 Structure and Signal transduction of Receptor Tyrosine Kinase

Regulation of Receptors Through Protein Tyrosine Phosphatases: The activity of receptor tyrosine kinase is regulated by protein tyrosine phosphatase enzymes. These enzymes remove phosphate groups from tyrosine residues of receptors. Therefore, these enzymes modify the actions of receptor tyrosine kinases by producing dephosphorylation of the activated phosphorylated tyrosine residues.

4. **Nuclear Receptors:** These receptors are not present on the cell surface; rather these are located inside the cytoplasm. The ligand is generally lipid soluble and it crosses the cell membrane to enter inside the cell and binds with these receptors. These receptors are called as nuclear receptors because after binding with a ligand, the ligand-receptor complex translocates from cytoplasm to the nucleus. The binding of these receptors to DNA portions results in alteration in gene expression. Thus, the onset of action of drugs acting through nuclear receptors is relatively slow. The drugs or steroidal hormones acting through these receptors include aldosterone, glucocorticoids, estrogen, progesterone etc. Structurally, the receptors generally possess:

(i) *C-Terminal Ligand-Binding Region:* Receptors have a ligand binding site at C terminal and thus, ligand binds to this site.

(ii) *Core DNA-Binding Domain (DBD):* This structural unit specifically binds to DNA. Infact, the receptor possesses two zinc fingers that are responsible for recognizing the DNA sequences specific to this receptor.

(iii) *N-Terminal Domain:* The domain at the N-terminal of these receptors interacts with cellular transcription factors in a ligand-independent manner. On the basis of these interactions, it modifies transcription of genes (Figure 19.2).

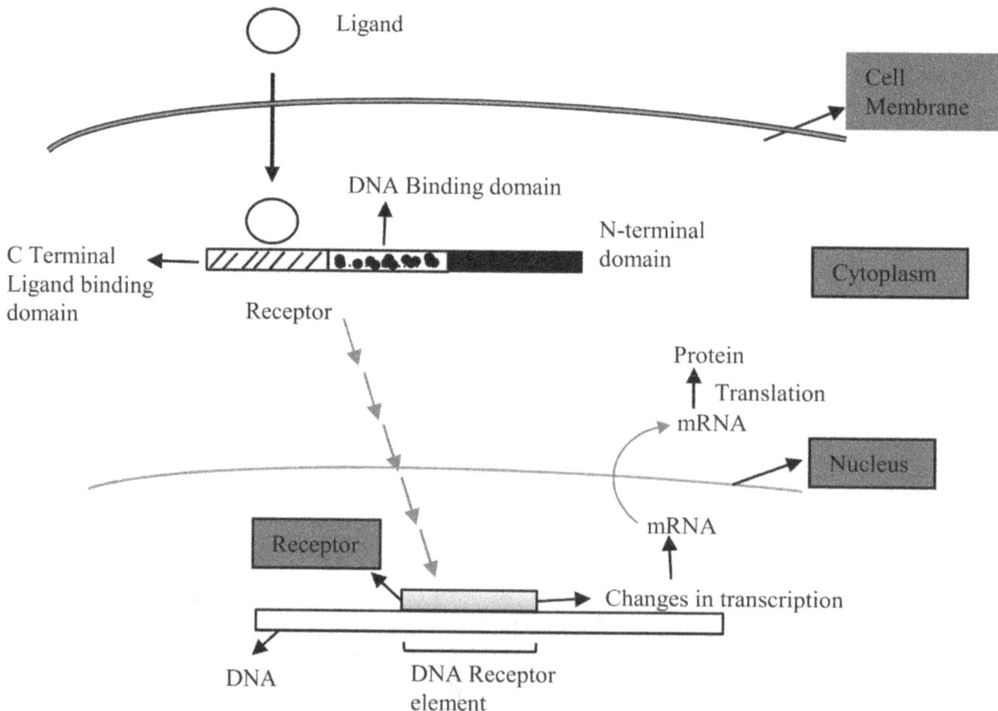

FIGURE 19.2 Signal transduction pathway of nuclear receptors

G-PROTEIN COUPLED RECEPTORS

G-Protein Coupled Receptors (GPCRs) constitute the largest family of cell surface receptors. These are membrane bound receptors which are coupled to the effector system (enzymes/channels) through guanosine triphosphate (GTP) binding proteins referred to as 'G-proteins'. There are hundreds of different GPCR proteins, which are important targets of drug action. About one third of currently available drugs act by binding to G-protein coupled receptors. The examples of these receptors include muscarinic receptors, adrenergic receptors, dopaminergic receptors, opioid receptors, serotonergic receptors, purine receptors etc. Apart from drugs, different endogenous peptide hormones and neurotransmitters also bind to these receptors.

STRUCTURAL FEATURES OF G-PROTEIN COUPLED RECEPTORS

These G-protein receptors have common structural features and all types of these receptors possess seven trans-membrane domains connected by three extracellular loops and three intracellular loops. The extracellular region possesses N-terminus and ligand binds to the extracellular region. On the other hand, the intracellular region possesses C-terminus region and interacts with G proteins, and other downstream effectors. Due to the binding of G proteins with intracellular domain of these receptors, these are termed as 'G-Protein Coupled Receptors'. G proteins are composed of three different subunits i.e., these proteins are heterotrimeric structures and these three subunits are α, β, and γ **(Figure 19.3)**.

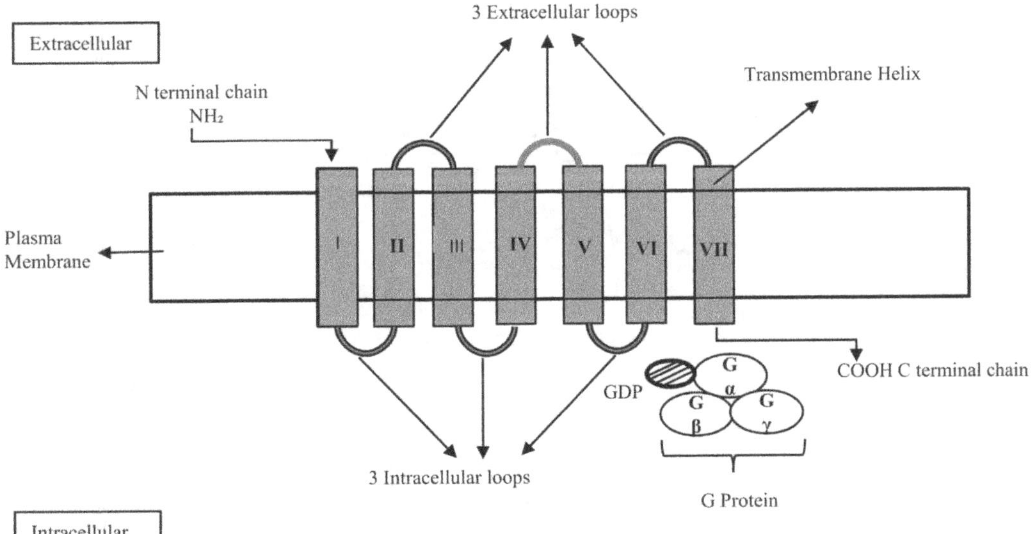

FIGURE 19.3 Structure of G-Protein Coupled Receptors

Depending on the functions of G proteins, there are different varieties of G-proteins i.e. Gs, Gi, Go and Gq. Since most of well known functions are performed by binding of α-subunit of G proteins with an effector, therefore, these G proteins are written along with a symbol of α. For example, Gs is also written as $G_{\alpha s}$, Gi as $G_{\alpha i}$, and Gq as $G_{\alpha q}$. Gs (s= stimulatory) produces stimulation of adenylyl cyclase to increase the levels of cAMP and it also leads to opening of Ca^{2+} channels. Gi (i = inhibitory) causes inhibition of adenylyl cyclase and decreases the levels of cAMP and it also leads to opening of K^+ channels. Go is involved in inhibition of Ca^{2+} channels; whereas Gq regulates phospholipase-C activity.

SIGNAL TRANSDUCTION

The different steps involved in signal transduction during activation of G protein coupled receptors include the following **(Figure 19.4)**:

1. In normal resting state i.e. in the absence of any stimulus/ligand, guanosine diphosphate (GDP) is bound to the α-subunit of the G proteins.
2. Upon activation of receptors by binding of a ligand, there is a conformational change in G proteins and GDP dissociates from α-β-γ subunit.

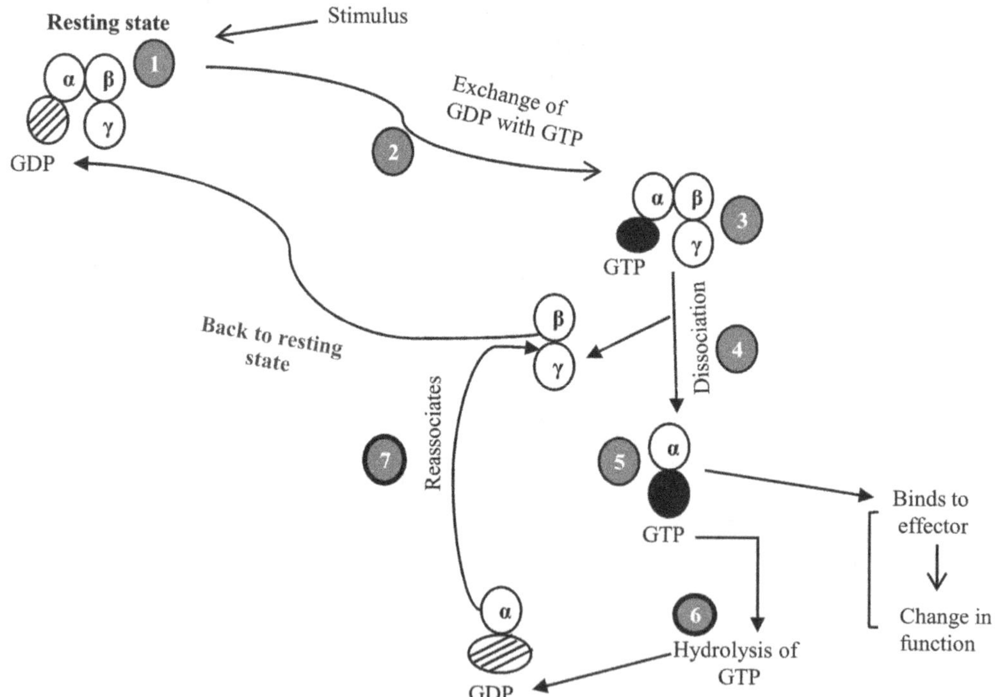

FIGURE 19.4 Signal Transduction Pathway in G- Protein Coupled Receptors. 1,2,3,4,5,6 and 7 are the steps explained in the text.

3. In the meanwhile, GTP associates with the α-subunit of the G proteins. In other words, ligand binding leads to exchange of GDP with GTP.

4. The binding of GTP activates the α-subunit and subsequently, α-GTP subunit dissociates from β and γ subunits.

5. The free α-GTP subunit binds to the effector/target protein and modulates its activity depending on the type of G proteins. Gs stimulates adenylyl cyclase to increase cAMP, opens Ca^{2+} channels; Gi inhibits adenylyl cyclase to decrease cAMP, opens K^+ channels; Go inhibits Ca^{2+} channels; Gq regulates phospholipase-C activity.

6. Due to intrinsic GTPase activity of α-subunit, GTP is hydrolyzed to GDP and the resulting α-GDP complex dissociates from the effector.

7. The α-GDP complex reassociates with the β-γ subunit to complete the cycle. It brings the cell back to normal resting state.

G-PROTEIN COUPLED EFFECTOR SYSTEMS

There are three main G-protein coupled effector systems including adenylate cyclase, phospholipase C and ion channels.

1. **Adenylate Cyclase:** This is an important effector system and has been linked with $G_{\alpha s}$ and $G_{\alpha i}$ proteins. Activation of $G_{\alpha s}$ proteins lead to activation of adenylate cyclase and increases the cAMP levels; while activation of $G_{\alpha i}$ proteins leads to inhibition of adenylate cyclase and decreases the cAMP levels. The details of cAMP signaling have been explained in Chapter 20. The β_1 adrenergic receptors in the heart are coupled to Gs proteins and activation of these receptors by norepinephrine and epinephrine leads to an increase in cAMP levels with increase in heart rate and heart contractility. On the hand, decrease in cAMP production due to activation of $G_{\alpha i}$-linked muscarinic receptors in heart produces decrease in heart rate and heart contraction.

2. **Phospholipase C:** In addition to $G_{\alpha i}$ and $G_{\alpha s}$ proteins, there is another important G protein, termed as $G_{\alpha q}$. Activation of $G_{\alpha q}$-linked receptors leads to activation of membrane enzyme, phospholipase C. It acts on phosphatidyl inositol 4,5-biphosphate (PIP_2) to generate inositol triphosphate (IP_3) and diacylglycerol (DAG). The details of these secondary messengers are explained below.

3. **Ion Channels:** In addition to well known effects of α-subunit of G proteins, it has been shown that βγ subunits of G proteins may also modulate the functioning of effectors. The most common target identified for Gβγ is G-

protein-regulated inwardly rectifying K^+ channels (GIRKs), which causes inward movement of K^+ ions. Other target modulated by $G\beta\gamma$ is Q- and N-type voltage-gated Ca^{2+} channels.

SECOND MESSENGERS

Second messengers are generated inside the cells in response to the binding of ligand to cell surface receptors. The ligands which bind to the extracellular portions of receptors are termed as 'first messengers'. The examples of first messengers include hormones, drugs or neurotransmitters such as norepinephrine, insulin, and histamine. On the other hand, the examples of second messenger molecules include cyclic AMP, cyclic GMP, inositol trisphosphate, diacylglycerol, and calcium. The main purpose of secondary messengers is to convey the signals from ligand, bound to the extracellular side of receptor, to inside the cells.

INOSITOL TRISPHOSPHATE (IP$_3$)

Inositol trisphosphate, also termed as inositol 1,4,5-trisphosphate, (also commonly known as triphosphoinositol) is an important secondary messenger and plays a key role in signal transduction. Structurally, it is composed of an inositol ring and three phosphate groups are attached at 1st, 4th, and 5th carbon positions. Moreover, three hydroxyl groups are attached at 2nd, 3rd, and 6th positions. IP$_3$ is soluble in cytoplasm and hence, it diffuses inside the cells.

BIOSYNTHESIS INSIDE THE CELLS

IP$_3$ is synthesized inside the cells along with diacylglycerol (DAG), from phosphatidylinositol 4,5-bisphosphate (PIP$_2$). PIP$_2$ is a phospholipid and it is an integral part of the plasma membrane. The binding of ligand to G protein-coupled receptors, coupled to a G_q protein, leads to activation of phospholipase C (PLC) enzyme. Indeed, α-subunit of G_q protein binds and activates PLC-γ isozyme. Phospholipase C acts on phosphatidylinositol 4,5-bisphosphate and it leads to its hydrolysis to release IP$_3$ and DAG. Moreover, activation of receptors linked with tyrosine kinase also leads to activation of PLC-γ, which may hydrolyze PIP$_2$ into DAG and IP$_3$. The binding of insulin to its receptor leads to activation of tyrosine kinase, with subsequent activation of PLC-γ and biosynthesis of DAG and IP$_3$ **(Figure 19.5)**.

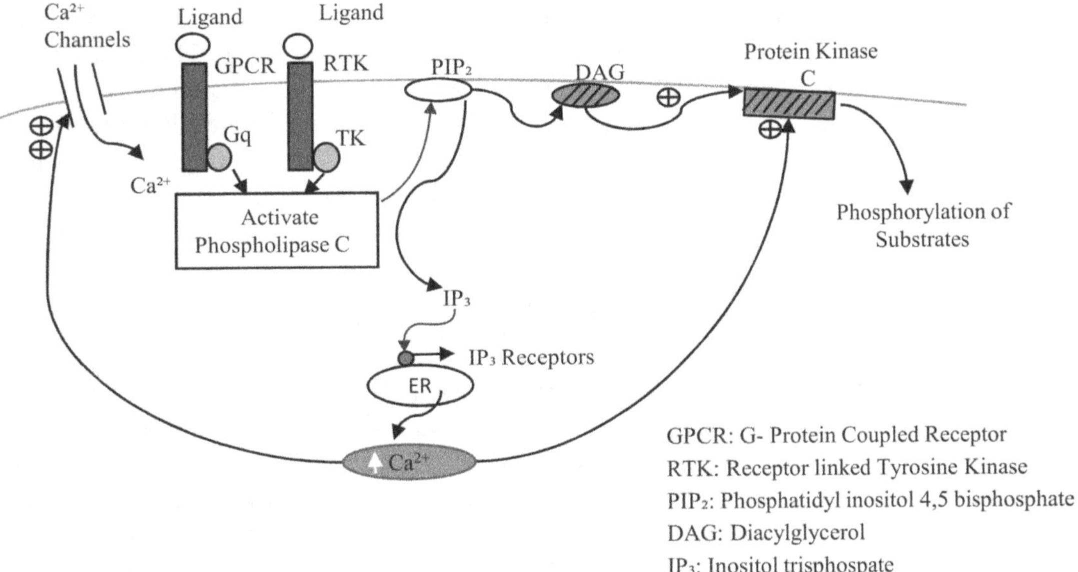

FIGURE 19.5 IP𝑓 and DAG as secondary messengers in cell signal transduction pathway

IP₃ SIGNALING PATHWAY

After formation of IP_3, it diffuses inside the cytoplasm and acts on Ins3P receptors located on the endoplasmic reticulum. Activation of Ins3P receptors leads to release of calcium from calcium store, endoplasmic reticulum and it is associated with an increase in the intracellular Ca^{2+} levels. In muscles, increase in calcium activates ryanodine receptor-operated calcium channels present on the sacroplasmic reticulum to release calcium from intracellular stores (discussed later).

DIACYLGLYCEROL (DAG)

Diacylglycerol is another important secondary messenger, which is generated along with IP_3 inside the cells **(Figure 19.5)**. However, DAG remains bound to cell membrane, which is in contrast to IP3, which diffuses in the cytoplasm. Structurally, diacylglycerol is a glyceride and it consists of two fatty acid chains attached to a glycerol molecule through ester bond.

SIGNALING PATHWAY

The main function of DAG is to activate protein kinase C and DAG is a physiological activator of protein kinase C. Indeed, DAG increases the activity of protein kinase C by increasing its affinity for calcium ions. Activation of protein kinase C leads to phosphorylation of serine/theorine residues of substrate molecules and produces a large number of physiological functions depending on the ligand and tissue/organ. Apart from activation of protein kinase C, DAG also performs other functions including production of prostaglandins, endocannabinoids and activation of transient receptor potential canonical (TRPC) cation channels.

CLINICAL USES OF PROTEIN KINASE C MODULATORS

Protein kinase C produces diverse actions and scientists have developed protein kinase C (PKC) inhibitors to manage diseases. Some of these inhibitors have been clinically approved. For example, ruboxistaurin has been found to be potentially useful in peripheral diabetic nephropathy. Bryostatin 1 is another PKC inhibitor and it has been tested for the management of cancer. Apart from PKC inhibitors, the PKC activators have also been evaluated for different diseases. Ingenol mebutate is a protein kinase C activator and it has been FDA-approved for the treatment of actinic keratosis. Another PKC inhibitor, bryostatin 1, has been investigated for Alzheimer's disease.

NITRIC OXIDE

INTRODUCTION AND BRIEF HISTORY

Nitric oxide (NO) is a volatile gas, which functions as a signaling molecule involved in many physiological and pathological processes. Being a volatile gas, it can freely diffuse across cell membranes and it has a very short half-life in the body. The half-life of NO in tissues is 3-6 seconds and in the blood, the half life is 1-2 seconds. Nitric oxide as a gas was discovered by Joseph Priestley in 1772 (two years after the discovery of oxygen). However, at that time it was known only for its toxic effects and it was found to produce death of several chemists by 'toxic-shock syndrome', due to accidental inhalation of large amounts of NO. In 1980, Furchgott and Zawadzki identified that endothelial cells secrete a molecules responsible for smooth muscle relaxation and they coined a term 'Endothelium-Derived Relaxing Factor' (EDRF). In 1987, Palmer, Ferrige and Moncada proposed that EDRF is actually a gaseous molecule i.e., NO, produced from L-arginine. In 1992, Malinski provide conclusive evidences that NO is the EDRF, which is released from endothelium and produces vasodilation.

SYNTHESIS OF NO BY NITRIC OXIDE SYNTHASE

NO is synthesized in the body by nitric oxide synthase (NOS), which oxidizes a guanidine nitrogen of L-arginine to release nitric oxide and citrulline **(Figure 19.6)**. There are three isoforms of NOS in the body: neuronal (nNOS or NOS-1), inducible (iNOS or NOS-2) and endothelial NOS (eNOS or NOS-3). The activities of nNOS and eNOS isoforms are dependent on calcium and these enzymes produce low amount of NO, which acts as physiological signaling molecule. On the other hand, iNOS-2 is calcium independent enzyme and it is responsible for production of large amounts of NO, which produces toxic effects.

FIGURE 19.6 Synthesis of NO from arginine with the help of NOS enzyme

KEY TARGETS OF NO

Nitric oxide acts on a number of targets in the body including 'thiol' groups. NO produces S-nitrosylation of thiols in which cysteine residues of proteins are reversibly modified by NO to form S-nitrosothiols. NO also leads to

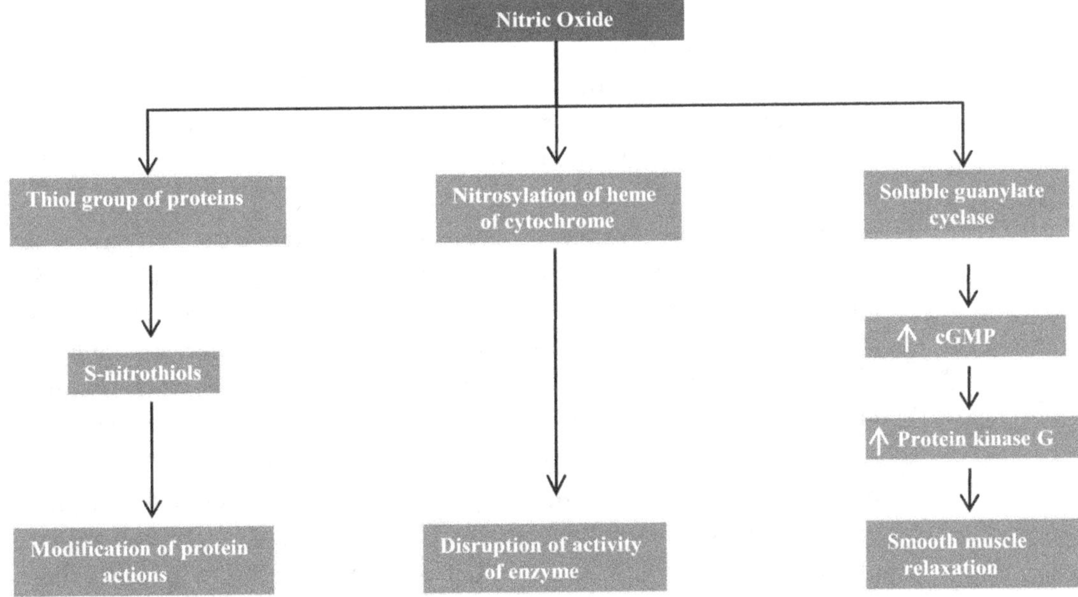

FIGURE 19.7 Key targets of nitric oxide in the body

nitrosylation of transition metal ion such as iron to form metal nitrosyl complex. For example, nitrosylation of heme proteins like cytochromes may disrupt the normal enzymatic activity. Hemoglobin is another heme containing protein that may be modified by NO. Guanylate cyclase is a heme-containing enzyme and it is activated by binding of NO with heme group of the enzyme. Activation of soluble guanylate cyclase leads to formation of cGMP, which is followed by activation of protein kinase G and smooth muscle relaxation **(Figure 19.7)** (details in chapter 20).

PHYSIOLOGICAL FUNCTIONS OF NO

Nitric oxide has dual role in the body. At low levels, production of NO due to eNOS and nNOS is responsible for a number of physiological functions. However, production of large amount of NO due to iNOS produces pathological actions (discussed later). The followings are the key physiological functions of NO in the body:

1. **Cardiovascular Functions:** Nitric oxide is an important molecule released by endothelial cells, which produces relaxation of vascular smooth muscles and blood vessel dilation. The basal release of NO from L-arginine in the presence of eNOS regulates the blood flow and vascular tone. Moreover, NO also helps in preventing platelet aggregation and blood clots. Approximately, 70–90% of endothelium derived NO passes in the blood to prevent platelet aggregation and blood clots. The remaining NO diffuses in the walls of arteries and veins (smooth muscle) to produce smooth muscle relaxation and vasodilation.

2. **Neurotransmitter in the Nervous System:** nNOS derived NO serves as an important neurotransmitter in the nervous system. In contrast to other neurotransmitters, it diffuses to other portions also (being a gas) and affect more than one cell.

   Central Nervous System: It has been identified that NO is a key neurotransmitter in a number of different brain portions and it controls neuronal morphogenesis, sexual and aggressive behaviors, food intake, pain perception, sleep, and cerebral blood flow. Its key role has been implicated in the hippocampus, which is key brain region in regulating learning and memory. NO is essential in establishing long-term potentiation required in formation of long term memory, not in short-term memory.

   Peripheral Nervous System: NO is a key neurotransmitter in the peripheral non-adrenergic non-cholinergic fibers (NANC). NANC is a general term of those nerve fibers, which do not belong to the sympathetic and parasympathetic branches. Indeed, NANC may be categorized as excitatory (eNANC) or inhibitory (iNANC) and nitric oxide is main neurotransmitter of iNANC system. Being a part of peripheral iNANC, nNOS derived NO inhibits gastrointestinal motility and relaxes sphincters, including lower esophageal sphincter, sphincter of Oddi, and anal sphincter. Since, iNANC also innervates bronchial airways and urogenital tract; therefore, NO relaxes bronchial muscles and regulates urogenital functions.

3. **Male Reproductive system:** Nitric oxide is considered as a physiological mediator of erection and one of the well described physiological effects of NO in the male reproductive system includes regulation of erection through NANC neurotransmission. The release and production of NO (nNOS) in the NANC and corpora cavernosa of the penis (eNOS) has been associated with erection.

4. **Immune and Antimicrobial System:** iNOS-derived NO modulate the functioning of immune system isoform. It acts to promote differentiation, proliferation and apoptosis of immune cells (B and T cells). Nitric oxide is generated by phagocytic cells including monocytes, macrophages, and neutrophils. A number of cytokines including interferon-gamma (IFN-γ) and tumor necrosis factor (TNF-α) activate iNOS present inside the phagocytic cells. NO combines with superoxide ion to form peroxynitrite (OONO$^-$), which is cytotoxic to bacteria and other microbes.

PATHOPHYSIOLOGICAL ROLE OF NO

Apart from physiological actions of NO, formation of large amount of NO may produce deleterious effects. Moreover, decrease in NO formation may also be deleterious.

1. **Ischemic Diseases:** During ischemic conditions such as myocardial infarction or stroke (decreased blood supply to brain), a massive release of NO may start reacting with superoxide anion to form cytotoxic peroxynitrite. It may contribute in producing serious and irreversible damage to heart and brain.

2. **Septic Shock:** Septic shock is a life threatening condition due to entry of bacterial toxin in the blood circulation. In this state, there is a massive release of NO, which produces extensive vasodilation to produce severe hypotension. A persistent and marked decrease in blood pressure may be responsible for death in septic shock patients.

3. **Atherosclerosis:** A persistently decrease in NO release due to endothelial dysfunction during diabetes mellitus, hypercholesterolemia, hypertension and smokers may be critical in the development of atherosclerosis.

4. **Diabetic Complications:** There is a decrease in the levels of nitric oxide in diabetic patients, which may result in diminished supply to different tissue including to lower extremities leading to development of neuropathy and non-healing ulcers.

CLINICAL USES OF DRUGS MODULATING NITRIC OXIDE

1. Nitroglycerin and nitrates are clinically employed in angina pectoris and congestive heart failure due to their vasodilatory actions.

2. Sodium nitroprusside is a NO donor and it has been clinically employed to mange hypertensive crisis and congestive heart failure.

CALCIUM SIGNALING

INTRODUCTION AND HISTORICAL DEVELOPMENT

Calcium is an important component of cell signaling cascade in virtually every cell of the body. The identification of calcium in signaling pathway was initiated by discoveries at the end of 1950s. Weber and his coworkers identified that the binding of calcium to myofibrils activates actomyosin. Ebashi and Lipmann identified that sarcoplasmic reticulum vesicles accumulate calcium using an ATP-energized system. Ebashi and Kodama identified the role of calcium in troponin and tropomyosin mediated myofibrillar contraction. The discoveries related to EDTA and its calcium chelating properties along with findings that removal of calcium by chelator (EDTA) leads to relaxation of muscle fibers. Presently, a lot of literature is available describing the role of calcium in cell signaling.

CHANNELS AND PROTEINS MODULATING CALCIUM LEVELS INSIDE THE CYTOPLASM

There are various proteins that influence the intracellular levels of calcium (**Figure 19.8**):

1. **Voltage or ligand gated calcium channels on the plasma membrane:** These channels open in response to voltage change or ligand binding and lead to inward movement of calcium inside the cell. Small increase in calcium due to movement of calcium from outside triggers the release of calcium

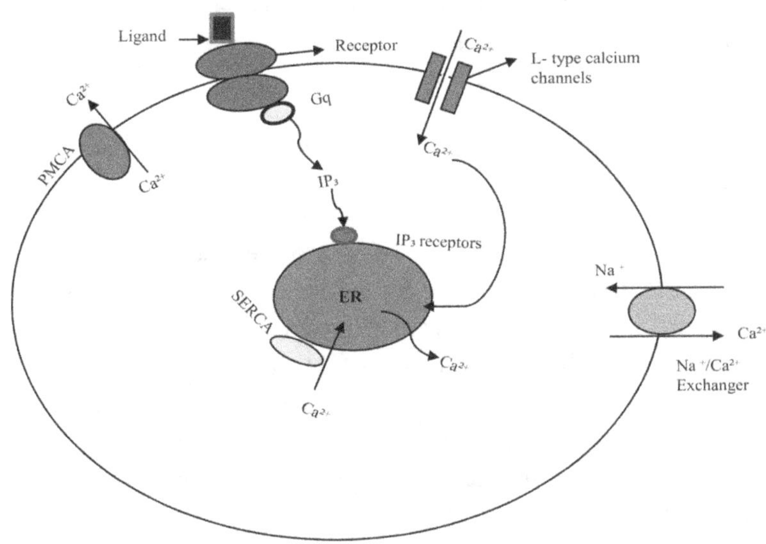

FIGURE 19.8 Channels and proteins modulating the calcium levels inside the cytoplasm. PMCA: Plasma Membrane Calcium ATPase; SERCA: Sarcoplasmic Reticulum Ca²⁺ATPase

from intracellular stores of calcium i.e. endoplasmic reticulum in almost all tissues and from sarcoplasmic reticulum from skeletal muscles. This phenomenon in which increase in calcium leads to release of calcium from intracellular stores is termed as 'calcium-induced calcium release'.

2. **Receptors on sarcoplasmic/endoplasmic reticulum:** Inositol 1-4-5 trisphosphate (IP_3) acts on IP_3 receptors located on endoplasmic reticulum to release calcium from internal stores (endoplasmic reticulum).

3. **Ca^{2+}APTase pumps:** These are present on the plasma membrane, termed as PMCA (plasma membrane calcium ATPase) and on endoplasmic/sarcoplasmic reticulum, termed as SERCA (Sarcoplasmic Reticulum Ca^{2+}ATPase). These pumps use ATP (energy) to move calcium against concentration gradient. PMCA tends to remove calcium from intracellular cytoplasm to outside. Ca^{2+}APTase pump removes excess calcium from the cytoplasm and moves inside the endoplasmic reticulum.

4. **Transporters such as Na^+/Ca^{2+} exchanger present on the cell membrane:** These transporters normally function in 'forward mode' to move calcium from cytoplasm to outside in exchange with sodium ion, which move inside the cell. However during ischemic conditions, these transporters

start operating in 'reverse mode'. In this mode, calcium moves inside the cell and sodium moves outside the cell.

CALCIUM AS SECONDARY AND TERTIARY MESSENGER

First messengers are defined to act on the plasma membrane receptors and induce the intracellular synthesis or release of second messengers. In turn, secondary messengers trigger changes to release or activate molecules and those released/activated molecules are termed as tertiary messengers. In most of cases, calcium has been described as a tertiary messenger as calcium is released from intracellular stores (endoplasmic reticulum) by the action of IP_3, which is a secondary messenger formed during activation of Gq protein. IP_3 mediated release of calcium has been described in earlier section **(Figure 19.9)**. However, calcium may also act as a secondary messenger. The opening of voltage or ligand gated calcium channels leads to inward movement of calcium and small increase in calcium triggers the release of calcium from intracellular stores of calcium. In this case, calcium released from intracellular stores acts as secondary messenger.

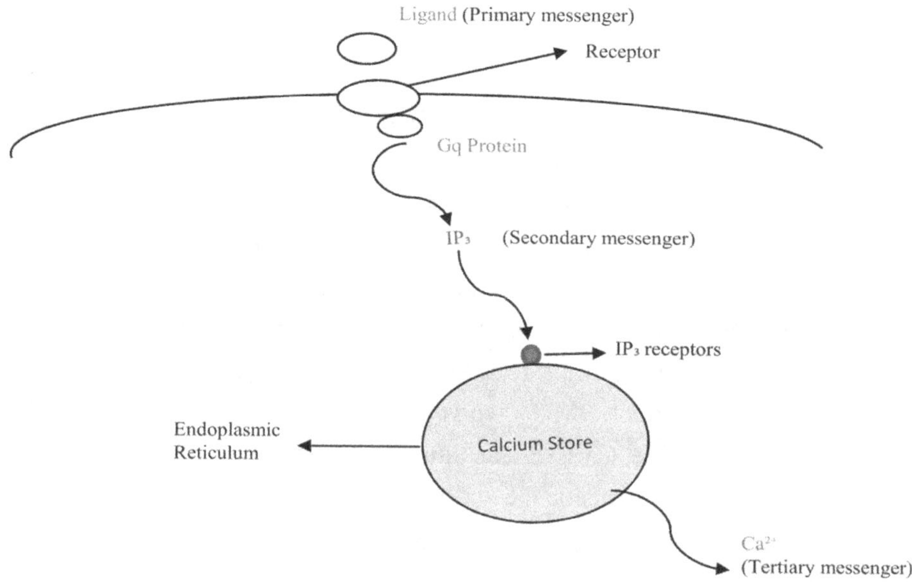

FIGURE 19.9 Calcium as tertiary messenger in cell signaling

INTRACELLULAR SIGNALING CASCADE

Calcium is involved in a number of signaling pathways, depending on the cells and tissues.

1. **Promotes Interaction with Actin-Myosin to Initiate Skeletal Muscle Contraction:** In skeletal muscles, there is an interaction between actin and myosin heads to promote skeletal muscle contraction. However in resting condition, myosin heads are covered with 'troponin-tropomyosin complex'. Calcium has very high affinity for protein, troponin. In response to rise in intracellular calcium levels, calcium binds to troponin and it is followed by displacement of 'troponin-tropomyosin complex' from myosin heads, making myosin heads free to interact with actin **(Figure 19.10).**

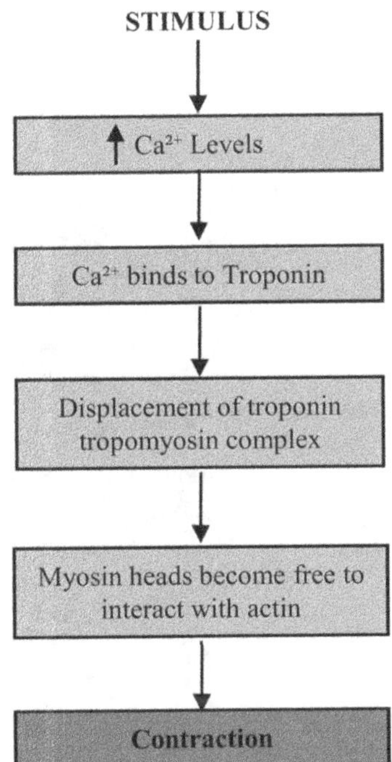

FIGURE 19.10 Role of calcium in promoting interaction between actin and myosin to initiate skeletal muscle contraction

2. **Interaction with Calmodulin to promote Smooth Muscle relaxation:** Calcium is also very important for smooth muscle contraction. An increase in calcium ions is followed by its binding to protein, calmodulin. Thereafter, calcium-calmodulin complex activates myosin light chain kinase (MLC kinase), which leads to phosphorylation of light chain of myosin. The phosphorylated form of myosin interacts with actin to promote smooth muscle contraction.

3. Changes in Gene Expression: *Involvement in cAMP dependent Alteration in Gene Expression*

An increase in calcium activates calmodulin kinase IV (CaMKIV), which phosphorylates and activates CREB (cAMP Response Element Binding Protein) (Discussed in chapter 20). In turn, phosphorylated CREB binds to cAMP response element (CRE) and Ca^{2+}-response element (CARE) to alter gene expression **(Figure 19.11)**.

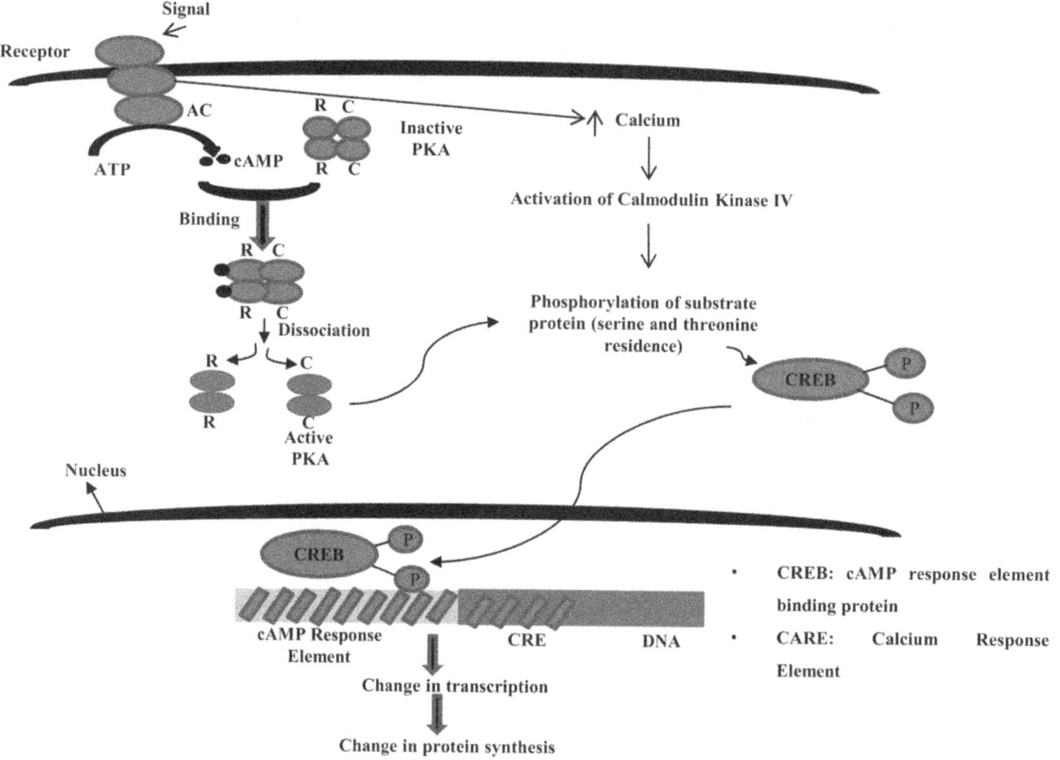

FIGURE 19.11 Role of calcium in cAMP dependent alteration in gene expression

Involvement in Calcineurin Mediated Alteration in Gene Expression:

It has been found that increase in calcium inside the cytoplasm leads to activation of calmodulin-dependent protein phosphatase, calcineurin. Calcineurin is an enzyme, whose primary function is to promote dephosphorylation of proteins. In T cells, activation of calcineurin leads to dephosphorylation of transcription factor, NFAT (Nuclear Factor of Activated T cells). The dephosphorylated form of NFAT translocates from the cytoplasm to the nucelus to increase the gene expression of IL-2 **(Figure 19.12).**

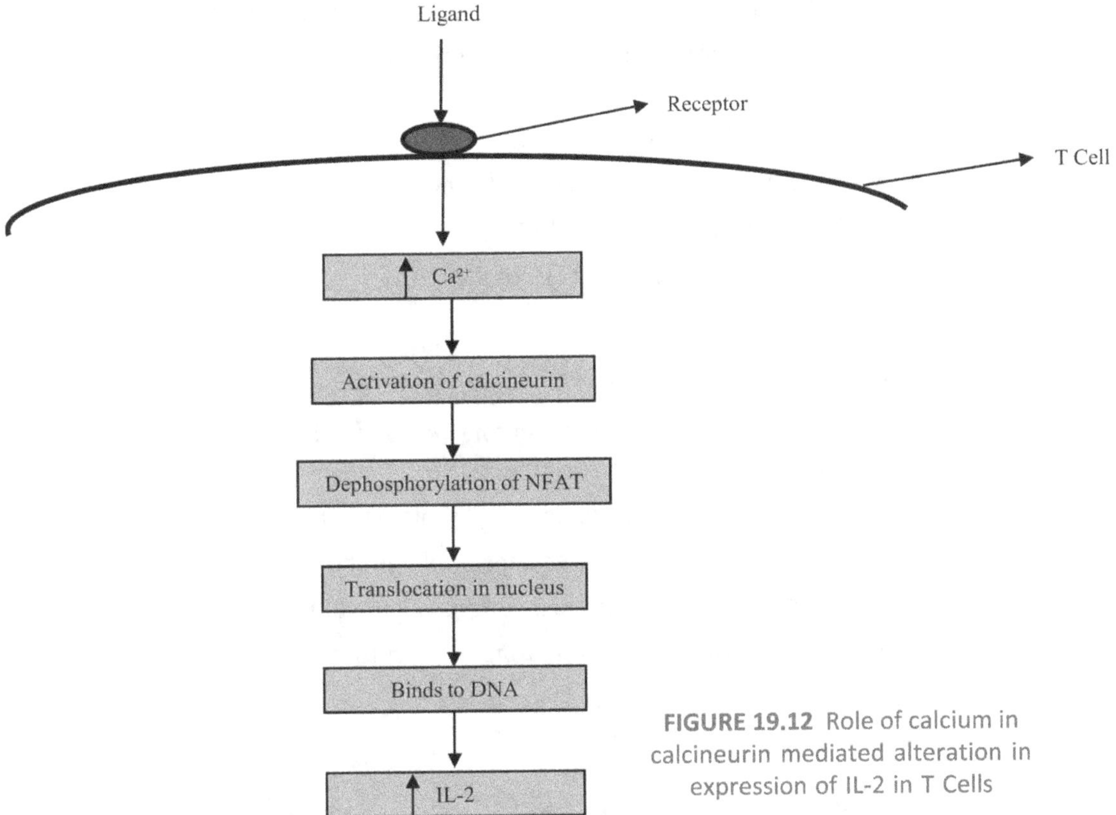

FIGURE 19.12 Role of calcium in calcineurin mediated alteration in expression of IL-2 in T Cells

4. **Long Term Potentiation (LTP):** Long Term potentiation (LTP) refers to an increase in synaptic transmission efficiency due to repeated high stimulation. LTP is well defined phenomenon in the memory formation. It has been defined that there is a key role of calcium activated calmodulin kinase II in LTP and memory formation in the hippocampus region.

REVIEW QUESTIONS

TWO MARKS QUESTIONS

1. What are the key structural features common to all G-protein coupled receptors (GPCRs)?
2. What do you understand by NANC?

3. What are receptor tyrosine kinases?
4. How steroidal hormones produce their actions?
5. What is the role of NO in the cardiovascular system?
6. Name different channels and pumps that regulate calcium levels inside the cell?
7. How is NO synthesized in the body?
8. How may NO be deleterious to the body?
9. What are the actions of DAG?
10. What is the function of IP_3 in the cell?

FIVE MARKS QUESTIONS

1. Write a note on nuclear receptors with special emphasis on its structural features and signal transduction.
2. Explain signal transduction of G protein coupled receptors.
3. What are physiological actions of NO in the body?
4. What are the physiological actions of calcium inside the cells?
5. Explain structure and signaling of receptor tyrosine kinase.

TEN MARKS QUESTIONS

1. Write a note on nitric oxide with special emphasis on its production, signaling, physiological and pathophysiological actions?
2. Write a note on calcium signaling with special emphasis on its regulators, signaling and actions.
3. What are receptors? Classify receptors. Explain G protein coupled receptors.

MULTIPLE CHOICE QUESTIONS

1. Which out of the following statements is true about G-protein couple receptors?
    (a) The N-terminal chain is extracellular and C-terminal chain is intracellular
    (b) It contains 5 trans-membrane hydrophobic sections

   (c) There are more extracellular loops than intracellular loops

   (d) None of above

2. Which of the following is a G-protein coupled receptor?
   - (a) Glycine receptor
   - (b) Adrenergic receptor
   - (c) NMDA receptor
   - (d) $GABA_A$

3. Which of the following catalyzes the hydrolysis of PIP2 to IP3 and diacylglycerol?
   - (a) Phosphokinase C
   - (b) Phospholipase C
   - (c) Lipokinase
   - (d) Phosphodiesterase C

4. A hormone or ligand is a
   - (a) First messenger
   - (b) Second messenger
   - (c) Third messenger
   - (d) Fourth messenger

5. Which of following second messenger releases Ca^{2+} from endoplasmic reticulum?
   - (a) IP_3
   - (b) 1,2 diacyl glycerol
   - (c) cAMP
   - (d) cGMP

6. The receptors for steroidal hormones are
   - (a) G protein coupled receptors
   - (b) Ligand gated Ion channels
   - (c) Nuclear Receptors
   - (d) None of above

7. Acetylcholine nicotinic receptors are
   - (a) G protein coupled receptors
   - (b) Ligand gated Ion channels
   - (c) Nuclear Receptors
   - (d) None of above

8. Insulin and growth factors act on
   - (a) G protein coupled receptors
   - (b) Ligand gated Ion channels
   - (c) Nuclear Receptors
   - (d) Receptor tyrosine kinase

9. Which of following is inducible and produces deleterious NO?
   - (a) eNOS
   - (b) nNOS
   - (c) iNOS
   - (d) All the above

10. The major neurotransmitter in NANC fibers is
    - (a) Calcium
    - (b) Adrenaline
    - (c) NO
    - (d) Acetylcholine

Intracellular Signaling Pathways

CHAPTER OUTLINE

cAMP
Definition, Synthesis and Degradation
Signaling Pathway
Physiological Functions of cAMP
Clinical Uses of cAMP Modulators

cGMP
Definition, Synthesis and Degradation
Signaling Pathway
Clinical Uses of cGMP Modulators
JAK-STAT Signaling
Mechanisms Involved in JAK-STAT
Signaling

Inhibitors of JAK-STAT Signaling
Functional Significance of JAK-STAT
Signaling and Clinical Uses of Inhibitors
Mitogen-Activated Protein Kinase
(MAP Kinase)

Activation Cascade of MAP Kinase
(Three-Kinase Module)
Inactivation of MAP Kinases

Types of MAP Kinases
Clinical Applications of MAP Kinase
Modulators

cAMP

DEFINITION, SYNTHESIS AND DEGRADATION

cAMP refers to cyclic 3',5' adenosine monophosphate and acts as an important secondary messenger in cell signaling pathway. In response to cell stimulus (hormone, neurotransmitter or drug), adenylate cyclase (adenylyl cyclase) is activated, which is located on the inner side of the plasma membrane. Activation of adenylate cyclase leads to synthesis of cAMP from ATP. The cAMP is hydrolyzed by cyclic nucleotide phosphodiesterases (PDE), which break the phosphodiester bond in the cAMP to form 5'-AMP **(Figure 20.1)**. There are different families of PDE, from PDE1 to 12. PDE4, 7 and 8 selectively hydrolyze cAMP; while PDE 1, 2, 3, 10, and 11 non-selectively hydrolyze cAMP as well as cGMP.

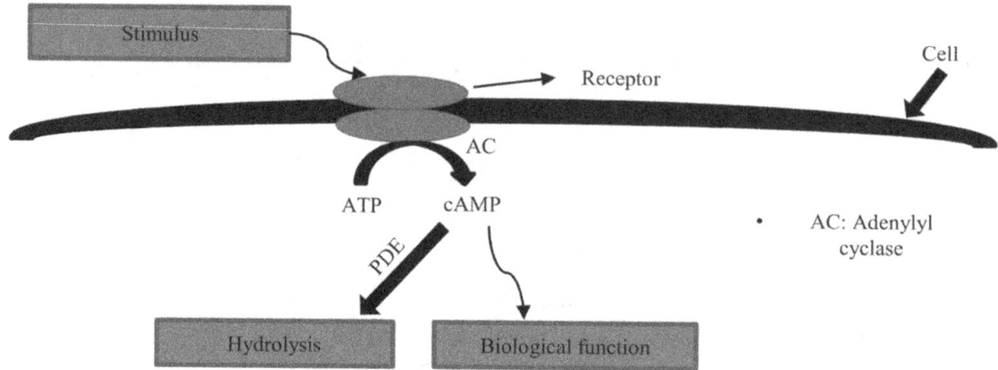

FIGURE 20.1 Steps in synthesis and degradation of cAMP

SIGNALING PATHWAY

Adenylyl cyclase enzyme is linked with G-proteins and its stimulation or inhibition depends on the type of G protein. In the presence of Gs protein, there is an activation of adenylyl cyclase and increase in cAMP takes place. However, in the presence of Gi protein, there is inhibition of adenylyl cyclase and decrease in cAMP takes place. An increase in cAMP levels may activate downstream signaling pathway and these include:

1. **Protein Kinase A dependent Signaling:** The majority of actions of cAMP are mediated through activation of cAMP-dependent protein kinase A (PKA). In normal inactive state, PKA exits in tetrameric form, with two catalytic and two regulatory units. Due to the presence of regulatory subunits, the catalytic units do not perform any biological action and protein kinase exists in inactive state. However, binding of two cAMP molecules with the regulatory subunits of PKA leads to dissociation of regulatory units from the catalytic subunits. This makes catalytic units free and these catalytic units subsequently induce phosphorylation of substrate proteins. In most of cases, there is phosphorylation of serine or threonine residues of substrate proteins. The phosphorylated proteins may act in a number of ways.

(i) In one the signaling pathways, these phosphorylated proteins may directly modulate the opening or closing of plasma membrane located ion channels.

(ii) Phosphorylated proteins may actually be CREB (cAMP Response Element Binding Protein). Phosphorylation of CREB may lead to its translocation inside the nucelus, where it may bind with cAMP response elements of DNA to alter transcription and translation **(Figure 20.2)**.

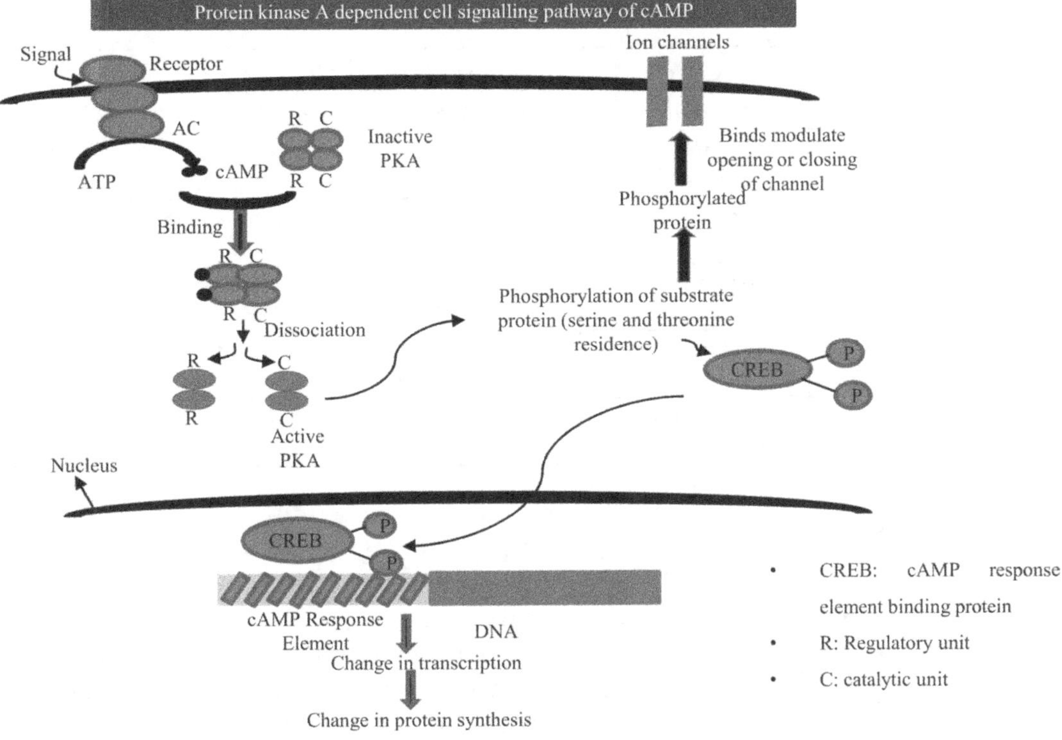

FIGURE 20.2 Protein kinase A dependent signaling pathway of cAMP

2. **Direct Actions:** In some cases, cAMP may act independent of protein kinase A and may directly modulate ion channels. For example, growth hormone-releasing hormone may increase cAMP levels, which directly activates calcium channels to produce biological actions.

3. **Guanine Nucleotide Exchange Factor (GEF):** It is also found that cAMP acts through guanine nucleotide exchange factor, independent of protein kinase A. In normal conditions, GEF remains in inactive state and it is covered by N terminal region. This covering region has cAMP binding domain. The binding of cAMP with this domain unmasks GEF and leads to its activation. The activated GEF activates small Ras-like GTPase proteins to produce biological actions.

PHYSIOLOGICAL FUNCTIONS OF cAMP

cAMP acts as a secondary messenger in intracellular cell signaling and its functions depends on drug/hormone or neurotransmitter as well on cells/tissues/ organs. The functions of cAMP have been represented in **Table 20.1.**

TABLE 20.1 Different functions of cAMP depending on ligands and tissues

S. No	Ligands	Tissues/Organs	Functions
1.	Adrenaline	Adipocytes	Lipolysis
2.	Adrenaline, noradrenaline	Heart	Increase in heart contraction
3.	Adrenaline	Smooth Muscles, blood vessels	Dilation, vasodilation
4.	Dopamine	Nucleus Accumbens	Activation of Reward
5.	Adrenaline	Juxtaglomerular cells of kidney	Renin release
6.	Adrenaline and glucagon	Liver	Glycogenolysis

CLINICAL USES OF cAMP MODULATORS

Amrinone (Inamrinone) and milrinone are clinically employed for the management of congestive heart failure. These drugs are selective inhibitors of phosphodiesterase 3, which leads to decrease degradation of cAMP. Due to increase in cAMP levels in heart, there is an increase in heart contraction (positive inotropic effect). Moreover, increase in cAMP levels in blood vessels leads to vasodilation. Both these pharmacological actions are beneficial to relieve the symptoms of CHF patients. Due to the dual activity on heart and blood vessels, these drugs are also termed as 'inodilators'.

cGMP

DEFINITION, SYNTHESIS AND DEGRADATION

cGMP refers to 3',5'-cyclic guanosine monophosphate and acts as an important secondary messenger in cell signaling pathway. In response to cell stimulus (hormone, neurotransmitter or drug), guanylate cyclase (guanyl cyclase, guanylyl cyclase, or GC) is activated, which is of two types. One type of enzyme is located on the inner side of the plasma membrane (type I) and second type of enzyme is freely present in cytoplasm (type II). The guanyl cyclase present in cytoplasm is also called as soluble guanyl cyclase (sGC). Nitric oxide acts on the cells to activate soluble guanyl cyclase and increase cGMP production. It has been identified that endothelium-derived relaxing factor is nitric oxide (NO), which stimulates soluble guanylyl cyclase (sGC) in the smooth muscle cells to synthesize cGMP and produce vasorelaxation.

Activation of guanyl cyclase leads to synthesis of cGMP from GTP in the presence of calcium ions. The cGMP is hydrolyzed by cyclic nucleotide phosphodiesterases (PDE), which break the phosphodiester bond in the cGMP to form 5'-GMP. There are different families of PDE, from PDE1 to 12. PDE 5, -6 and -9 selectively hydrolyze cGMP; while PDE 1, 2, 3, 10, and 11 hydrolyze both cAMP as well as cGMP **(Figure 20.3)**.

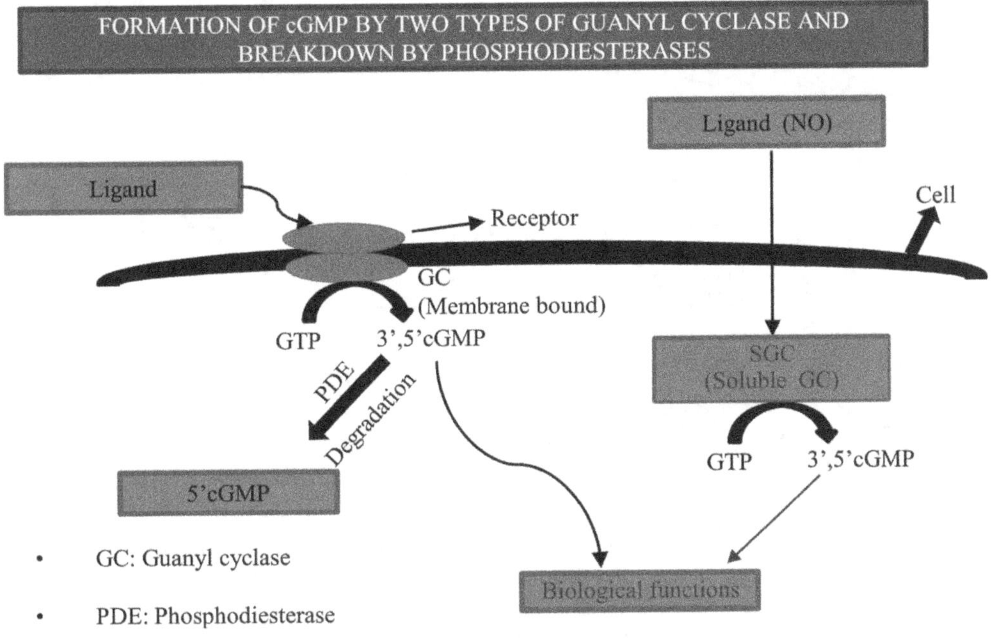

FIGURE 20.3 Formation of cGMP by two types of guanyl cyclase and breakdown by phosphodiesterases

SIGNALING PATHWAY

An increase in cGMP levels may activate downstream signaling pathway, including cGMP-dependent protein kinases (PKG). Two different types of PKG have been identified:

1. PKG type I (PKG-I) is predominantly present in the cytoplasm of cells. These enzymes are mainly localized in the smooth muscle cells, platelets, fibroblasts, hippocampus, cerebellar Purkinje cells and dorsal root ganglia.

2. PKG type II (PKG-II) is predominantly bound to plasma membrane and these are present in the renal cells, intestinal mucosa, pancreatic ducts, parotid and submandibular glands, chondrocytes, and several brain nuclei.

Activation of PKG modulates a number of physiological functions including smooth muscle relaxation, platelet function, sperm metabolism and cell division etc. Activation of PKG may activate myosin phosphatase enzyme, which dephosphorylates myosin light chain to reduce its interaction with actin. This is manifested in the form of smooth muscle relaxation. Apart from these actions, PKG may promote the opening of calcium-activated potassium channels, leading to hyperpolarization and relaxation. It may also block the enzymatic activity of phospholipase C to reduce the intracellular levels of inositol triphosphate and it is manifested in the form of decrease in intracellular calcium release **(Figure 20.4).**

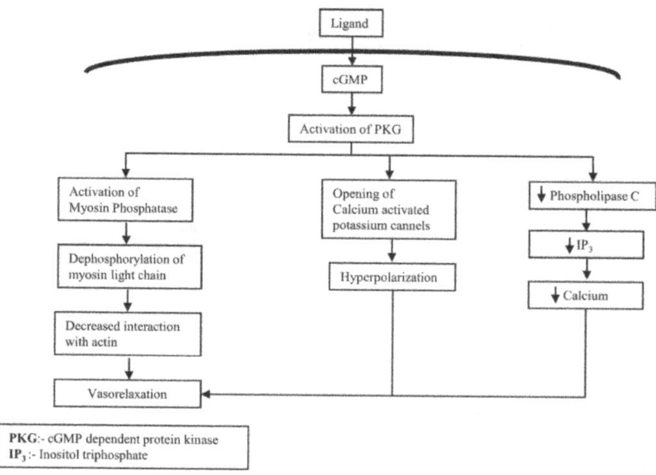

FIGURE 20.4 cGMP-mediated activation of protein kinase G to produce vasorelaxation

CLINICAL USES OF cGMP MODULATORS

1. Selective inhibition of PDE5 has been shown to produce vasodilatory effects within the corpus cavernosum and this property has been clinically used in the management of erectile dysfunction. The drugs employed for this purpose include sildenafil (Viagra) and tadalafil, latter being more selective inhibitor of PDE 5.

2. Nitrates, employed in cardiovascular disease such as angina pectoris and congestive heart failure, produce therapeutic effect (vasodilation) by activating cGMP signaling pathway.

JAK-STAT SIGNALING

JAK-STAT signaling is an important part of intracellular signal transduction pathway and this signaling plays a key role in physiological processes including immunity, cell division, and tumor formation. A defect in this signaling leads to development of a number of diseases of skin, immune system and cancer. A number of endogenous molecules utilize JAK-STAT signaling to produce their actions e.g. erythropoietin. There are three important parts of this signaling pathway:

1. **Receptors:** Various ligands such as drugs or cytokines including interferons and interleukins bind to receptors present on the surface of cell and it leads to activation of signaling pathway.

2. **Janus Kinase (JAK):** There are 4 different types of JAK proteins i.e. JAK1, JAK2, JAK3 and TYK2. These proteins have common structural features and these possess a FERM domain, SH2-related domain, kinase domain and pseudokinase domain. Amongst these different domains, 'kinase domain' is important for JAK activity and it is responsible for phosphorylation of STAT proteins.

3. **Signal Transducer and Activator of Transcription proteins (STATs):** There are 7 STAT proteins i.e., STAT1, STAT2, STAT3, STAT4, STAT5A, STAT5B and STAT6. These proteins also possess common structural features and SH2 domain is the most conserved structural unit of STAT proteins. The other important domains include transcriptional activation domain (TAD) and DNA-binding domains.

MECHANISMS INVOLVED IN JAK-STAT SIGNALING

The different steps involved in cell signaling pathway include the followings **(Figure 20.5)**:

1. **Dimerization of Receptors and Binding of JAK to Receptors:** The process starts after binding of different ligands to cell-surface receptors. The binding of ligand leads to dimerization of receptors and JAK proteins bind to dimerized form of receptors.

2. **Phosphorylation and Activation of JAK Proteins:** The binding of JAK to receptors is followed by phosphorylation of tyrosine residues of JAK proteins. This process is called as 'transphosphorylation' and it increases the kinase activity of JAK proteins.

3. **Phosphorylation of Receptors and Binding of STAT to Receptors:** The activation of JAKs causes phosphorylation of tyrosine residues of receptors. Thereafter, STAT proteins bind to the phosphorylated form of receptors using their SH2 domains.

4. **Phosphorylation of STAT proteins and Dissociation from Receptors:** Subsequently, JAK proteins cause phosphorylation of tyrosine residues of

STAT proteins. The phosphorylated form of STAT proteins dissociate from receptors.

5. **Dimerization of phosphorylated form of STAT and translocation from cytoplasm to Nucleus:** The activated STAT proteins (phosphorylated) form homodimers and after dissociation from receptors, the dimer of STAT moves from cytoplasm to nucleus.

6. **Transcriptional Changes:** The dimer form of STAT enters in the nucleus and binds to DNA to bring transcriptional changes.

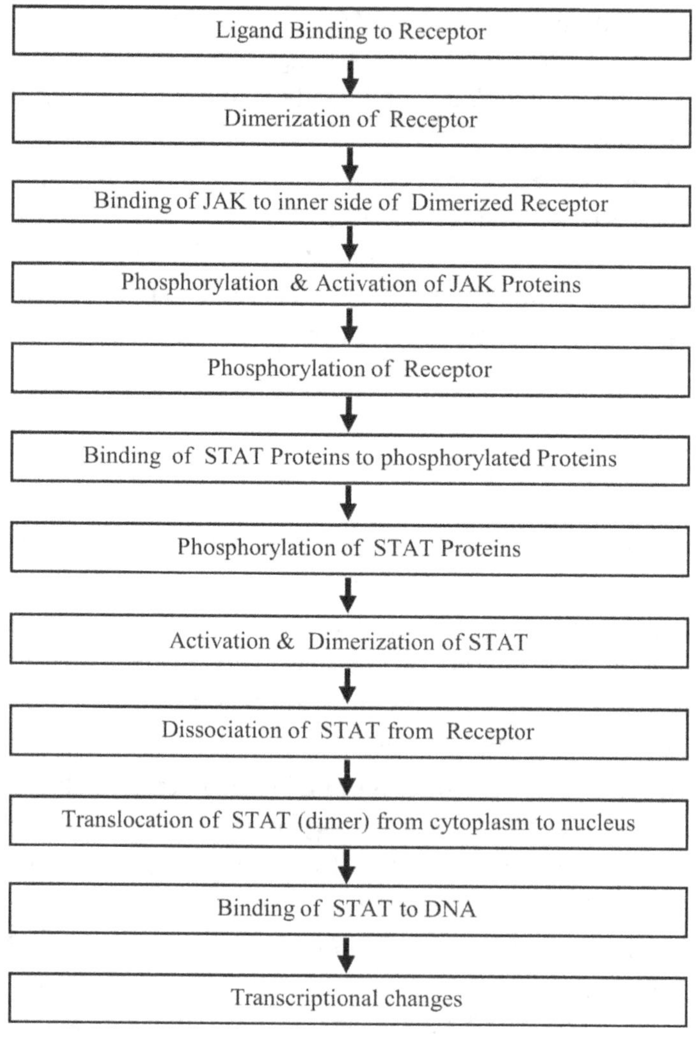

FIGURE 20.5 Sequence of events involved in JAK-STAT Signaling Pathway

INHIBITORS OF JAK-STAT SIGNALING

There are three levels of inhibition that has been employed by different scientists. These include:

1. **Protein Inhibitors of Activated STATs:** These inhibitors block phosphorylation of STATs, prevent their dimerization and translocation to nucleus. These may also prevent the binding of STAT to DNA and inhibit transcriptional changes.

2. **Protein Tyrosine Phosphatases:** These are the enzymes that remove phosphate groups from tyrosine residues. Since, phosphorylation of receptors, JAK and STAT play a key role in JAK-STAT signaling, therefore, dephosphorylation may inhibit a large number of steps in this form of cell signaling.

3. **Suppressors of cytokine signaling (SOCS):** There are eight members of this SOCS family and these tend to inhibit JAK-STAT signaling by inducing degradation of protein molecules including of JAK, receptors and STAT proteins. The proteins of SOCS family induce protein digestion by activating endogenous ubiquitin-proteasome system, which causes breakdown.

FUNCTIONAL SIGNIFICANCE OF JAK-STAT SIGNALING AND CLINICAL USES OF INHIBITORS

1. **Development of Immune System:** It is well known that JAK-STAT signaling is very important in signaling of IL-2, IL-4, IL-15, IL-21 and other cytokines. In turn, these cytokines helps in maturation and development of functional immune system. Therefore, mutations in JAK3 proteins lead to defective immune system in humans and non-functional JAK3 has been associated with development of Severe combined immunodeficiency disease (SCID). Similarly, mutations in STAT1 and STAT2 increase the susceptibility to bacterial and viral infections, and mutation in STAT4 is associated with autoimmune diseases such as rheumatoid arthritis. Tofacitinib is JAK1 and JAK 3 inhibitor and it has been approved for the management of psoriasis and rheumatoid arthritis.

2. **Skin Disorders:** It has been reported that defects in JAK-STAT signaling pathway produces skin disorders. For example, overexpression of STAT3 has been associated with psoriasis, an autoimmune disease associated with red, flaky skin.

3. **Cancer:** Since, JAK-STAT signaling controls cell proliferation; therefore, excessive activation of JAK-STAT signaling may lead to cancer formation. Particularly, excessive activity of STAT3 and STAT5 activation may lead to

development of tumors such as melanoma (skin cancer), prostate cancer, and breast cancer. Moreover, mutations in JAK2 may also lead to different cancers such as leukaemia and lymphoma. Accordingly, JAK2 inhibitor (Ruxolitinib) has been developed and FDA approved to manage myelofibrosis.

MITOGEN-ACTIVATED PROTEIN KINASE (MAP KINASE)

MAP kinases constitute an important class of intracellular signaling cascade system. These belong to the class of serine/threonine protein kinase and specifically phosphorylate serine and threonine residues. These kinases are activated by a diverse range of stimuli including growth factors, mitogens, osmotic stress, heat shock and inflammatory cytokines etc.

ACTIVATION CASCADE OF MAP KINASE (THREE-KINASE MODULE)

MAP kinases remain in an inactive state inside the cells and under in the influence of particular stimuli, these enzymes are activated by phosphorylation. The unique feature of MAP kinases is that activation of these enzymes requires two upstream protein kinases. It means there exists a three kinase system working in tandem (Figure 20.6).

1. **MAP Kinases (MAPK):** MAP kinases possess the 'activation loop' and activation of MAP kinase require phosphorylation of threonine/serine and tyrosine residues.

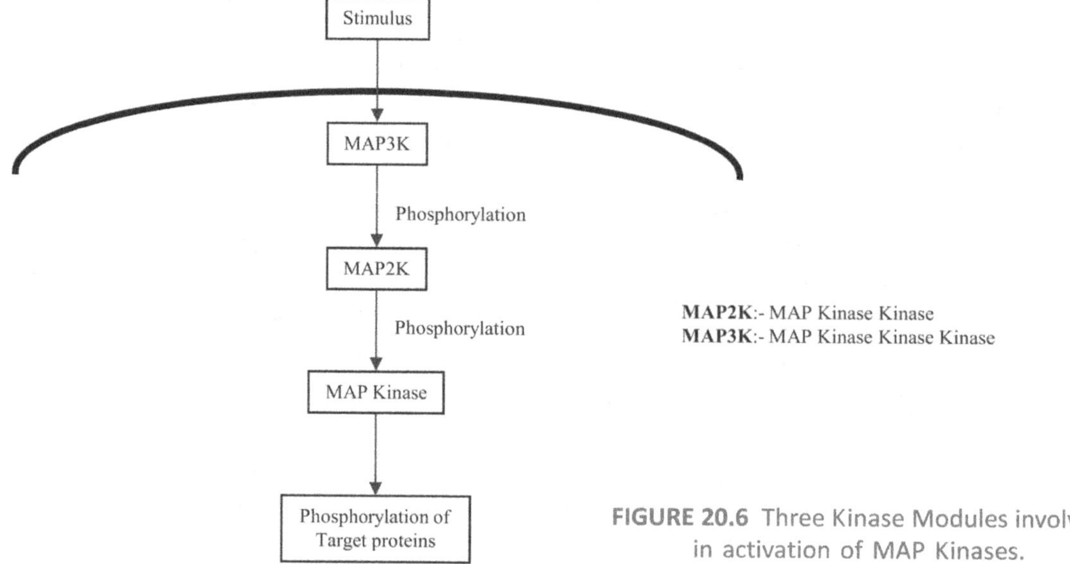

FIGURE 20.6 Three Kinase Modules involved in activation of MAP Kinases.

2. **MAP Kinase Kinase (MAPK Kinase, MAP2K, MKK, MEK):** These enzymes directly phosphorylate and activate MAP kinases. These are immediately upstream of MAP kinase. MAP2K activate MAP kinase by phosphorylation of hydroxyl groups of serine/threonine and tyrosine residues of MAP kinase.

3. **MAP Kinase Kinase Kinase (MAPKK Kinase, MAP3K, MEKK):** These kinases are upstream of MAP2K and MAP3K phosphorylate serine/threonine residues of MAP2K kinases to trigger their activation.

INACTIVATION OF MAP KINASES

Following activation of signaling cascade, MAP kinases are inactivated by a number of phosphatases, called as MAP kinase phosphatases. These phosphatases hydrolyze the phosphate group from phosphotyrosine and phosphothreonine residues of MAP kinases. The removal of phosphate groups reduces MAP kinase activity. Apart from MAP kinase phosphatase, tyrosine phosphatases are also involved in inactivating MAP kinases.

TYPES OF MAP KINASES

MAP kinases are of classified into three main types:

1. **Extracellular signal–regulated kinases (ERK)**

   ERK1 and ERK 2 are the best-characterized MAP kinases in mammals. These are ubiquitously expressed and activation of these kinases require the phosphorylation of tyrosine and threonine residues in the activation loop. In response to growth factors, there is activation of MAP3K (MEKK) (mostly, Raf proteins such as A-Raf, B-Raf or c-Raf), which phosphorylate and activate MAP2K (MEK). More specifically, ERK1 and ERK2 are activated by a pair of closely related MEKs, MEK1 and MEK2. Following MEK-mediated phosphorylation and activation, ERK1/2 activates intracellular signaling cascade involving phosphorylation of substrates required for cell proliferation, cell cycle progression, cell division and differentiation **(Figure 20.7)**.

2. **p38 Kinase:** This is another MAP kinase which is activated in response to cytokines, ultraviolet irradiation, heat and osmotic shock and its activation helps the organism to adapt to stress. In response to stimuli, there is activation of enzymes MAP3K (mainly, MEKK1 and MEKK4), which phosphorylate and activate MAP2K (mainly, MEK3, MEK4 and MEK6). Thereafter, there is activation of p38α and p38β isoforms of p38 MAP kinase **(Figure 20.7)**.

3. c-Jun N-terminal kinases (JNK)

There is considerable overlap at the level of MEKK in activating p38 and JNK. Like p38 MAP kinase, the upstream activator of JNK at MAP3K level is MEKK1 and MEKK4. Moreover, MAP2K enzymes like MKK4 may activate both p38 and JNK. However, other MAP2K such as MKK7 selectively activate JNK. Therefore, stimuli that activate p38 MAP kinase may also activate JNK. Activated form of JNK phosphorylates a number of targets including c-Jun and NFAT4 **(Figure 20.7)**.

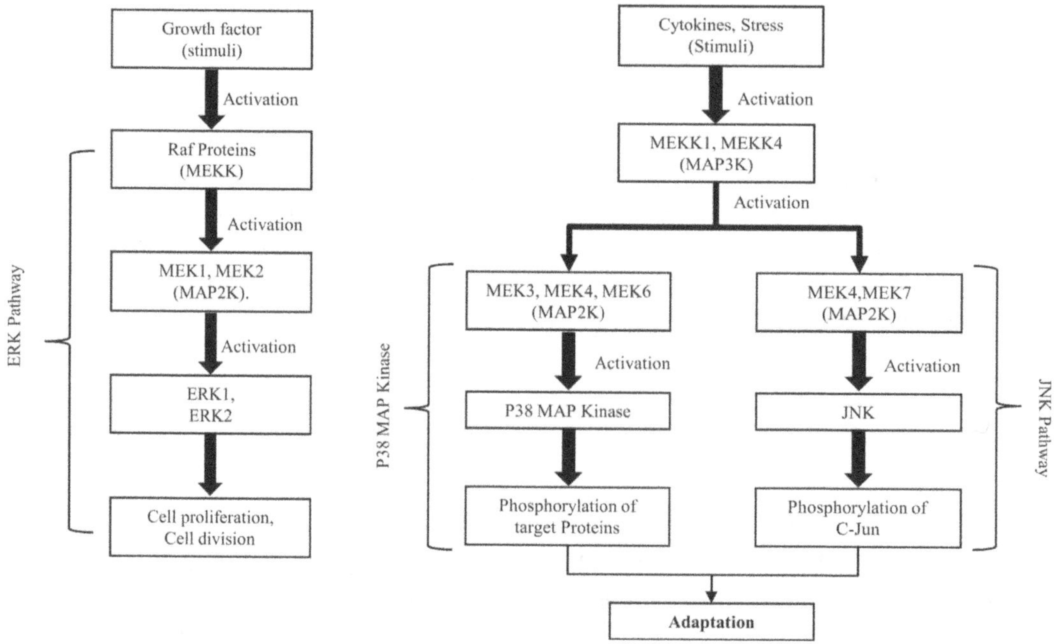

FIGURE 20.7   Activation and Role of three types of MAP Kinases in the mammalian cells

CLINICAL APPLICATIONS OF MAP KINASE MODULATORS

1. **Anti-neoplastic drugs:** Since ERK signaling pathway is involved in promoting cell proliferation and cell division, therefore, ERK1/2 inhibitors have been projected as antineoplastic agents. Presently, ERK1/2 inhibitors are in different stages of preclinical and clinical testing before their use in patients. However, Raf kinase inhibitor including Sorafenib has been employed as antineoplastic agent in various types of cancer.

2. **To Overcome Insulin Resistance in Diabetes Mellitus:** It is suggested that JNK kinases are involved in the development of insulin resistance in obese individuals and JNK inhibitors have been shown to decrease insulin

resistance in animal models. However, these agents have not shown efficacy in humans till now.

3. **Loss of Hearing:** A peptide-based JNK inhibitor (AM-111, also termed as XG-102) is under clinical trials for the treatment of sensorineural hearing loss.

4. **Anti-inflammatory Drugs:** Studies have shown the important role of p38 MAP kinase in the development of inflammation in animal models. However, clinical studies have not shown the effectiveness of p38 MAP kinase inhibitors in humans. Moreover, the clinical utility of presently available p38 inhibitors is limited due to hepatotoxicity.

REVIEW QUESTIONS

TWO MARKS QUESTIONS

1. What is cAMP? How is it formed?
2. What is cGMP? How is it formed?
3. What do you mean by three tier activation of MAP kinases?
4. What are clinical uses of ERK inhibitors?
5. What are phosphodiesterases?
6. What is protein kinase A and protein kinase G?
7. What are the endogenous inhibitors of JAK-STAT pathway?
8. What are clinical uses of JAK-STAT inhibitors?
9. What are different types of MAP kinases?
10. How MAP kinases are inactivated in the body?

FIVE MARKS QUESTIONS

1. What is cAMP? How is it formed? What are its actions?
2. What do you understand by MAP kinase signaling?
3. What are the clinical uses of MAP kinase inhibitors?
4. What are the clinical uses of JAK-STAT signaling?
5. Explain cGMP-mediated signaling pathway.

TEN MARKS QUESTIONS

1. Write a note on JAK-STAT signaling pathway.
2. Write a note on cGMP signaling.

MULTIPLE CHOICE QUESTIONS

---

1. Which of following is a target of cAMP
   (a) Protein kinase A
   (b) Ion channels
   (c) Guanine nucleotide exchange factor
   (d) All the above

2. In inactive state, protein kinase exists as
   (a) Tetramer   (b) Dimer
   (c) Trimeric   (d) As a single unit

3. Amrinone increases cAMP levels to
   (a) Increase heart contraction (d) Vasoconstriction
   (c) Decrease heart contraction (d) None of above

4. NO acts on following to increase cGMP levels
   (a) GC   (b) sGC
   (c) PKG   (d) None of above

5. Which of following are the targets of PKG?
   (a) Myosin phosphatase enzyme
   (b) Calcium-activated potassium channels
   (c) Phospholipase C
   (d) All the above

6. Sildenafil has more affinity for following enzymes
   (a) PDE1   (b) PDE2
   (c) PDE3   (d) PDE5

7. Which of following pathway is utilized by erythropoietin?
   (a) cAMP   (b) cGMP
   (c) JAK-STAT   (d) None of above

8. Which of following are inhibitors of JAK-STAT pathway?
   (a) Suppressors of cytokine signaling
   (b) Protein Tyrosine Phosphatases
   (c) Protein Inhibitors of Activated STATs
   (d) All the above

9. Which of following is MAP kinase?
    (a) ERK   (b)   p38 kinase
    (c) JNK   (d)   All the above
10. Which of following is clinical use of MAP kinase inhibitors?
    (a) Anti-inflammatory   (b)   Anticancer
    (c) Insulin Resistance   (d)   All the above

Answers

CHAPTER 1

1. (a)	2. (c)	3. (c)	4. (a)	5. (b)
6. (b)	7. (a)	8. (b)	9. (d)	10. (a)

CHAPTER 2

1. (a)	2. (a)	3. (b)	4. (c)	5. (a)
6. (c)	7. (a)	8. (a)	9. (a)	10. (d)

CHAPTER 3

1. (c)	2. (d)	3. (a)	4. (b)	5. (d)
6. (b)	7. (a)	8. (a)	9. (b)	10. (b)

CHAPTER 4

1. (a)	2. (a)	3. (c)	4. (a)	5. (d)
6. (b)	7. (c)	8. (b)	9. (b)	10. (a)

CHAPTER 5

1. (d)	2. (d)	3. (d)	4. (b)	5. (a)

CHAPTER 6

1. (b)	2. (c)	3. (a)	4. (a)	5. (d)
6. (d)	7. (c)	8. (a)	9. (c)	10. (a)

CHAPTER 7

1. (a)	2. (a)	3. (b)	4. (d)	5. (b)
6. (b)	7. (a)	8. (b)	9. (b)	10. (d)

CHAPTER 8

1. (a)	2. (b)	3. (a)	4. (b)	5. (a)
6. (d)	7. (c)	8. (d)	9. (c)	10. (b)

CHAPTER 9

1. (a)	2. (b)	3. (a)	4. (c)	5. (d)
6. (b)	7. (d)	8. (a)	9. (a)	10. (c)

CHAPTER 10

1. (b)	2. (a)	3. (c)	4. (b)	5. (d)
6. (c)	7. (b)	8. (b)	9. (b)	10. (d)

CHAPTER 11

1. (b)	2. (a)	3. (a)	4. (a)	5. (a)
6. (a)	7. (b)	8. (b)	9. (a)	10. (b)

CHAPTER 12

| 1. (c) | 2. (a) | 3. (d) | 4. (a) | 5. (a) |

CHAPTER 13

| 1. (c) | 2. (a) | 3. (d) | 4. (b) | 5. (a) |
| 6. (d) | 7. (c) | 8. (c) | 9. (d) | 10. (b) |

CHAPTER 14

| 1. (b) | 2. (a) | 3. (a) | 4. (c) | 5. (d) |
| 6. (c) | 7. (a) | | | |

CHAPTER 15

| 1. (b) | 2. (b) | 3. (b) | 4. (b) | 5. (c) |
| 6. (d) | 7. (c) | 8. (d) | 9. (a) | 10. (d) |

CHAPTER 16

| 1. (a) | 2. (d) | 3. (c) | 4. (b) | 5. (b) |
| 6. (d) | 7. (a) | 8. (d) | 9. (d) | 10. (a) |

CHAPTER 17

| 1. (b) | 2. (d) | 3. (b) | 4. (a) | 5. (d) |

CHAPTER 18

| 1. (c) | 2. (c) | 3. (b) | 4. (c) | 5. (a) |
| 6. (c) | 7. (d) | 8. (d) | | |

CHAPTER 19

1. (a)	2. (b)	3. (b)	4. (a)	5. (a)
6. (c)	7. (b)	8. (d)	9. (c)	10. (c)

CHAPTER 20

1. (d)	2. (a)	3. (a)	4. (b)	5. (d)
6. (d)	7. (c)	8. (d)	9. (d)	10. (d)

Index

A

ABC transporters 232
Acrylamide 130
Actin 13
Adeno-associated virus 150
Adenosine deaminase 157
Adenovirus 149
Adenylate cyclase 317
Agarose gel 127
Alkaline phosphatase 108
Alpha-complementation 117
Anaphase 88
Anchorage dependent culture system 272
Anchorage independent culture system 273
Animal cell culture 279
Annealing 170
Annexin 69
Annotation 243
Apoptosis 60
Apoptosome 64
Array hybridization 194
ATP Assay 295
Automated fluorescence sequencing 81
Autophagosome 50
Autophagy 49
Autoradiography 205

B

Bacterial artificial chromosomes 98
Bacteriophage 98
Bidirectional blotting 203
Biologics 263
Biosafety cabinet 273
Biosimilars 263

Biotin streptavidin system 206
Blocking 181
Blood bank screening 191
Blotting 203
Blunt ends 104
Bromophenol blue 132

C

Ca2+APTase pump 325
Calcium influx assays 296
cAMP 333
Capillary blotting 200
Caspases 67
Cell 3
Cell cycle 86
Cell viability assays 291
Cellular therapy 262
cGMP 336
Chaperones 51
Chemiluminescent 181
Chimeric DNA 95
Chimeric monoclonal antibodies 258
Chromatosome 22
Cisternae 9
c-Jun N-terminal kinases (JNK) 344
Cloning of genes 213
Cloning vector 97
Coagulative Necrosis 47
Cold CaCl$_2$ method 110
Comparative genomics 244
Competitive ELISA 188
Complimentary DNA (cDNA) 97
Conjugation 111
Constitutive genes 30
Coomassie brilliant blue 136
Copper staining 137
Cosmids 98
Coulter counter 281

Cyclin dependent kinases 89
Cyclin-dependent kinase inhibitors 90
Cyclins 88
Cystic fibrosis 159
Cytochrome P450 227, 229
Cytoplasm 6

D

Death receptors 62
Denaturation 170
Detection system 193
Diacylglycerol (DAG) 319
Dideoxynucleotides 78
Diffusion blotting 200
Digoxigenin-antidigoxigenin system 206
Direct ELISA 180
DNA chips 192
DNA polymerase 168
DNA-Coated gold particles 152
Drug metabolism 227
Duchene muscle dystrophy 161
Duplicated genes 24

E

Eagle's minimum essential medium 279
Electroblotting 201
Electroelution 138
Electrophoretic blotting 201
Electrophoretic mobility 126
Electroporation 110
Electrospray ionization 241
ELISA 179
Emphysema 158
Endogenous metabolites 246
Endoplasmic reticulum 7
Epigenetics 30
Epigenomics 244
Erlenmeyer flasks 273
Euchromatin 22
Evans Blue 295

Ex vivo gene therapy 144
Exogenous metabolites 246
Exometabolomics 246
Exons 29
Exonucleases 101
Expression proteomics 238
Extension 170
Extracellular signal–regulated kinases (ERK) 343
Extrinsic (death receptor) Pathway 62

F

Field flow fractionation 240
First dimension separation 240
Flow cytometry 301
Fluid mosaic model 4
Fluorescent labeled antibodies 284
Fully human monoclonal antibodies 260
Functional cloning 214
Functional genomics 243
Functional proteomics 238
Functionomics 250
Fura 2 ester 297
Fusion proteins 261

G

G0 phase 87
G1 phase 86
Galactosidase 101
Gangrene 47
Gas chromatography-mass spectrometry (GC-MS) 245
Gel electrophoresis 68
Gene cloning 95
Gene critical region 216
Gene expression 27
Gene gun 152
Gene mapping 213
Gene therapy 287
Genetic polymorphism 217

Genetic variations 221
Genetics 242
Genome 21
Genome analysis 242
Genomic medicine 244
Genomics 242
Germ line gene therapy 145
Glasgow's minimum essential media 279
Glucose-6-phosphate dehydrogenase 219
Golgi apparatus 9
G-Protein coupled receptors 221
Guanine Nucleotide Exchange
Factor (GEF) 335
Guanylate cyclase 322

H

Haemocytometer 280
Hanging drop technique 270
Heat shock protein 51
Herpes simplex 151
Heterochromatin 22
High Performance
Liquid Chromatography (HPLC) 246
Histone proteins 21
HITES medium 279
Horse radish peroxidase 181
Human genome project 242
Humanization of antibodies 257
Humanized antibodies 257
Hybridoma cells 256, 275
Hybridoma technology 120

I

Immunoassays 241
Immunotherapeutic agents 255
Immunotherapy 255
In situ hybridization 40
In vivo gene therapy 143
Indirect ELISA 182
Inducible genes 30
Inositol trisphosphate (IP3) 318

Integral proteins 5
Intermediate filaments 13
Intermediate metabolizer phenotype 229
Interphase 86
Intrinsic (Mitochondrial) pathway 63
Introns 29
Inverse PCR 173
Ion exchange membranes 205
Isocaudamers 106
Isoelectric focusing 240
Isoelectric point 240
Isoschizomers 106
Isozymes 284

J

JAK-STAT signaling 338
Jumping genes 26

K

Karyolysis 48
Karyorrhexis 48
Karyotyping 283
Klenow fragment 168

L

Lac Z 115
Laminar flow hood 273
Lentivirus 150
Ligand gated ion channels
(Ionotropic receptors) 312
Ligases 106
Liposomes 153
Liquefactive necrosis 47
Long Interspersed Elements (LINES) 24
Long Term Potentiation (LTP) 329
Lysosomal membrane proteins 54
Lysosomes 11

M

MALDI 241
MAP kinases 342
Mass spectrometry 241
Mass spectrometry (MS) 247
Maxam-gilbert sequencing 75
Melting 23
Metabolomics 245
Metagenomics 244
Metaphase 88
Microarray technology 192
Microfilaments 13
MicroRNAs 31
Microtubules 54
Missense mutation 218
Mitochondria 10
Mitochondrial outer
Membrane permeabilization 63
Mitochondrial permeability
transition pore 63
Mitogen-Activated Protein
Kinase (MAP Kinase) 342
Molecular cloning 95
Monitoring of cell lines 283
Monoclonal antibodies 256

N

N-Acetyltransferases 231
Necrosis 45
Neutral SNPs 218
Nitric oxide 320
Nitric oxide synthase (NOS) 321
Nitroblue tetrazolium 184
Nitrocellulose 204
Non-adrenergic Non-cholinergic
Fibers (NANC) 322
Non-radioactive labels 182
Nonsense mutation 218
Non-viral vectors 37
Normal cells 67
Northern blotting 199
Nuclear Magnetic Resonance (NMR) 247

Nuclear receptors 314
Nucleolus 15
Nucleosome 21
Nucleus 15
Nutrigenomics 248
Nutriome 248
Nylon (Polyamide) 205

O

Oncogenes 160
Organic cation transporter 233
Ornstein and Davis model
of discontinuous buffer system 133
Oxysomes 11

P

p38 MAP kinase 344
Palindrome sequence 102
Passage number 276
pBR vector 99
Perforin-granzyme system 62
Peripheral proteins 5
Peroxisomes 12
Personalized medicine 244
Pharmacogenetics 216
Pharmacogenomics 219
Phase I metabolism 227
Phase II metabolism 231
Phosphatidylinositol
4,5-bisphosphate 318
Phosphodiester bond 333
Phosphodiesterases (PDE) 333
Phospholipase C 317
Physical mapping 40
Plasma membrane 4
Plasmids 98
Poly(A) Tail 28
Polyacrylamide gels 130
Polyclonal antibodies 256
Polymerase Chain Reaction (PCR) 165
Polyvinylidenedifluoride (PVDF) 205

Poor metabolizer phenotype 228
Positional cloning 214
Post translational modifications 29
Primary antibodies 188
Primary cell culture 275
Primary metabolites 246
Primers 167
Probes 193
Promoter 27
Prophase 87
Propidium iodide based cell
viability assay 294
Protease activity based viability
assay 294
Proteasomes 12
Protein chips 241
Protein kinase A 334
Protein kinase C 320
Protein tyrosine phosphatases 341
Proteome 237
Proteomics 237
Pseudogenes 25
pUC vector 100
Pyknosis 48

R

Radioimmunoassay 179
Radiolabeling 205
Real Time-Polymerase Chain
Reaction (RT-PCR) 172
Receptor tyrosine kinase
(Enzyme-Linked receptor) 313
Recircularization of vector 108
Recombinant cytokines 261
Recombinant DNA technology 95
Recombinant vaccines 120
Repetitious DNA 25
Resazurin reduction assay 293
Resolving gel 134
Restriction endonucleases 102
Restriction point 87
Retrotransposons 26
Retroviruses 146
Ribosomes 9

RNA polymerase 28
RNA splicing 29
Ryanodine receptor-operated
calcium channels 319

S

S phase 87
Sandwich ELISA 185
Sanger's chain termination
method 78
SCID 341
SDS–PAGE (discontinuous
buffer system) 135
Second dimension separation 240
Second messengers 318
Secondary antibodies 205
Secondary cell culture 276
Secondary metabolites 246
Selection 115
Semidry blotting 202
Short interspersed elements (SINES) 24
Signal transduction 313
Silent SNPs 218
Silver staining 137
Simple-sequence DNA 24
Single copy DNA 24
Single Nucleotide
Polymorphism (SNP) 217
Small Interfering RNAs 32
Sodium dodecyl sulphate 132
Solitary genes 24
Soluble cytokine receptors 262
Solute Carrier (SLC) transporters 233
Somatic cell gene therapy 145
Southern blotting 199
Spacer DNA 24
Splice sites 218
Stacking gel 134
Sticky ends (cohesive ends) 103
Stop codon 218
Structural genomics 243
Structural proteomics 238
Sub-culturing 274

T

T4 DNA ligase 107
Tandemly repeated genes 25
Taq polymerase 168
Telophase 88
Tertiary messenger 326
Tetrazolium reduction assays 291
Thiopurine
Methyltransferase (TPMT) 231
Tracking dye 132
Transcription 27
Transfer methods 200
Transformation 109
Transformed cell culture 277
Transgenic animals 119
Transgenic plants 120
Translation 29
Transposable element 26
Transposons 26
Trypan blue test 295
Tubulin 14
Tunel staining 68
Two dimensional-gel
electrophoresis 240

U

UDP Glucuronyltransferases (UGTs) 231
Ultrarapid metabolizer phenotype 228
Untranslated regions 218

V

Vacuum blotting 201
Viral vectors 145

W

Western blotting 199

X

Xenometabolites 246

Y

Yeast artificial chromosomes 99

Z

Zymogram 284
Zymography 284